Migraine and Epilepsy

Migraine and Epilepsy

Edited by

Frederick Andermann, M.D., FRCP(C)

Professor of Neurology, Department of Neurology and Neurosurgery, McGill University, Director of the Epilepsy Service, The Montreal Neurological Hospital and Institute, Montreal, Quebec, Canada

Elio Lugaresi, M.D.

Professor of Neurology and Director of the Neurological Institute, University of Bologna, Bologna, Italy

With a foreword by Henri Gastaut, M.D.

Butterworths
Boston London Durban Singapore Sydney Toronto Wellington

Every effort has been made to ensure that the drug dosage schedules within this text are accurate and conform to standards accepted at time of publication. However, as treatment recommendations vary in the light of continuing research and clinical experience, the reader is advised to verify drug dosage schedules herein with information found on product information sheets. This is especially true in cases of new or infrequently used drugs.

Library of Congress Cataloging-in-Publication Data

Migraine and epilepsy.

  Includes bibliographies and index.
  1. Migraine.   2. Epilepsy.   I. Andermann, Frederick.
II. Lugaresi, Elio. [DNLM: 1. Epilepsy. 2. Migraine.
WL 344 M6355]
RC392.M57 1986   616.8′53   86-21636
ISBN 0-409-95083-1

Butterworth Publishers
80 Montvale Avenue
Stoneham, MA 02180

10 9 8 7 6 5 4 3 2 1

Printed in the United States of America

We dedicate this book to our wives,
Eva and Maria Rosa
and to our children
Lisa, Anne, Mark, Allessandra, and Nicola

Contents

II.   ICTAL HEADACHE

Contributors

Gary M. Abrams, MD
Assistant Professor, Department of
Neurology, College of Physicians and
Surgeons of Columbia University;
Assistant Attending Neurologist,
Presbyterian Hospital of the City of
New York, New York, NY

Jean Aicardi, MD
Director of Investigation, INSERM
(Institut National de la Santé et de la
Recherche Médicale); Director, Child
Neurology Unit, Hôpital des Enfants
Malades, Paris, France

Eva Andermann, MD, PhD
Associate Professor, Department of
Neurology and Neurosurgery and the
Center for Human Genetics, McGill
University; Head, Neurogenetics Unit,
Montreal Neurological Institute and
Hospital, Montreal, Quebec

Frederick Andermann, MD, FRCP(C)
Professor of Neurology, McGill
University; Director of the Epilepsy
Service and the Epilepsy Clinic,
Montreal Neurological Institute and
Hospital, Montreal, Quebec

G. Andrighetto, MD
Research Fellow in Pediatric
Neurology, Department of Pediatrics,
University of Verona, Verona, Italy

Wolfgang Baier, MD
Assistant Medical Director,
Department of Neuropediatrics,

Christian-Albrechts University of Kiel,
Federal Republic of Germany

Anna Baldrati, MD
Research Fellow, Neurological
Institute of the University of Bologna,
Bologna, Italy

Anne Beaumanoir, MD
Lecturer in Oto-Neuro-Ophthalmology,
Faculty of Medicine, University of
Geneva; Chief, Division of Clinical
Neurophysiology, Hôpital Cantonal
Universitaire, Geneva,
Switzerland

Sabah Bekhor, MB ChB, FRCP(C)
Assistant Professor of Neurology,
Department of Neurology and
Neurosurgery, McGill University;
Director of Neurology, St. Mary's
Hospital, Montreal, Quebec

Samuel F. Berkovic, MD, FRACP
Research Fellow, Department of
Neurology, Austin Hospital,
Melbourne, Australia

Peter F. Bladin, MD, FRACP, MRCP (Edin)
Professorial Associate, Department of
Medicine, Melbourne University;
Director, Department of Neurology,
Austin Hospital, Melbourne, Australia

Warren T. Blume, MD, CM, FRCP(C)
Professor of Neurology, Department of
Clinical Neurological Sciences,

University of Western Ontario;
Co-Director, Epilepsy Unit, University
Hospital, London, Ontario

Guy Bouvier, MD, FRCS(C)
Professor of Neurosurgery, University
of Montreal; Head, Department of
Neurosurgery, Hôpital Notre-Dame,
Montreal, Quebec

G. Capovilla, MD
Research Fellow in Pediatric
Neurology, Department of Pediatrics,
University of Verona, Verona, Italy

Piero De Carolis, MD
Research Fellow, Neurological
Institute of the University of Bologna,
Bologna, Italy

Stirling Carpenter, MD
Professor of Neurology and
Neurosurgery and Pathology, McGill
University; Chief of Neuropathology,
Montreal Neurological Institute and
Hospital, Montreal, Quebec

Fabio Cirignotta, MD
Assistant Professor of Neurology,
University of Bologna; Neurologist,
Neurological Institute of the University
of Bologna, Bologna, Italy

V. Colamaria, MD
Assistant Professor of Pediatric
Neurology, Department of Pediatrics,
University of Verona, Verona, Italy

Pietro Cortelli, MD
Research Fellow, Neurological
Institute of the University of Bologna,
Bologna, Italy

Bernardo Dalla Bernardina, MD
Professor of Pediatric Neurology,

Department of Pediatrics, University of
Verona, Verona, Italy

Roberto D'Alessandro, MD
Assistant Professor of Neurology,
University of Bologna; Neurologist,
Neurological Institute of the University
of Bologna, Bologna, Italy

Hermann Doose, MD
Professor of Neuropediatrics and Head
of the Neuropediatric Department,
Christian-Albrechts University of Kiel,
Federal Republic of Germany

Gary S. Dvorkin, MD, FRCP(C)
Neurologist, Verdun General Hospital,
Verdun, Quebec

M. Egli, MD
Medical Director and Professor,
Schweizerische Epilepsie-Klinik,
Zurich, Switzerland

E. Fontana, MD
Research Fellow in Pediatric
Neurology, Department of Pediatrics,
University of Verona, Verona, Italy

Henri Gastaut, MD
Honorary Professor of Clinical
Neurophysiology, Director of the
Institute for Neurological Research,
W.H.O. Collaborating Center for
Research in Neurosciences, Faculty of
Medicine, Marseilles, France

Giuseppe Gobbi, MD
Research Fellow, Department of
Pediatric Neurology, Neurological
Institute of the University of Bologna

Eduna Grandjean, MD
Division of Clinical Neurophysiology,
Hôpital Cantonal Universitaire,
Geneva, Switzerland

Hansruedi Isler, MD
Lecturer in Neurology, University of
Zurich; Senior Registrar, Department
of Neurology, University Hospital,
Zurich, Switzerland

J. C. Jacob, FRCP(C)
Clinical Professor, Departments of
Medicine and Pediatrics (Neurology),
Memorial University Medical School;
Neurologist, Department of Medicine
(Division of Neurology), St. John's
General Hospital, St. John's,
Newfoundland

Mira Jekiel, MD
Division of Clinical Neurophysiology
Hôpital Cantonal Universitaire,
Geneva, Switzerland

Pierre Laplante, MD, FRCP(C)
Associate Professor of Neurology,
University of Montreal; Neurologist,
Maisonneuve Rosemont Hospital,
Montreal, Quebec

Martin Lauritzen, MD
Senior Research Fellow, Department of
Medical Physiology A, Panum
Institute, University of Copenhagen;
Senior Research Fellow, Department of
Neurology, Rigshospitalet, University
of Copenhagen, Copenhagen, Denmark

Elio Lugaresi, MD
Professor of Neurology, University of
Bologna; Director, Neurological
Institute of the University of Bologna,
Bologna, Italy

Daune L. MacGregor, MD, FRCP(C)
Associate Professor of Pediatrics,
University of Toronto; Neurologist,
Hospital for Sick Children, Toronto,
Ontario

Gian Camillo Manzoni, MD
Associate Professor, Institute of

Neurology, University of Parma,
Parma, Italy

Elizabeth Matthew, MD, FRCP (C)
Assistant Professor, Department of
Neurology and Neurosurgery, McGill
University; Neurologist, Montreal
Neurological Institute and Hospital,
Montreal, Quebec

Denis Melanson, MD
Associate Professor, Departments of
Neurology and Neurosurgery, and
Radiology, McGill University;
Associate Neuroradiologist, Montreal
Neurological Institute and Hospital,
Montreal Quebec

Pasquale Montagna, MD
Research Fellow, Neurological
Institute of the University of Bologna,
Bologna, Italy

Richard Newton, MD, MRCP, DCH
Consultant Pediatric Neurologist to
Booth Hall and the Royal Manchester
Children's Hospitals, Pendlebury,
England

Shunsuke Ohtahara, MD
Director, Department of
Developmental Neuroscience and
Child Neurology, Institute for
Neurobiology, Okayama University
Medical School, Okayama, Japan

C. P. Panayiotopoulos, MD, PhD
Professor and Head, Division of
Neurology, King Saud University,
College of Medicine; King Khalid
University Hospital, Riyadh, Saudi
Arabia

Liborio Parrino, MD
Research Fellow, Institute of

Neurology, University of Parma,
Parma, Italy

Paolo Pazzaglia, MD
Professor of Neuropathology and
Psychopathology, University of
Bologna; Neurologist, Neurological
Institute of the University of Bologna,
Bologna, Italy

Luis F. Quesney, MD, PhD
Associate Professor, Department of
Neurology and Neurosurgery, McGill
University; Chief, Department of EEG
and Clinical Neurophysiology,
Montreal Neurological Institute and
Hospital, Montreal, Quebec

Paola Giovanardi Rossi, MD
Professor of Pediatric Neurology,
University of Bologna; Director of
Pediatric Neurology, Neurological
Institute of the University of Bologna,
Bologna, Italy

J. Chris Sackellares, MD
Associate Professor of Neurology,
University of Michigan; Director,
Clinical Neurophysiology Laboratories,
University Hospital, Ann Arbor,
Michigan

Tommaso Sacquegna, MD
Assistant Professor of Neurology,
University of Bologna; Neurologist,
Neurological Institute of the University
of Bologna, Bologna, Italy

Margherita Santucci, MD
Research Fellow, Department of
Pediatric Neurology, Neurological
Institute of the University of Bologna,
Bologna, Italy

Jean-Marc Saint-Hilaire, MD, FRCP(C)
Professor of Neurology, University of

Montreal; Chief, Department of
Neurology, Hôpital Notre-Dame,
Montreal, Quebec

Allan L. Sherwin, MD, PhD, FRCP(C)
Professor of Neurology, Department of
Neurology and Neurosurgery, McGill
University; Head, Neuropharmacology,
Montreal Neurological Institute and
Hospital, Montreal, Quebec

Carlo Alberto Tassinari, MD
Professor of Neurology, University of
Bologna; Chief of the Second
Neurological Service, Neurological
Institute of the University of Bologna,
Bologna, Italy

Tomoyuki Terasaki, MD
Department of Development
Neuroscience and Child Neurology,
Institute for Neurobiology; Okayama
University Medical School, Okayama,
Japan

Mario Giovanni Terzano, MD
Professor of Clinical Neurophysiology,
Institute of Neurology, University of
Parma, Parma, Italy

Paolo Tinuper, MD
Research Fellow, Director of the EEG
Laboratory, Neurological Institute of
the University of Bologna, Bologna,
Italy

E. Trevisan, MD
Research Fellow in Pediatric
Neurology, Department of Pediatrics,
University of Verona, Verona, Italy

Nico M. van Gelder, PhD
Professor of Physiology, Department of
Physiology, Centre de recherche en
sciences néurologiques, University of
Montreal, Montreal, Quebec

Simon Verret, MD, FRCP(C)
Professor of Neurology (Medicine),
Chairman, Department of Pediatrics,
Faculty of Medicine, Laval University,
Québec, Quebec

Heinz-Gregor Wieser, MD
Lecturer, Department of Neurology,
University of Zurich, Oberarzt, Head of
EEG Department, Department of
Neurology, University Hospital,
Zurich, Switzerland

Arnold J. Wilkins, D Phil
Scientist, MRC Applied Psychology
Unit, Cambridge, England

John Willoughby, MD, FRACP
Associate Professor of Medicine,
Flinders University of South Australia;
Consultant Neurologist, Flinders
Medical Center, Adelaide, Australia

Yasuko Yamatogi, MD
Department of Developmental
Neuroscience and Child Neurology,
Institute for Neurobiology, Okayama
University Medical School, Okayama,
Japan

G. Bryan Young, MD, FRCP(C)
Associate Professor, Department of
Clinical Neurological Sciences,
University of Western Ontario;
Director of EEG/Evoked Response
Laboratory, Victoria Hospital, London,
Ontario

Benjamin G. Zifkin, MD, CM, FRCP(C)
Assistant Professor, Department of
Neurology, State University of New
York, Health Sciences Center at
Brooklyn, New York; Head, Epilepsy
Unit, New York State Institute for
Basic Research in Developmental
Disabilities (OMRDD), Staten Island,
New York

Foreword

When I originally accepted Prof. Lugaresi's invitation to present my recent work on benign occipital epilepsy of childhood as part of his annual epilepsy course, I little anticipated that I would later be asked to contribute a foreword to this handsome volume. When the course was given, it had developed into a joint meeting of the Center for Epilepsy Studies at the Neurological Institute in Bologna and the Italian Society for the Study of Headache on the topic of "Migraine and Epilepsy"; and included keynote addresses by Prof. Andermann and myself and more than 10 other related communications.

At that time, it was decided to publish a monograph on this subject under the editorial stewardship of Profs. Andermann and Lugaresi, but there was nothing to suggest that the final result of their effort and inspiration would be a sizeable book of 27 chapters written by 64 authors representing 10 countries and exploring all facets of the current state of knowledge of the possible relations between migraine and epilepsy. I am sure that it will become an indispensable reference for those seeking authoritative discussions of these topics.

Both Hughlings Jackson and Gowers found certain cases of migraine and epilepsy difficult to distinguish and were intrigued by the coexistence of the two disorders. However, they never lost sight of the different nature of the two conditions. In his great textbook, Gowers never considered migraine in the differential diagnosis of epilepsy as he did syncope and hysteria, and Hughlings Jackson rigorously separated migraine and epilepsy on the practical grounds of symptoms, diagnosis, and treatment. In his inimitable style, he noted, ". . . it would be as absurd to classify [migraine] along with ordinary cases of epilepsy for practical purposes as to classify whales with other mammals for purposes of practical life. A whale is in law a fish, in zoology it is a mammal."

The history of some of these difficult issues, and my own clinical experience, led me to approach this topic with caution. I was, therefore, particularly pleased that the editors took great pains to ensure that the many similarities and recently demonstrated relationships between migraine and epilepsy did not obscure the fundamental differences between them.

Every neurologist since the days of Jackson and Gowers has been confronted with puzzling cases which seem to present features of both these common conditions. This book is a modern effort to clarify these clinically vexing syndromes and to draw from them valuable lessons on the underlying nature of the two diseases. "Migraine and Epilepsy" is both faithful to history and an authoritative volume for today and the future. Andermann and Lugaresi merit the gratitude of all, and I am proud to have been involved in their work.

Dr. Henri Gastaut
Marseille

Preface

". . . I have seen cases intermediate in type between migraine, epileptiform seizures and epilepsy proper ("Missing Links")."

JOHN HUGHLINGS JACKSON, 1888

"Some surprise may be felt that migraine is given a place in the borderland of epilepsy, but the position is justified by many relations, and among them by the fact that the two maladies are sometimes mistaken, and more often their distinction is difficult."

WILLIAM R. GOWERS, 1907

Migraine and epilepsy are distinct disorders with characteristic clinical features. The diagnosis of the two entities is based mainly on the availability of a detailed and accurate history. Though both were historically thought of as paroxysmal disorders, there was no reason to expect an overlap between the two. I was therefore surprised to see, as a junior resident in neurology, a young boy known to have classical migraine who developed a partial seizure at the time of a migraine attack. This apparent overlap or coexistence of the two disorders did not seem to surprise my clinical supervisor who had had experience with similar patients. The literature revealed that the relationship between migraine and epilepsy had puzzled neurologists since the days of pioneers like Jackson (1875) and Gowers (1907). Over the years the subject has been discussed by Ely (1930), Brain (1953), Barolin (1966), Ziegler and Wong (1967), Slatter (1968), Basser (1969), and Ninck (1970), and it has been the focus of at least two editorials, in *Lancet* (1969) and *Hemicrania* (1972).

The relationships of migraine to epilepsy remained largely unresolved, though some authors suggested that the migrainous aura, probably caused by spreading depression, might cause a seizure (Basser, 1969), and that cerebral damage caused by the migraine might lead to epilepsy (Barolin, 1966; Slatter, 1968; Ninck, 1970).

Recent reviews (Lance, 1981; Moskowitz, 1984) summarize opinions and evidence on the nature of migraine, including studies that demonstrate oligemia during the classical migraine aura (Olesen et al., 1981; Lauritzen et al., 1983a; Lauritzen et al., 1983b; Lauritzen, Chapter 22, this volume). Ischemia associated with migraine, which can be severe enough to lead to infarction, could certainly also be sufficient to lead to epileptic discharge, particularly in younger individuals whose seizure threshold is lower.

This monograph assimilates clinical information about the various interfaces of migraine and epilepsy. Eight migraine epilepsy syndromes are identified:

1. Epileptic seizures induced by a classical migraine aura
2. Epilepsy with seizures no longer triggered by migrainous aura
3. Epilepsy due to gross cerebral lesions caused by migraine
4. Benign occipital epilepsy of childhood and the spectrum of the occipital epilepsies
5. Benign rolandic epilepsy
6. Malignant migraine, related to mitochondrial encephalomyopathy
7. Migraine attacks following partial complex seizures
8. Alternating hemiplegia of childhood

Certain patients have epileptic seizures during a classical migraine aura only (Andermann, Chapter 1, Terzano et al., Chapter 3), others then go on to develop epilepsy independent of migrainous auras (Andermann, Chapter 1). Benign epilepsy with occipital spike wave complexes represents a form of primary partial childhood epilepsy (Gastaut and Zifkin, Chapter 3; Terasaki et al., Chapter 7) with a high incidence of migraine and a family history of migraine. The occipital epilepsies of childhood, though they share certain clinical and electrographic features, are not always benign (Andermann, Chapter 1; Gastaut and Zifkin, Chapter 2; Aicardi and Newton, Chapter 6; Terasaki et al., Chapter 7) and there is evidence for a wide spectrum of occipital epilepsies ranging from the mainly genetic to the mainly acquired or symptomatic. This finding is in keeping with current views on the multifactorial nature of the epilepsies.

Benign rolandic epilepsy is also migraine related (Bladin, Chapter 9), though Giovanardi Rossi et al. (Chapter 21) present a dissenting opinion. Epilepsy may result after migraine-related strokes. Migraine may occur following complex partial seizures (D'Allessandro et al., Chapter 18). A characteristic syndrome of classical migraine, intractable epilepsy and multiple strokes related to mitochondrial encephalomyopathy with lactic acidosis is presented by Dvorkin et al. (Chapter 14). Migraine is a constant feature in parents of children with alternating hemiplegia (Dalla Bernardina et al., Chapter 13; Andermann, personal observations). Migraine and epilepsy may be associated in this disorder, also.

Difficulties in distinguishing between occipital epileptic and migrainous manifestations are discussed by Panayiotopoulos (Chapter 2) and the electrographic abnormalities encountered over occipital regions are described by

Beaumanoir and Grandjean (Chapter 5). The reactivity of normal and abnormal occipital EEG rhythms to light and darkness is presented by Cirignotta et al. (Chapter 8). Rhythmic spike discharge recorded over occipital regions during the classical migraine aura (Beaumanoir and Jekiel, Chapter 10, Sacquegna et al., Chapter 11) represents epileptic discharge, a finding important for our understanding of migraine-epilepsy relationships. A fatal case of migraine and epilepsy with pathological evidence of mesial temporal sclerosis is presented by Bladin and Berkovic (Chapter 12).

Ictal pain is discussed by Blume and Young (Chapter 15) and recording with depth electrodes shows that at least one type of ictal headache results from epileptic discharge arising from mesial temporal structures (Isler et al., Chapter 16; St. Hilaire et al., Chapter 17).

The epidemiological difficulties which beset studies of migraine and epilepsy are reviewed by Andermann and Andermann, (Chapter 19). There is no evidence for a common genetic basis of the two disorders in general, though in certain epileptic syndromes (benign rolandic epilepsy, benign occipital epilepsy, and perhaps primary generalized epilepsy with absence attacks (Baier and Doose, Chapter 20)) such a genetic relationship may be present.

Current studies of cerebral blood flow and spreading depression (Lauritzen, Chapter 22), visual sensitivity in relation to cerebral hyperexcitability (Wilkins, Chapter 23), calcium mobility and glutamic acid release (Van Gelder, Chapter 24), the role of peptides (Matthew and Abrams, Chapter 25), and of a dopaminergic mechanism in relation to photosensitivity (Quesney and Andermann, Chapter 26) provide a background against which these clinical problems unfold.

This book is aimed at neurologists, pediatric neurologists, and clinical neurophysiologists as well as all those interested in migraine and epilepsy and the puzzling relationship between them. We hope that it will prove to be a step forward in the century-old quest for resolution of this clinical enigma.

REFERENCES

Anonymous. Migraine and epilepsy. Lancet 1969;2:527–8.

Barolin G. Migraines and epilepsy—a relationship? Epilepsia 1966;7:53–66.

Basser LS. The relation of migraine and epilepsy. Brain 1969;92:285–300.

Brain W. Diseases of the nervous system. London: Oxford University Press, 1953.

Ely FA. The migraine-epilepsy syndrome: a statistical study of heredity. Arch Neurol Psychiat 1930;24:943–9.

Gowers WR. The borderland of epilepsy: faints, vagal attacks, vertigo, migraine, sleep symptoms, and their treatment. London: Churchill, 1907.

Jackson JH. Hospital for the epileptic and paralyzed: case illustrating the relation between certain cases of migraine and epilepsy. Lancet 1875;2:244–5.

Lance JW. Headache. Ann Neurol 1981;10:1–10.

Lauritzen M, Olsen TS, Lassen NA, Paulson OB. Changes in regional cerebral blood flow during the course of classic migraine attacks. Ann Neurol 1983;13:633–41.

Lauritzen M, Olsen TS, Lassen NA, Paulson OB. Regulation of regional cerebral blood flow during and between migraine attacks. Ann Neurol 1983;14:569–72.

Moskowitz MA. The neurobiology of vascular head pain. Ann Neurol 1984;16:157–68.

Ninck B. Migraine and epilepsy. Eur Neurol 1970;168–78.

Olesen J, Larsen B, Lauritzen M. Focal hyperemia followed by spreading oligemia and impaired activation of rCBF in classic migraine. Ann Neurol 1981;9:344–52.

Slatter KH. Some clinical and EEG findings in patients with migraines. Brain 1968;91:85–98.

Whitty CWM. Migraine and epilepsy. Hemicrania 1972;4:2–4.

Ziegler DK, Wong G Jr. Migraine in children: clinical and electroencephalographic study of families, the possible relation to epilepsy. Epilepsia 1967;8:171–87.

Acknowledgments

Inspiration for studies on migraine and epilepsy came from Francis McNaughton and Preston Robb, who stressed accuracy of neurological diagnosis and the concept that seizures are a symptom and not a disease. Peter Camfield carried out our initial study on migraine–epilepsy relationships. The conclusions of that study intrigued Henri Gastaut and rekindled his long-standing interest in the occipital epilepsies of childhood. This in turn led to his formulation of the concept of "benign occipital epilepsy of childhood with spike-wave paroxysms."

Discussion of these studies at the Neurology and Epilepsy congresses in Kyoto resulted in the planning of an international workshop on Migraine and Epilepsy held in Bologna, generously supported by Sigma Tau. This was followed by the decision to summarize current knowledge in a monograph. Sandoz Canada provided support for clerical help.

Dr. Benjamin Zifkin selflessly contributed his neurological knowledge coupled with considerable linguistic and stylistic skill; he greatly facilitated the task of the editors of this book.

Our editor at Butterworth, Ms. Nancy Megley, was an invaluable provider of expert advice and encouragement based on her excellent judgment and experience with the vagaries of medical writers.

To the collaborators in this volume we express our thanks for the high quality of their contributions, their unflagging cooperation, and also for their patience. Our wives, and especially our children, very generously and without complaint accepted our additional time commitment and preoccupation with this book.

I

Clinical and EEG Studies

1

Clinical Features of Migraine-Epilepsy Syndromes

Frederick Andermann

When the clinical patterns of epilepsy and migraine were described in detail in the last century, the coexistence of the two conditions in some individuals presented a mysterious and puzzling problem (Jackson 1875, 1888). Gowers (1907), after considering the many interrelationships of the two disorders, as well as the difficulties at times encountered in distinguishing between them, finally concluded that the two conditions were fundamentally different.

The clinical observations that migraine and epilepsy may at times occur in the same individual, have been interpreted along three lines of thought: first, migraine and epilepsy are both relatively common in the general population and therefore must occur together by chance in a number of people; second, migraine and epilepsy may share a pathophysiological or genetic basis explaining their occasional coexistence; and third, the two conditions might be at times causally related, one leading to the other in certain individuals.

There is no doubt that, despite the epidemiological difficulties and uncertainties which exist in assessing the prevalence of these disorders, migraine and epilepsy at times do coexist on a random basis. A mathematical expression of this association can be formulated, and differing prevalence figures generated, depending on one's assumption of the individual prevalences of migraine and of epilepsy in the general population. Such an exercise, however, fails to take into account the specific clinical circumstances of the occurrence of this association in many patients, which often suggest a more specific rather than a random association. Although random association must also occur, even then the two disorders may interact and influence each other's course.

It is unlikely that the two conditions are genetically related (Andermann E. and Andermann F., Chapter 19, this volume) or that their fundamental physiological and neurochemical mechanisms are identical (van Gelder, Chapter 24, this volume; Quesney and Andermann, Chapter 26, this volume;

Matthew and Abrams, Chapter 25, this volume; Lauritzen, Chapter 22, this volume). Clinical observations, however, do suggest a number of specific relationships between migraine and epilepsy, and these are the subject of this and other chapters which constitute the first section of this volume.

Several years ago, we studied four adolescents with basilar migraine, seizures, and severe epileptiform electroencephalogram (EEG) abnormalities (Camfield et al., 1978). Although these four young people had similar clinical and EEG findings, it rapidly became clear that there were a number of other clinical situations in which migraine and epilepsy overlapped or were causally related. Furthermore, in many of those cases the interictal EEGs were normal, in marked contrast to the cases we initially reported.

It therefore seemed appropriate to examine a greater number of patients with both migraine and seizures in order to attempt to clarify the clinical aspects of the relationship between these two common conditions. We investigated 25 patients either as inpatients or as outpatients at the Montreal Neurological Hospital. The selection and age range of the patients reflect the profile of the author's interest in epilepsy and pediatric neurology. No attempts were made to collect all patients presenting at the hospital, and no specific questionnaires were used in this study.

The patients appeared to fit into several clinical categories. The majority developed seizures during a classical migraine aura. A few then went on to develop seizures independently of the migraine. A third group, children with occipital epilepsy, also had migraine or a family history of migraine; this appeared to be a risk factor in the development of epilepsy in these patients.

CLASSICAL MIGRAINE WITH SEIZURES OCCURRING ONLY DURING THE AURA IN ADOLESCENTS AND YOUNG ADULTS

CASE 1   A boy developed attacks of autonomic dysfunction, then classical migraine, and later an unusual aura with stereotyped complex auditory hallucinations lasting many minutes. Following such auras, he often had a partial or generalized seizure. Seizures occurred only in the context of migrainous attacks and appeared to be caused by the migraine. His sister, mother, grandmother, and a cousin had severe classical migraine.

This 15-year-old had developed recurrent abdominal pains at age 3. Later he had attacks of blurred vision followed by severe headache. At age 7, he developed episodes that he described as dreams, in which he heard male and female voices arguing, talking, or screaming at him. These attacks usually occurred during the night and were associated with a sensation that the surroundings were strange. One of his hands felt altered; it became very long and distant from his body. Very occasionally he would see zigzag lines. Prolonged attacks culminated in nausea, retching, vomiting, and pounding headache. Shorter attacks led to a queasy feeling and mild headache.

At the height of the attacks, while retching and having severe headache, his eyes rolled up and his jaws clenched. He developed tonic stiffening of one arm, and this was followed by clonic movements and, at times, by a generalized seizure.

He was diagnosed to have seizures originating in the temporal lobe and was treated with phenytoin, carbamazepine, and phenobarbital. At age 11, his attacks ceased, and medication was discontinued. He had a searching electrographic study, including seven records with sphenoidal recordings. There was no epileptogenic discharge, and only mild diffuse slow abnormalities were found. A computerized tomography (CT) scan was normal. His verbal IQ was 96 and performance IQ 120 (full-scale IQ was 108).

He remained seizure-free for almost a year. Migraine attacks and seizures recurred, and the latter were controlled by high average doses of phenytoin and primidone. Medication exacerbated behavioral and cognitive problems that had improved greatly when pharmacologic treatment was not required.

His sister had attacks of classical migraine with an aura of distortion of time wherein things seemed to be moving very fast: for example, bread was being cut very fast, or people were talking very quickly. His mother and grandmother had severe classical migraine. A maternal cousin also had classical migraine, and his EEG showed diffuse epileptogenic abnormalities.

CASE 2 This young man developed migraine and seizures late in the first decade. The seizures were partial simple occipital attacks with spread and secondary generalization. The epileptic manifestations were probably triggered by the migrainous aura. The seizures eventually ceased, but he remained with attacks of classical and probably basilar migraine. His mother also had classical migraine.

This 27-year-old man developed seizures and migrainous manifestations before age 10. Initially it was difficult to distinguish between migraine and seizures. The attacks started with flashes of yellow light that resembled a glittering screen moving in the horizontal plane. Later this was followed by involuntary blinking, stiffness with wringing of the hands, loss of consciousness, or a generalized tonic-clonic seizure. Most attacks occurred while he was in the sun.

At age 15 he described his attacks as follows: "A pressure in the head, as if it is going to open, followed by colored spots of light moving to the left." His head and eyes followed the spots as if he were focusing on them, and he could not see anything else. These visual changes lasted for many minutes, and he remained conscious. He was dizzy and nauseated and developed severe generalized pounding headaches that lasted for hours.

At age 16 he again had focal seizures after seeing geometric figures. In these attacks there was adversion of the eyes, followed by clonic jerking of the left arm and of the head to the left. He frequently had after-images. His neurologic examination and CT scan were normal. EEGs at that time showed bioccipital slow activity predominating on the left and bitemporal sharp waves not amounting to clear foci of epileptogenic discharge.

The patient improved spontaneously and for 10 years had no further seizures. Off antiepileptic medication for 7 years, he continued to have migraine attacks about once a month. He felt tired, saw black when he blinked, and then perceived bright light spots in the periphery of the visual field, followed by headache of variable severity.

His mother had had classical migraine for many years. Her attacks were preceded by distortion of vision that could last for 1 day: looking at a sign showing two children at a street crossing, she would see six legs. During an aura in a restaurant, when she looked at the waiter she could see just his abdomen.

CASE 3   A young woman had a long history of attacks of classical migraine starting with an intense and prolonged aura of déjà vu or déjà vécu. She had a strong family history of classical migraine. She developed three generalized tonic-clonic seizures; two were preceded by her typical migrainous aura. A searching study failed to demonstrate clear epileptic discharge in her EEGs, and the attacks were easily controlled by small doses of carbamazepine.

A 27-year-old executive secretary had a generalized seizure while jogging at age 23. A second tonic-clonic attack was preceded by an intense and prolonged feeling of familiarity, as if she had been in these surroundings before.

From the ages of 8 to 22 she had severe migraine attacks. These were usually preceded by the same aura and led to bioccipital pounding headache, nausea, vomiting, and photophobia.

Neurologic examination was normal. CT scan showed a minimally larger left ventricle, and EEGs demonstrated only generalized paroxysmal discharges without spike and wave. She had a recurrence 3 years later, again preceded by déjà vu and déjà vécu, when her carbamazepine was stopped.

She had a strong family history of migraine. A maternal aunt had had attacks preceded by a prolonged feeling that she described by saying: "I knew I had never been there, but it was as if I had been there before," or "It seems as if it had happened before." This was followed by tingling in her fingers and on one side of her mouth, usually the right. Her father had common migraine and so did her mother; there were other relatives with classical migraine on her mother's side, as well.

Comment

These three young people all had classical migraine and a family history of classical migraine. There was a striking intrafamily similarity in the features of the migrainous aura: an unusual aura of familiarity suggesting temporal lobe involvement was found in Case 3 and in her aunt, and distortions of both body image and time were seen in Case 1 and in his sister. The epileptic manifestations occurred at the height of the migrainous aura. Initially the sequence of events was not entirely clear, and, given the history of isolated attacks out of context, the relationship of the seizures to the migraine was not immediately obvious, as in Case 3, for instance. Distinguishing between migrainous and epileptic manifestations was initially difficult, as in Case 2, but description of subsequent attacks was helpful in clarifying this question.

CLASSICAL MIGRAINE WITH SEIZURES OCCURRING ONLY DURING THE AURA IN ADULTS

CASE 4   A man with worsening classical migraine often had hemianopia preceeding the headache. The first aura which involved bilateral visual loss followed sleep deprivation and fatigue, and triggered a brief generalized tonic-clonic seizure. When last seen, he had had no recurrence for 2 years.

> A sensitive, intelligent, 28-year-old man who had been adopted as a child had a long history of recurrent throbbing headaches lasting 1 to 2 days. These had worsened over the last 2 years; he had a visual aura that he described as a fog or a haze in the periphery of the visual field on all sides with retained central vision. Another pattern was that of hemianopic visual loss, half of the time on the right and half of the time on the left, but never involving both sides in one attack. The headache was already present at the beginning of the aura and then increased. At times he also had tingling of his whole body.
>
> After being awake for more than 24 hours, and having worked a double shift, he felt his visual aura coming on, with blurring in the left visual field. This then became bilateral, so that his vision was dim on both sides. He remembered being told by one of his coworkers to move his car, in which he was sitting; then he lost consciousness and had a tonic-clonic seizure. His neurologic examination was normal except for color blindness. CAT scan and EEG were normal. When last seen he had had no further seizures for 2 years.

CASE 5   A single generalized seizure was triggered by a classical visual migrainous aura in a man who drank to excess in order to control his essential tremor.

> A 38-year-old man had a long history of essential tremor. He became aware that alcohol would relieve this and drank beer to excess. He had rare classical migraine attacks with a visual aura. One Sunday morning, having drunk a great deal of beer the preceding evening, he went out on the dock to look at the lake in front of his cottage and developed a migrainous aura, quite typical of his usual attacks. He then lost consciousness and was seen to have a tonic-clonic seizure. Neurologic examination revealed only his familial tremor. An EEG was normal.

Comment

A migrainous aura is less likely to lead to a cerebral seizure in adults, probably because of their higher seizure threshold. In both these cases, the circumstances of the aura leading to a seizure were rather unusual, including obvious fatigue, sleep deprivation, and alcohol intake. The aura leading to the seizure was more severe than usual, and qualitatively different, in Case 4. The bilateral visual loss suggested basilar involvement, which the patient had not experienced previously.

In these two patients, there was no EEG abnormality some days after the acute event, and there was no tendency to recurrence of seizures.

CLASSICAL OR COMMON MIGRAINE WITH SEIZURES OCCURRING DURING THE ATTACKS IN CHILDREN

CASE 6   A boy had migraine and complex attacks that included features of both epilepsy and classical migraine. The sequence of events did not point to a clear causal relationship. These attacks did not respond to antiepileptic treatment but improved spontaneously. The boy had a family history of both common and classical migraine and seizures.

A 7-year-old boy had been born with a face presentation but had normal developmental milestones. He developed his first seizure at age 2½. His arms and legs jerked but his parents thought he was responsive and he could talk, though in a stuttering manner. During or before these attacks, he had nausea and headache, and saw balls of flashing light. During the night, he had episodes of crawling about the bed and speaking, of which he had no recollection. He also had a history of pounding headaches, associated with sleepiness, that occurred at other times.

He was referred with the suspicion of temporal lobe epilepsy, since right and then left temporal spikes had been noted at different times.

Investigation revealed active generalized spike and multiple spike and wave discharges that were greatly enhanced by sleep. Despite numerous recordings with sphenoidal electrodes and sleep, no localized temporal epileptic discharges were found and no attacks were recorded. A CT scan showed mild diffuse atrophy.

The mother had severe common migraine and her sister had classical migraine. The boy's uncle had had two seizures at age 7.

CASE 7   A boy presented with cerebral seizures of multiple types. Attacks started with prolonged irritability, aggressiveness, and right-sided headache, and evolved to generalized tonic-clonic seizures. In another type of attack, the initial manifestations gave way to striking hallucinatory phenomena followed by headache and mood change. The history suggested acquired cerebral dysfunction, and there was a family history of febrile convulsions. A searching electrographic investigation showed no interictal epileptogenic discharge. The history suggested that the epileptic manifestations were preceded by migrainous events.

A 9-year-old boy had a brief generalized seizure in association with tonsillitis and fever at the age of 20 months. Seizures recurred, and he had 11 hospital admissions for investigation and treatment of these by age 5.

He had several different types of attacks: in some, there was prolonged irritability, aggressiveness, and right-sided headache, followed by a generalized tonic-clonic seizure. In others, there was again irritability and aggressiveness; then he would see bumblebees that he would try to avoid, or swat, using one or the other hand. It was uncertain whether these visual hallucinations were in one or both halves of the visual field. He became drowsy or vomited. It was difficult to tell whether the attacks were epileptic or migrainous in nature. In addition, he had a history of brief absence attacks, apneic spells, and drop attacks; but these did not occur in the hospital, even on reduced antiepileptic medication.

The mother had had one abortion before his conception. When carrying this child, she bled during the first trimester, and was treated with Provera. Labor lasted more than 24 hours. A Caesarian section was performed for fetal distress and a footling breech presentation. His milestones were entirely normal, and his mental functioning was in the bright normal range without significant discrepancies. He was in the 3rd percentile for height, and his weight was at the 10th percentile. His head circumference was in the 50th percentile. He had a grade 2/6 systolic ejection murmur over the left sternal border of the benign flow type, and two patches of hypopigmentation on the left shin and the right thigh. Investigation included 10 EEGs that showed moderate biposterior slow dysrhythmia but no interictal epileptogenic discharge. A muscle biopsy specimen showed some excess lipid but no mitochondrial abnormality. Skin and nerve biopsy specimens were normal. His brother had had a single febrile convulsion. No family history of migraine was recorded. He was treated with carbamazepine and propranolol.

CASE 8   A girl developed seizures and migraine at age 3. Some seizures were preceded by nausea and followed by headache. When migraine increased in frequency, seizures were likely to occur. She had a strong family history of migraine and a family history of epilepsy. A more clear-cut causal relationship between the migraine and seizures could not be established.

A 6-year-old girl had her first seizure at age 3. At a time when she was quite well, she awoke during the night and went to the bathroom to vomit. The mother, who was holding her, described her as being very red. She collapsed into the bowl and then had a seizure involving the right side of the body, including the face, arm, and leg; it lasted 10 minutes. She remained unresponsive for 1.5 hours. She developed another form of nocturnal seizure before age 6; during these seizures the mother found her having clonic movements of the right arm and vomiting.

Migraine attacks also started at age 3. They often occurred in the morning. She had severe, usually lateralized headache, vomited, and went back to sleep. Although she had nausea before the first seizure, this was not noted in every subsequent attack.

In one episode, she woke in the morning, vomited, and developed twitching of the right arm; she then fell asleep. When she awoke she complained of a bad headache. In another attack she was unresponsive, but kept repeating "Mummy, don't leave me." She then vomited and complained of a bad headache. The mother believed that the child was liable to have a seizure when she had a buildup of headaches or migraine attacks. When she was tired, she dragged the right leg. The neurologic examination and CT scan were normal. Her EEGs showed active epileptiform abnormality over the left occipital region and also the centroparietal and temporal areas. At times, the presence of an independent left anterior temporal focus was suspected.

The mother had severe migraine with nausea and vomiting for 9 years. The maternal grandfather had severe migraine. The child's father had severe lateralized migraine associated with swelling of either eyelid. There was a family history of seizures.

Comment

Two of these children had visual hallucinations, nausea, and headache as prominent features of their attacks. The third had a similar history but no visual aura. All three had motor manifestations that could not be explained on a migrainous basis and were manifestly epileptic in nature. No inquiry was made regarding a family history of migraine in Case 7, but a strong family history of migraine was present in the other two families. No seizures occurred independently of the attacks of nausea, vomiting, and headache in two of the patients, although a history of undocumented absence and drop attacks was mentioned in Case 7. There was, however, no evidence that a secondarily generalized and self-sustained epileptic process had developed in this boy.

Electrographic abnormalities in this group of children ranged from generalized or focal occipital epileptic discharges to diffuse nonepileptic changes.

From children in this age group, a subjective history was necessarily difficult to obtain, and the sequence of events as well as the causality of the migraine-epilepsy relationship was more difficult to establish.

BASILAR MIGRAINE AND SEIZURES OCCURRING DURING THE ACUTE ATTACK IN ADOLESCENTS

CASE 9   A boy with basilar migraine developed partial or secondarily generalized seizures that started during the migrainous aura. EEG abnormalities were abundant and severe. Migraine improved spontaneously and seizures ceased. Phosphenes continued to occur following fatigue and eye closure. Striking EEG abnormalities persisted at age 25.

A 27-year-old man began to experience migraine at age 11. A dazzling white, round, multifaceted light began to appear in his left visual field and spread to the right, rendering him completely blind for 2 to 15 minutes although he remained fully conscious. Sometimes a tingling sensation developed on the left side of his body. On rare occasions, starting during his early migraine attacks, he became confused but not unconscious and then developed tonic-clonic adversive seizures involving the left side of the face, with jerking of the head and eyes to the left for several minutes. Whether or not a seizure developed, these episodes terminated with a severe posterior pounding headache, sometimes with copious vomiting followed by sleep for 1 to 2 hours.

Both his mother and father had classical migraine, with a scintillating scotoma in one visual field followed invariably by headache. One brother also had classical migraine, with concentric fortification spectra and retained central vision. Another brother had common migraine.

At age 11 neurologic examination was normal. Carotid and vertebral angiograms were normal, and a pneumoencephalogram showed minimal dilatation of the right lateral ventricle. Attacks gradually abated, and antiepileptic medication was stopped at age 18. At age 27 he was a successful interior decorator. He had occasional phosphenes when he was tired and closed his eyes.

His EEG at age 12 showed almost continuous spike, sharp-wave, and slow activity, the latter at 1.5 to 2 Hz, from the right posterior temporal and parieto-occipital areas (Figures 1.1 and 1.2). At age 18 continuous, sometimes rhythmic slow-sharp-wave activity, blocking with eye opening, was seen in the same distribution. Background activity showed mild disorganization with traces of alpha at 9 Hz (Figure 1.3). Abnormalities were similar but of lower voltage at age 25 (Figure 1.4).

CASE 10   During childhood this young woman developed basilar migraine, at times leading to unresponsiveness and hypotonia. From time to time, during this state, she developed generalized tonic-clonic seizures. Migraine improved spontaneously, and her attacks no longer evolved to unconsciousness or seizures. Abundant bioccipital spike and wave discharges were found initially; these also remitted spontaneously.

A 21-year-old woman developed attacks at age 9. In these she saw circular lights of many colors over the entire visual field, although occasionally only to the left. They resembled the after-image that results from pressing or rubbing the eyes. A buzzing sensation in her ears would follow. After about 10 minutes, everything would suddenly go black. The attack might stop at this point, with vomiting and gradual clearing of vision over a period of 1 to 15 minutes.

On rare occasions the attack progressed to a gradual fading of consciousness. She slowly sat or lay down and became flaccid for as long as 40 minutes, with saliva running from her mouth. On some occasions such episodes were associated with a headache that lasted 1 to 2 hours. This headache generally was bitemporal, although occasionally it consisted of a unilateral pressure sensation. Her father

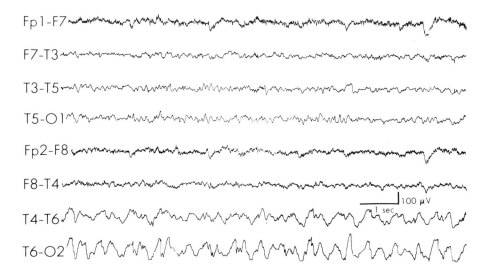

Figure 1.1   Case 9, age 12. Continuous sharp and slow wave activity from the right posterior temporal and occipital areas.

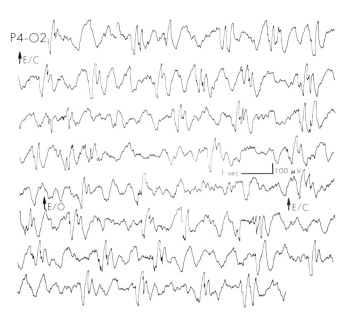

Figure 1.2   Case 9, age 12. Continuous recording showing spike, sharp and slow activity from the right parieto-occipital areas, attenuating with eye opening, (E/O). (E/C = eye closure.)

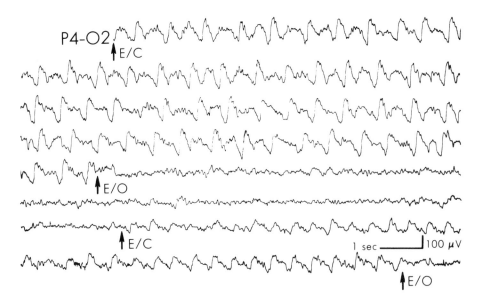

Figure 1.3   Case 9. At age 18, continuous, sometimes rhythmic slow sharp activity from the right parieto-occipital region blocked by eye opening (E/O) and returning gradually after eye closure (E/C).

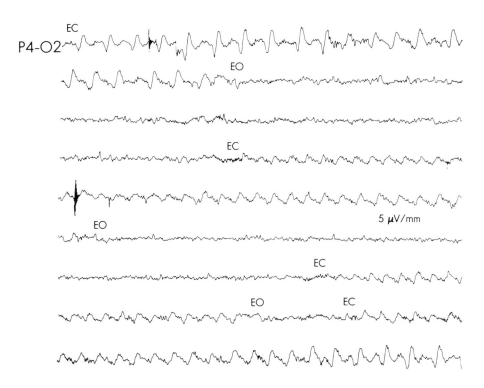

Figure 1.4 Case 9. At age 25, rhythmic slow activity is still present but of lower voltage. (EC = eyes closed; EO = eyes open.)

had common migraine. Several times a year he was sick for a day at a time with pounding headache and nausea.

She was a pleasant, intelligent adolescent with a normal neurologic examination. CT scan suggested mild cerebellar atrophy, inferred from an increase in the size of the fourth ventricle. She was treated with phenytoin and phenobarbital.

EEGs at ages 10 and 11 demonstrated striking and very active bilaterally synchronous, sharp-and-slow-wave, and spike and wave epileptogenic discharges at 1.5 to 2 Hz over posterior head regions (Figure 1.5). These were enhanced by hyperventilation and during drowsiness were replaced by repetitive and at times rhythmic spikes blocked by arousal or eye opening (Figure 1.6). Whenever epileptogenic activity was not present, the background activity was normal. An EEG taken at age 14 was almost completely normal.

When last seen, at age 21, she had had no further seizures and only occasional migraine attacks. Her examination remained normal, and she had received no antiepileptic medication for 8 years.

CASE 11 A young woman had classical migraine suggesting basilar involvement starting in childhood. Rare nocturnal seizures occurred, not clearly related in time to her visual symptoms; her only diurnal attack was preceded by the dizziness that habitually ushered in her migrainous aura.

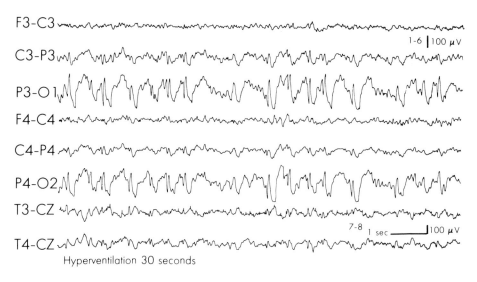

F3-C3
C3-P3
P3-O1
F4-C4
C4-P4
P4-O2
T3-CZ
T4-CZ

1-6 | 100 µV

7-8 | 1 sec _____ | 100 µV

Hyperventilation 30 seconds

Figure 1.5   Case 10; age 11. Spike and slow wave activity over both occipital regions.

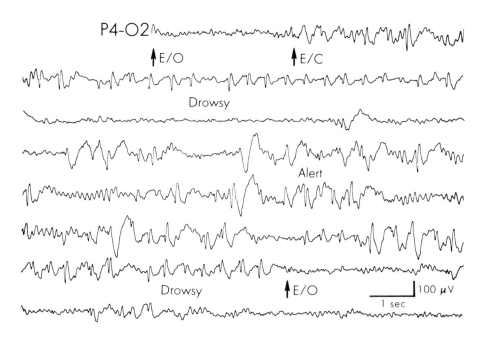

P4-O2

↑E/O   ↑E/C

Drowsy

Alert

Drowsy   ↑E/O | 100 µV
                                1 sec

Figure 1.6   Case 10, age 10. Continuous recording, showing spikes, sharp waves, and spike and wave complexes blocking with eye opening (E/O). (E/C = eyes closed.)

A 26-year-old woman had migrainous symptoms which began at age 10. In association with febrile illnesses, she had attacks of severe dizziness and persistent vomiting, lasting 1 hour to as long as several days. These attacks terminated abruptly with sudden complete loss of vision ("Everything goes black") that lasted from 1 to 10 minutes but were not associated with any impairment of consciousness. Severe generalized pounding headache preceded or followed the visual loss. On one occasion, instead of losing her vision, she described yellow vision lasting for 5 hours. On three occasions, at ages 11, 14, and 17, she had generalized nocturnal tonic-clonic seizures. A single diurnal seizure was preceded by her usual feeling of intense dizziness. The ictus consisted of generalized stiffening. Her physical examination was completely normal at age 18.

Her mother and a grandmother had common migraine.

CT scan was normal. EEGs showed rhythmic sharp-and-slow-wave discharges, maximally over the left posterior temporal region, activated by hyperventilation and blocking with eye opening (Figure 1.7). During sleep, the morphology of the wave forms changed, with the appearance of spikes in the same region. Alpha activity was poorly regulated and of low voltage.

CASE 12 A boy with basilar migraine developed a seizure during a migrainous aura. He had abundant focal and generalized epileptic abnormalities and a family history of both common migraine and epilepsy.

At age 4, this boy began having frequent prostrating headaches. Many of these were accompanied by nausea and vomiting as well as some form of visual distortion. At age 7, an EEG showed a very active epileptic abnormality from the right

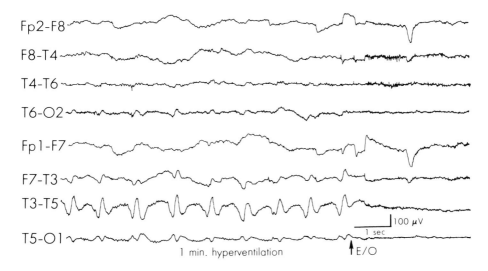

Figure 1.7 Case 11, age 17. Continuous sharp-and-slow-wave discharges over the left posterior temporal region, activated by hyperventilation and blocking with eye opening (E/O).

posterior temporal and occipital regions. He was treated with phenobarbital, but his headaches did not abate. At age 9, he had, with the headache, hallucinations of monsters that he could draw convincingly during and after the attack.

At age 9 he also had his first and only seizure. While watching television he developed sudden complete visual loss. This was followed about 5 minutes later by loss of consciousness and then by a brief seizure beginning in the left arm and becoming generalized. His EEG the next day showed continuous generalized irregular spike and wave discharge blocking almost completely on eye opening. Occasional sporadic spikes and spike-and-wave complexes originated in the right posterior temporal area. The background was normal.

His neurologic examination and CT scan were normal. At age 9½, he was an excellent student. He was treated with phenytoin, but his EEG continued to show prolonged trains of generalized spike and wave activity that blocked on eye opening.

His father had seizures following a severe head injury and also common migraine with severe headaches, photophobia, and vomiting.

Comment

These patients had classical migraine that, because of total visual loss, was suggestive of involvement of the basilar territory (Bickerstaff 1961a, 1961b). In three patients, the seizures clearly started during an acute migrainous event or aura. In the fourth, no information was available about the nocturnal seizures, but the single diurnal attack was preceded by the dizziness that ushered in the patient's habitual migraine attacks.

It is not entirely clear why this group of patients with involvement of the basilar territory had more abundant or striking interictal epileptic EEG abnormalities than did adolescents with classical but, as far as one could tell, nonbasilar migraine and seizures. The prognosis appeared to be similar in the two groups.

All had seizures that were easily controlled, and all remained normal despite their ongoing and very active EEG abnormalities. In two cases, these were temporo-occipital and lateralized, in one they were bioccipital, and in the fourth they were generalized with some independent temporo-occipital focal discharges. These epileptogenic abnormalities consisted of spikes, sharp and slow waves, and spike and wave discharges, at times activated by hyperventilation and often blocked by eye opening. All had a family history of migraine, classical in one and common in the other three. These patients were previously presented, in part, by Camfield et al. (1978).

CONFUSIONAL MIGRAINE WITH SEIZURES DURING THE CONFUSIONAL PERIOD

CASE 13   A young man with a strong family history of classical migraine developed common migraine evolving to confusional migraine. Several years later, the prolonged confusional episodes culminated in brief tonic-clonic seizures that were readily controlled by medication. Only minor electrographic abnormalities were found.

> A 20-year-old premedical student had common migraine since childhood. A brother had classical migraine with hemianopia and a sister had, in addition, prolonged confusion or amnesia during an attack. The father, paternal grandmother, and great-grandmother had severe migraine.
>
> Migraine attacks evolving to a confusional or amnestic state lasting hours started at age 11. One attack developed in a restaurant; the father, who was a physician, took the boy outside and told him to sit on the curb. He did not know where the curb was and could not find it.
>
> At age 18, he developed one Saturday morning, a mild headache and nausea: "It was the same feeling I get with my migraine." He was confused the whole morning but remembered going to the college cafeteria and having a glass of juice. He went to watch TV and had a brief generalized seizure. Further seizures, always during confusional migraine attacks, occurred on Mother's Day, Father's Day, and the father's birthday. The attacks began with extreme nausea and dizziness; he did not know where he was but seemed aware of his surroundings.
>
> The EEGs showed generalized but asymmetrical slow activity during hyperventilation only. He had no attacks for a year while taking carbamazepine and pyzotiline, but he had a recurrence when he stopped taking his medication.

Comment

The mechanism of confusion and amnesia in such patients is probably similar to that of transient global amnesia and implies a disturbance in the distal territory of supply of the basilar system on both sides. The prolonged confusion is probably analogous to the classical or basilar migrainous aura, although this cannot be proved (Gascon and Barlow, 1970).

Genetic evidence in this family clearly linked the confusional episodes to classical migraine. This boy had seizures only during the confusional episodes, and successful preventive treatment of the migraine resulted in cessation of the epileptic manifestations as well.

CLASSICAL MIGRAINE WITH PROLONGED POSTMIGRAINOUS AND POSTICTAL DEFICIT

CASE 14 During a time of stress, a young woman with a family history of migraine developed increasingly severe classical or complicated migraine with persistent neurologic symptoms. Acoustic distortion and numbness suggested predominantly temporal and parietal involvement.

She developed a seizure followed by persistent facial and arm numbness and hemianopia that disappeared over 2 weeks. She did not remember a migrainous aura to the seizure; there was, on the other hand, a striking resemblance between her postictal deficit and her habitual migrainous aura.

The 27-year-old daughter of a physician had a congenital renal anomaly and recurrent pyelonephritis.

She developed migraine at age 24. She noticed an alteration in the quality of sound, which increased in resonance as if she were in a cavern. Then she developed tingling in the left corner of the mouth. This tingling involved the upper and lower lips and the side of the tongue, and it spread gradually to the side of the face and to the left arm. The duration of spread of the paresthesiae from the corner of the mouth to the hand was 10 minutes; their total duration was about an hour. They disappeared first from the territory where they had appeared last. She dropped things from the left hand and also had minor visual halucinations described as zigzag lines in the center of the visual field. Afterward, she had bitemporal headaches with nausea and repeated vomiting.

When the aura and the headache were severe, she sometimes had residual numbness of the face that lasted up to a whole day.

After a week of great pressure, she went to the theater, usually a source of relaxation to her. She lost consciousness, tensed, cried out, and had a generalized seizure. She awoke in the hospital with numbness of the left face and, to a lesser extent, of the left arm, and with a left homonymous hemianopia. These abnormalities disappeared over 2 weeks.

Her examination and CT scan were normal; her EEGs were reported at another center to show bitemporal independent epileptic discharges. Her brother and several relatives on her father's side had a history of migraine. There was also a family history of seizures. Treatment with carbamazepine and pizotyline was advised.

Comment

This patient with classical migraine had prolonged neurologic deficits following severe attacks, and these were attributed to ischemia occurring during the migrainous aura. The relationship of her single epileptic seizure to the migrainous aura was suggested by the similarity of the neurologic sequelae in the two types of attacks. It is possible that she was amnestic for the aura or that she had no aura to her epileptic seizure. The more severe and prolonged deficit following her seizure may have been caused by a mechanism similar to that of the migrainous aura, such as ischemia, or perhaps to a vascular occlusion. The EEG abnormalities described were difficult to explain but were not confirmed on repeat examination.

CLASSICAL MIGRAINE AND LATER DEVELOPMENT OF TEMPORAL LOBE EPILEPSY— RIPENING OF EPILEPTOGENIC AREAS OWING TO CEREBRAL DAMAGE CAUSED BY THE MIGRAINE?

CASE 15   This patient initially had classical migraine leading to epileptic manifestations during migrainous auras only. She had right posterior temporal and occipital EEG slow wave abnormalities and epileptogenic discharges. In her early 20s she developed minor attacks of temporal lobe epilepsy. At that time there was additional evidence of independent bitemporal anterior and inferomesial epileptogenic abnormalities. She had a family history of migraine and epilepsy.

The independent bitemporal epileptogenic discharges were most likely a manifestation of secondary epileptogenesis related to the original right posterior temporal and occipital epileptic abnormalities, which in turn appeared to be related to her classical migraine.

A 27-year-old woman was followed from age 9. At that time she developed attacks in which she saw colored lights starting in either the left or the right visual field, followed by headache and nausea. Following these visual manifestations, she occasionally turned her head or developed jerking of the head to the left, leading to secondary generalization. Her intelligence progressively deteriorated. Her global IQ was 92 at age 8 and 72 at age 15.

When she was 19, slow and slow sharp wave discharges were recorded from the right posterior temporal and occipital head regions. At age 22, she developed absence attacks with staring and automatism. At age 24, serial EEGs with sphenoidal electrodes showed active, independent anterior and inferomesial bitemporal epileptogenic discharges, as well as independent right posterior temporal epileptic discharge and right posterior temporal and occipital slow activity.

This young woman had a sister with retardation and seizures, and her mother had common migraine.

In later years, it was no longer possible to obtain from her the history of migraine auras leading to seizures that was so characteristic of her early attacks.

CASE 16   A woman with a family history of classical migraine developed common migraine followed by prominent acephalgic migraine with striking separation in time of somatosensory and visual attacks. She then developed recurrent symptoms of temporal lobe dysfunction. The duration and clustering of these attacks suggested an epileptic etiology, and on one occasion she went on to have a major seizure. The repeated migrainous auras may well have led to ripening of a temporal focus of epileptogenic discharge. It is less likely that her experiential hallucinations, evolving on one occasion to an epileptic attack, were migrainous.

A 38-year-old nursing administrator had common migraine from the age of 18. At age 30 she started to have episodes of acephalgic migraine with numbness moving up from the fingers to the face, including the lip, and at times spreading to the leg. The numbness developed over a 5-minute period, remained for an additional 5 minutes, and disappeared in the order in which it had come on. The duration was often shorter, and at times she was lightheaded. A second form of acephalgic migraine attack consisted of visual symptoms: these included hemianopic, quadrantic, or altitudinal defects containing zigzag or jacquard patterns, at times resembling fireworks. They tended to move slowly from one side of the visual field to the other. At times she also had monocular visual changes. On at least one occasion the visual changes went on to a full-fledged migraine attack with headache and other autonomic symptoms.

At age 36, she developed episodes when, stimulated by a word she heard, she would have the impression that she knew what the next word was going to be, how the discussion was going to end, or what her mood was going to be when the discussion ended. She denied prescience as such and considered these experiences to resemble a remembered scene or experience. She relived an experience that had occurred between the ages of 13 and 15 when she had been friendly with a neighboring family and had spent a great deal of time with them. They had had a toy doghouse with toy bassets, one for every member of the family, and anyone who misbehaved would "go to the doghouse." She was told she had visited there so often that she merited inclusion in the family and a toy dog of her own. In association with this experience she had a sensation of discomfort or fear. She found the attacks bothersome and waited for them to pass. They occurred in clusters or bouts of seven or eight and at times woke her during the night. Afterward, she felt washed-out or tired. Once these feelings continued after the usual 1 to 2 minutes and evolved to a major tonic-clonic seizure.

She had mild hypertension. Her neurologic examination and CT scan were normal. She did not have a searching EEG study. Her father, a psychiatrist, had classical migraine with visual changes similar to her own. A brother had migraine of undetermined type. Treatment with carbamazepine and propranolol was suggested.

CASE 17   A young woman with classical migraine and a family history of classical migraine developed a right quadrantic field defect and, later, temporal lobe epilepsy originating on the left side. At operation, hippocampal gliosis and sclerosis of the third temporal gyrus were found. She remained seizure-free after temporal lobectomy but continued to have classical migraine attacks. Classical migraine may explain both the field defect and seizures of this patient.

A 24-year-old graduate student developed classical migraine during adolescence. During the migrainous aura, she saw shining or shimmering lights in a hemianopic distribution followed by perioral numbness that spread to the fingers and the arm, usually on the left side but at times on the right. This was followed by severe headache. Her sister had classical migraine with hemianopia, but there were no other affected family members. She then developed seizures at age 19. The aura contained very rich and varied temporal manifestations with sexual feelings, uncinate symptoms, and mixed pleasure and fear, as well as various experiential feelings, mainly déjà vu. Occasionally she had secondarily generalized attacks.

On examination she was found to have a right quadrantic field defect. Electrographic investigation showed left anterior and inferomesial temporal epileptic abnormality. At operation she was found to have a sclerotic third temporal gyrus as well as an abnormal fusiform gyrus and hippocampal sclerosis. Following surgery she had several neighborhood attacks but no further seizures. She continued, however, to have attacks of classical migraine, with the aura most often suggesting involvement of the right hemisphere.

Comment

The first patient had a clear history of seizures occurring during migrainous auras only. Over the years this pattern was no longer apparent, but she developed temporal lobe epilepsy. The original temporo-occipital EEG abnormalities persisted and coexisted with her temporal foci. The second patient had no epileptic manifestations during her migrainous attacks; her seizures started late, at age 36, and no etiological factors other than her complicated migraine could be identified. The third patient had a quadrantic field deficit most likely caused by a vascular occlusion, perhaps related to migraine. There was no evidence for vascular abnormality other than migraine to explain this, and the pathologic changes were not specific.

In these three patients, the temporal epileptogenic process most likely ripened in response to repeated cerebral insults caused by complicated migraine.

CLASSICAL MIGRAINE FOLLOWED BY TEMPORAL LOBE EPILEPSY AND PEDUNCULAR HALLUCINOSIS

CASE 18   A young woman with classical migraine developed seizures, suggesting posterior temporal localization, in her teens. Later, prolonged hallucinations resembling peduncular hallucinosis started. The temporal relationships between these different disorders and the family history could not be clarified because of emotional and cultural factors.

> A 22-year-old woman had a history of severe pounding, mainly occipital headaches since childhood, preceded or accompanied by seeing white or flashing spots.
>
> At age 15 she developed seizures that started with vivid visual hallucinations of a person she could not identify. This person was dressed in white, flowing robes and told her she was bad. The attacks became generalized and were not clearly related in time to the migraine. They responded to carbamazepine.
>
> At age 21 she developed prolonged visual and auditory hallucinations that occurred while she was studying or reading quietly. She saw a crowd of more than 100 people; some were dressed in white. She could not identify them or their racial background. They talked rapidly, and she could not understand what they were saying; they were neither pleasant, unpleasant, nor threatening. These hallucinations could last for many minutes and were not associated with migrainous symptoms. They disappeared when she changed her activity or put on some music.
>
> Her EEGs showed bioccipital spike and multiple spike and slow wave and sharp and slow complexes in brief bursts, becoming almost continuous during hyperventilation. The abnormality was also photosensitive. At other times, independent bioccipital epileptogenic foci with left-sided predominance were seen. Background activity was normal, and the epileptic discharges tended to block with eye opening.

Comment

Like the previous three patients, this young woman developed temporal lobe epilepsy after a history of classical migraine going back several years. Later, however, she also developed peduncular hallucinosis, a nonepileptic disorder suggesting midbrain dysfunction. This disorder is occasionally encountered in patients with complicated migraine.

CLASSICAL MIGRAINE AND EPILEPSY: AN UNUSUALLY LONG FOLLOW-UP

CASE 19   An elderly woman had a 56-year history of prolonged visual attacks associated with severe headache and, at times, convulsions. She had a clear history and family history of migraine. Attacks improved with age, but she still had a tendency to seizures, which were controlled by small doses of antiepileptic medication.

> A 69-year-old woman began to have attacks at age 13. These started with lights in the right visual field that lasted up to 30 or 40 minutes and were followed by severe headache. At times the visual changes were associated with convulsions, and she also developed seizures not preceded by migrainous symptoms. Over the years the attacks improved, but at age 66 she had four seizures with loss of consciousness. Over the years she also had recurrent throbbing headaches without aura. Her intelligence was normal, but her early history was vague. Her sister had a history of migraine of undetermined type.
>
> She had an unusual posture, stooped, with the neck flexed and the head tilted, but she had no field defect. A CT scan showed moderate diffuse cerebral atrophy, maximal posteriorly; an EEG, while she was receiving medication, showed only minimal diffuse slow irregularities.

Comment

This woman illustrates the difficulty of retrospectively evaluating the nature and relationship of prolonged visual symptoms, headaches, and seizures. Most likely the prolonged visual manifestations were migrainous, leading to seizures during the aura and eventually to the ripening of a focal epileptogenic area. In this case, however, because of the lapse of time and the lacunae in the history, the proposed sequence remains speculative.

OCCIPITAL EPILEPSY ASSOCIATED WITH COMMON MIGRAINE OR A FAMILY HISTORY OF MIGRAINE

CASE 20   This boy developed occipital and temporal epileptic manifestations but had no clear-cut migraine history. He had, however, a strong and probably significant family history of classical migraine. There was also a less striking family history of epilepsy.

> An 11-year-old boy had developed episodes of blindness lasting 1 minute, not accompanied by alteration of consciousness, at the age of 7. At age 8 he developed absence attacks. These were ushered in by left-sided multicolored whirling, flashing lights that lasted 10 to 20 seconds. This experience was followed by an insecure, frightened feeling of being far from home and unable to get back. Then he became unresponsive for 20 to 30 seconds, and would sleep for an hour. EEGs

showed slow spike and wave discharge, maximal over the right posterior temporal region.

His mother and his maternal aunt had infrequent classical migraine, with hemianopic blurring and zigzag lines. The visual loss then became generalized. The paternal grandfather had common migraine, and a maternal uncle had a history of cerebral seizures.

CASE 21 A boy with common migraine and a family history of common migraine developed bioccipital epileptic foci and seizures. Bioccipital hypodense lesions in the parenchyma correlated with the epileptogenic process. The etiology of these lesions remained unexplained, but a relationship to the migrainous process could be suspected.

A 12-year-old boy with common migraine and a family history of common migraine started to have seizures at age 8. Lightning-like flashes progressed to clonic movements of the right arm and secondary generalization. He also had minor attacks with staring and fluttering of the lids. He developed a severe behavioral disturbance, and seizures did not respond to medication. Neurologic examination was normal. The CT scan showed bilateral occipital nonenhancing hypodense lesions. EEGs showed occipital independent epileptogenic abnormalities shifting from side to side with maximum background disturbance over the left.

CASE 22 A boy experienced two different types of occipital seizures. One form of attack originated on the right; it was unclear whether the second type originated on the same or on the opposite side, where an independent focus of interictal epileptic discharge had also been found. His mother's prolonged labor was probably etiologically significant. The patient, his mother, and his grandmother had common migraine, and his father had classical migraine. The role of the migraine and of the family history of classical migraine in the production of his seizures remains speculative.

This 14-year-old boy was born after a prolonged labor. His developmental milestones were normal. He developed seizures at age 3. In the initial attacks, he stopped all activity, sank to the ground, and became unresponsive for 30 to 60 seconds. Attacks stopped spontaneously for a year. At age 5 he had seizures in which his eyes, head, and trunk turned to the left and he had clonic movements of the left arm. He had two different visual auras: one consisted of a small spot in the left visual field, the other of waving elementary colors in the right field.

Neurologic examination was normal. An attack that started with his seeing small white lights was recorded—he yelled "Seizure!" and seemed to be looking at something; then he yelled "Over!" Electrographic seizure activity remained confined to the right occipital region, but there was generalized background attenuation as well. Interictal epileptic foci were recorded from the right temporo-occipital area and, independently, from the left. The right-sided focus was more active. There was an excess of slow activity over both these areas.

Visual evoked responses showed increased latency on the left (116–120) as compared with the right (109–115). A CT scan showed minor asymmetry of the lateral ventricles, the left being larger than the right. He had superior intelligence. He was treated with carbamazepine and valproic acid, but the seizures continued.

His father had classical migraine with zigzag lines and blurring of vision in the left visual field. He could not see to the left during this aura, which would last about 20 minutes; he would be unable to park his car. The boy's mother and maternal grandmother had common migraine. The patient had intermittent headaches, and these were severe enough to make him lie down.

CASE 23   A boy with common migraine and a family history of both common and classical migraine developed a lacunar occipital lesion, probably at the time of a mild head injury with brief concussion. He then developed occipital seizures that sometimes became secondarily generalized. In addition to the head injury, abnormal vascular reactivity caused by the patient's migraine and family history of migraine was suspected to be important in the causation of the occipital lesion. There was little or no relationship in time between the patient's epileptic visual symptoms and his migrainous attacks with headache and nausea.

At age 12, starting 5 to 10 minutes after a brief concussion, this boy could not see the lower half of the visual field for about 15 minutes. Clinically, this may have represented footballer's migraine or, less likely, the effect of contusion. Sometime later he began to have attacks with the sensation of a light flashing in the left lateral corner of the visual field for 5 to 15 minutes. This was followed by loss of vision in that area. At times the visual changes were followed by unconsciousness, and he was found retching or vomiting. He also had a history of fairly severe headaches associated with vomiting. The mother had had an episode of numbness of the hand, face, mouth, and tongue on the right side when she was a child. She remembered dropping a glass of soda given to her by her mother. She had similar attacks on other occasions and severe headaches preceded by hemianopic visual loss at least once. Her father and paternal grandmother had severe recurrent headaches.

The boy's alternating finger movements on the left were slower than expected in a left-handed individual. A CT scan showed a small hypodense lesion in the right occipital region. An attack lasting 55 seconds was recorded during the EEG following hyperventilation. Right occipital spikes were recorded during the initial 15 seconds of the attack. He complained of his usual flashes of light and of a blind spot in the left upper visual field. Later he had a transient left hemianopia. His EEGs also showed a generalized paroxysmal abnormality. The hypodense lesion found on the CT scan resolved progressively.

He was still complaining monthly, 6 years later, of flashes of yellow light followed by a scotoma in the left upper field but not by headache or loss of consciousness.

CASE 24   Partial occipital simple seizures developed following a mild head injury in a boy with macrocrania and a family history of macrocrania. Later the attacks progressed to include prominent clinical evidence of temporal lobe involvement. He had recurrent frontal headaches, and his mother had mild infrequent headaches that were compatible with mild common migraine. The relationship of the epilepsy to the migraine and the macrocrania is uncertain, but the coexistence of these disorders is probably not merely coincidental.

A 12-year-old boy weighed 4,950 grams at birth. He had macrocrania (head circ., 59 cm), and a family history of macrocrania (mother's head circ., 59 cm). Following a brief concussion at age 9, he developed partial simple visual seizures consisting of white, red, purple, and blue flashing lights in the left visual field, lasting 10 to 20 seconds. At age 11 he developed a secondarily generalized nocturnal seizure and partial complex attacks with adversion, twitching of the left side, and unconsciousness.

A CT scan showed no focal abnormality. His EEG showed almost continuous right posterior temporal and occipital sharp and slow wave complexes activated by hyperventilation (Figure 1.8). The response of this abnormality to eye opening and closure was not assessed during this recording.

A year later, partial simple attacks were still present, and at times he saw coloured geometric shapes resembling octagons. In about a third of those attacks he would become unresponsive, and would chew, swallow, and speak inappropriately. Once, when asked, he said he saw someone on a seesaw that he was moving with his leg. He complained of recurrent frontal headaches; his neurologic examination remained normal.

His mother had occasional mild recurrent headaches.

Comment

These five children had occipital epilepsy as well as a striking family history of classical migraine in three and common migraine in all five. They themselves

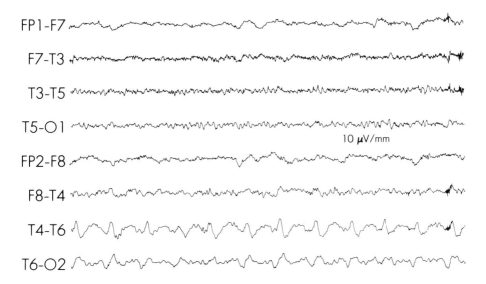

Figure 1.8   Case 24, age 11. Continuous right posterior temporal sharp-and-slow wave complexes.

all had common migraine, but no classical migraine aura leading up to their seizures. Single or bilateral occipital hypodense lesions, prolonged labor, trauma, and macrocrania were underlying abnormal findings.

FOCAL CEREBRAL DAMAGE IN A PATIENT WITH PRIMARY GENERALIZED EPILEPSY AND CLASSICAL MIGRAINE: A FACTOR CONTRIBUTING TO DIFFICULTY IN OBTAINING SEIZURE CONTROL

CASE 25   A man with primary generalized epilepsy and a history of classical migraine with hemianopic auras was found to have a homonymous quadrantanopia. The presence of an additional cerebral lesion may have been responsible for the difficulty in controlling his attacks for many years. The seizures finally yielded to good therapeutic levels of valproic acid.

The quadrantanopia may have been caused either by the migraine or by a vascular lesion of other cause perhaps related to his prematurity, but this alternative seems less likely.

A 38-year-old man had a history of seizures since childhood. Major attacks ceased at age 27, but he continued to have brief episodes of jerking of the face and, at times, of the hands. These occurred mainly in the morning and when he was eating. The jerks corresponded to brief bursts of generalized spike and wave discharge that lasted 1 to 4 seconds, and he was probably briefly unresponsive during these periods. These minor attacks thus represented absences with myoclonic component.

He had been born after a premature delivery at 37 weeks' gestation weighing 4 pounds. On examination he had a right lower homonymous quadrantic field defect. He had classical migraine with a hemianopic visual aura since adolescence; these attacks remitted in the third decade.

A CT scan showed mild diffuse cortical atrophy, and an arteriogram was normal. EEGs showed moderately active, generalized epileptogenic abnormality of spike and polyspike and wave type, correlating with his clinical attacks. There was also a mild disturbance of cerebral activity over the left frontotemporal region. His verbal IQ was 136 with a significantly lower performance IQ. His attacks were fully controlled by valproic acid.

Comment

Seizures in patients with generalized epilepsy who have focalization of their discharge or a focal structural abnormality often do not respond well to antiepileptic treatment. This patient illustrates well the multifactorial nature of the epilepsies (Andermann, 1982).

DISCUSSION

Three forms of association between migraine and epilepsy emerge from review of this group of patients.

Most numerous are those patients who, during a classical migraine aura, go on to develop an epileptic seizure. This occurs more commonly in children and adolescents but also in adults: Of the 25 patients in this group 14, or 56% of the total, presented in this way (Cases 1 – 14). The diagnosis is based on the history, particularly on the march of the migrainous aura. This is of necessity clearer in older children and in adults, since these patients do not have seizures independent of their migraine attacks. The mechanism of the epileptic events thus appears to be attributable to the spreading depression or oligemia that characterizes the classical or basilar migraine aura and confusional migraine attacks. Electrographic abnormalities are more striking in childhood and adolescence; adults more commonly have normal EEGs. This age-dependent relationship is not unexpected, and it corresponds to what is known to occur in many epileptic EEG abnormalities, such as the rolandic spike and the 3/sec spike and wave, for instance. Most of these patients appear to have a benign course and eventually remit; their EEG abnormalities also tend to disappear. In some, however, the persistence of electrographic abnormality suggests that the process may be responsible for some permanent cerebral dysfunction.

Control or prevention of the migraine may be expected to prevent recurrence of the seizures. It is less clear whether or not these patients should also be treated with anticonvulsants. Antimigraine preventive agents are not always effective. Breakthrough attacks may still lead to seizures, and these may be prevented, shortened, or otherwise modified by the use of antiepileptic drugs. For these rather theoretical reasons, we have been inclined to use anticonvulsants, generally carbamazepine or phenytoin, when the attacks continue despite preventive antimigrainous treatment.

One might expect a greater genetic predisposition to epilepsy or a lower seizure threshold in this group of patients; this is suggested by a family history of epilepsy in some. A more formal controlled study would be valuable.

It is not clear whether there is an increased prevalence of history or findings suggesting preexistent cerebral dysfunction in this group of patients. This was not obvious, but again no controlled studies were available.

The second, much smaller group of patients (4 patients or 16%) consists of those with classical or complicated migraine who go on to develop epilepsy involving preferentially the temporal lobe (Cases 15 – 18). The sequence from classical migraine to seizures occurring only during the migraine aura and to the eventual ripening of a temporal epileptic process has been clearly documented over the years in Case 15. *Pari passu* she developed striking temporo-occipital surface EEG changes and later bilateral, inferomesial, epileptogenic foci. Even in this patient, the sequence of earlier events could not be reconstructed from the history that she gave in adult life. It is likely that a similar sequence occurred in the other patients; the quadrantanopia of Case 17 may have been caused by a vascular complication of classical migraine.

A preferential occipitotemporal pathway has been demonstrated to facilitate secondary epileptogenesis (Olivier et al., 1982), and such a mechanism may be present in these patients. Permanent ischemic changes in the territory of the posterior cerebral artery could also lead to the development of temporal lobe epileptic discharge. Rémillard et al. (1974) have suggested this in patients who, in association with occlusion of the posterior cerebral artery or its branches, later develop temporal lobe epilepsy.

Whether classical or complicated migraine is more frequently an etiological factor in the development of temporal lobe epilepsy remains speculative. Certainly further historical inquiry along these lines and other longitudinal observations would be valuable in the absence of measurable markers.

Complicated migraine may cause a fixed neurologic deficit, and this may also affect an underlying generalized epileptic process. This was suggested by Case 25, whose quadrantic field defect may well have been related to his classical migraine. This man's primary generalized epilepsy was very difficult to control; in our experience, this tends to correlate with the obviousness and severity of the acquired component in patients with generalized epilepsy.

The third group consists of children or adolescents with occipital epilepsy who have common migraine and a family history of classical or common migraine. Cases 20–24 (five of our patients, or 20%), were in this group. They did not have a history of classical migraine aura. We wondered if this could not be documented because of their age; however, this seems unlikely since children will usually talk about a prolonged visual aura and because some of the patients in this group were older children or adolescents who could be expected to give a clear history. In this group there was a high prevalence of both acquired dysfunction and structural abnormalities. Of the children in this group, 2 children had hypodense occipital lesions demonstrated by the CT scan.

A high prevalence of headache in patients with occipital epilepsy has been confirmed by Gastaut and Zifkin (Chapter 3, this volume) and by Aicardi and Newton (Chapter 6, this volume). In our group of patients, common migraine and a positive family history of migraine were present in all, with classical migraine occurring in close relatives in three families. This high prevalence of migraine in children with focal epilepsy was unusual, though it is also seen in patients with benign rolandic epilepsy (Chapter 9, this volume).

Migraine, and particularly a genetic predisposition to classical migraine, may predispose to the development of vascular lesions in the posterior circulation and may prove to be a significant factor in the development of occipital epilepsy. This hypothesis requires confirmation by the study of larger series of patients with this form of epilepsy, including complete genetic histories based on uniform criteria of diagnosis of classical, common, and other varieties of migraine.

The histories of these children do not suggest that their headaches derive from brain stem vasomotor disturbance caused by the occipital epileptic discharge, as Gastaut and Zifkin (Chapter 3, this volume) have suggested; this could hardly explain the positive family history of migraine in these patients.

Migraine and epilepsy are also found in association in patients with malignant migraine and mitochondrial encephalopathy or encephalomyopathy. Our patients with this syndrome are presented separately by Dvorkin et al. (Chapter 14, this volume). In this condition migraine, generally classical and with a

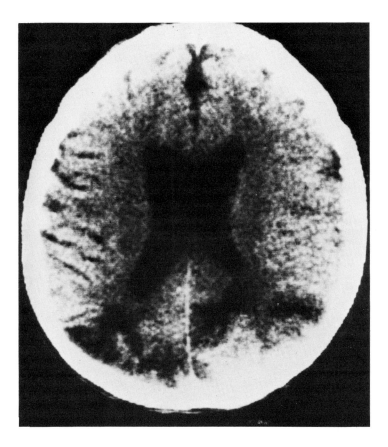

Figure 1.9   CT scan of a patient with malignant migraine, epilepsy, and mitochondrial encephalomyopathy showing irregular bilateral hypodensities caused by strokes, mainly in the territory of the posterior circulation.

positive family history, is associated with or leads to epilepsy followed by status epilepticus, multiple strokes (Figure 1.9), increasing neurologic deficit, and death. The syndrome is associated with mitochondrial myopathy and lactic acidosis in some. Not all our patients had ragged red fibers when biopsied, and the process may have been more marked in brain than in muscle in these individuals; the clinical course, however, was quite characteristic. The relationship of the migraine present (and genetically determined) in other family members to the abnormality in energy metabolism demonstrated, only in some of these patients, remains unknown. Many features were those of the MELAS (mitochondrial encephalomyopathy, lactic acidosis, and stroke) syndrome identified by Pavlakis et al. (1984). However, the short stature, deafness, and myopathic features of that syndrome may be missing, and patients may present with either occipital epilepsy or progressively severe migraine.

SUMMARY

We conclude that four migraine epilepsy syndromes may be identified:

1. Patients who have seizures only when triggered by a classical migrainous aura, and where the epileptic manifestation was attributed to ischemia or spreading depression or oligemia.
2. Patients who later go on to develop epilepsy originating in the temporal lobe, presumably by a mechanism of secondary epileptogenesis.
3. Patients with occipital epilepsy. Migraine and a positive family history of migraine, are common in children with occipital epilepsy. Migraine may predispose to the development of vascular lesions in the posterior circulation and prove to be a significant risk factor in the development of occipital epilepsy.
4. Patients with mitochondrial disease. Migraine and a positive family history of migraine, epilepsy, and multiple strokes, are cardinal features of mitochondrial encephalopathy with or without mitochondrial myopathy and lactic acidosis.

Identification of these syndromes brings us a step closer to solving the enigma first recognized by Hughlings Jackson more than a century ago.

REFERENCES

Andermann E. Multifactorial inheritance of generalized and focal epilepsy. In: Anderson VE et al., eds. Genetic basis of the Epilepsies. New York: Raven Press, 1982:355–74.

Bickerstaff ER. Basilar artery migraine. Lancet 1961;1:15–7.

Bickerstaff ER. Impairment of consciousness in migraine. Lancet 1961;2:1057–9.

Camfield PR, Metrakos K, Andermann F. Basilar migraine, seizures and severe epileptiform EEG abnormalities: a relatively benign syndrome in adolescents. Neurology 1978;28:584–8.

Gascon G, Barlow C. Juvenile migraine, presenting as an acute confusional state. Pediatrics 1970;45:628–35.

Gowers Sir William R. The borderland of epilepsy: faints, vagal attacks, vertigo, migraine, sleep symptoms, and their treatment. London: Churchill, 1907.

Jackson J. Hughlings. Hospital for the epileptic and paralyzed: case illustrating the relation betwixt certain cases of migraine and epilepsy. Lancet 1875;2:244–5.

Olivier A, Gloor P, Andermann F, Ives J. Occipitotemporal epilepsy studied with stereotaxically implanted depth electrodes and successfully treated by temporal resection. Ann Neurol 1982;11:428–32.

Pavlakis SG, Phillips PC, Di Mauro S, De Vivo DC, Rowland L. Mitochondrial myopathy, encephalopathy, lactic acidosis, and stroke-like episodes: a distinctive clinical syndrome. Ann Neurol 1984;16:481–8.

Rémillard GM, Éthier R, Andermann F. Temporal lobe epilepsy and perinatal occlusion of the posterior cerebral artery. A syndrome analogous to infantile hemiplegia and a demonstrable etiology in some patients with temporal lobe epilepsy. Neurology 1974;24:1001–9.

2

Difficulties in Differentiating Migraine and Epilepsy Based on Clinical and EEG Findings

C. P. Panayiotopoulos

Migraine and epilepsy, according to our present status of knowledge, are two different disorders with recurrent and paroxysmal—and usually brief and abrupt—manifestations of disturbed brain function. Their pathophysiology is entirely different: migraine is a vasomotor disease whereas epilepsy is a disorder of the electrical properties of the brain. The clinical symptomatology of migraine, with the cardinal feature of headache, is also quite different from that of epilepsy, in which convulsions and disturbed consciousness are the main manifestations. Headache is usually a minor and neglected sequel of an epileptic attack.

The question of a possible relationship between migraine and epilepsy has arisen mainly from cases of migraine associated with, followed by, or interposed with epileptic attacks, which may also occur independently in the same subject (see Chapter 1). A link between the two diseases has been the subject of numerous studies on genetic, electroencephalographic (EEG), and statistical correlations between migraine and epilepsy patients; but most of these results and views are still in conflict. At the present time, it does not seem possible to formulate definite conclusions regarding the existence or nonexistence of a relationship that will be generally accepted.

The purpose of this chapter is to emphasize the clinical and electroencephalographic difficulties that are sometimes encountered when trying to make a definite diagnosis of migraine or epilepsy in certain cases. These difficulties have been postulated by many masters of neurology such as Gowers (1907):

> Some surprise may be felt that migraine is given a place in the borderland of epilepsy, but the position is justified by many relations and among them by the

fact that the two maladies are sometimes mistaken and more often their distinction is difficult.

It should be emphasized from the beginning that in presenting separately some of the patients' symptoms, there is no deviation from the golden rule of medicine — an accurate diagnosis utilizes every piece of information regarding heredity, history, age, symptoms and signs, sequence of events, timing, etc., as well as the results of carefully screened laboratory investigations. This method of presentation has been chosen because some of these features are predominantly related to "epilepsy" or "migraine" and may cause some bias in our final judgment.

IMPAIRMENT OR LOSS OF CONSCIOUSNESS— CONVULSIONS

Impairment or loss of consciousness, which is the cardinal symptom in epilepsy, occurring usually in an abrupt, instantaneous manner, has also been described in migraine. It is seen in the juvenile form as protracted confusional episodes (Gascon and Barlow, 1970), but more frequently in the so-called basilar artery migraine, which has been brought into focus by Bickerstaff (1961a; 1961b; 1962). The latter form of migraine has been attributed to transient dysfunction in the territory of the basilar artery, and affects mainly adolescents, more often girls than boys, with a frequent family history of other forms of migraine. The clinical prodrome phase is manifested by visual symptoms, teichopsia throughout both visual fields, and blurring or total loss of vision associated with vertigo, ataxia, tinnitus, bilateral peripheral dysesthesias, and other brain stem and occipital lobe symptoms. This is followed by severe, throbbing, posterior bilateral headache.

In one-fourth of the cases impairment or loss of consciousness may appear, usually between the prodrome phase and the headache, although unconsciousness preceding the other symptoms also occurs. It is usually brief, from 1 to 10 minutes, with features distinguished from epilepsy, as described by Bickerstaff (1961b, 1058):

> The loss of consciousness was always curiously slow in onset — never abrupt, and never causing the patient to fall or to be injured. A dreamlike state sometimes preceded unconsciousness. The degree of unconsciousness was never profound and the patients were never unrousable; on vigorous stimulation they could be aroused to good cooperation but they returned to unconsciousness when the stimulation ceased.

The disturbance of consciousness, with slow onset and no convulsions, is more likely a stupor attributable to transient vasomotor ischemia of those parts of the brain stem that subserve consciousness. The train of symptoms and the other features described distinguish this disorder from epilepsy and syncope.

The EEG has usually been reported as normal (Bickerstaff, 1961a; 1962), but gross EEG abnormalities have also been known (Lapkin et al., 1977).

The situation, however, is not always so clear. There are reports of severe, long-lasting neurologic symptoms and stupor, probably reflecting more severe vasoconstriction, and instances of abrupt loss of consciousness or associated generalized tonic-clonic seizures that may follow the sequence of prodromal events or occur independently (Slatter, 1968; Lee and Lance, 1977; Swanson and Vick, 1978; Manzoni et al., 1979).

HEADACHE

Headache, the cardinal symptom of migraine, is not uncommon as a postictal event in epilepsy, although it is admittedly a minor and neglected sequel of an epileptic attack. Its severity is usually found to be in proportion to the severity of the attack itself. Headache as a prodromal symptom, hours or days prior to an epileptic attack, has been reported in many patients (Penfield and Kristiansen, 1951). There are rare reports of headache as an ictal manifestation of epilepsy, but the "headache" is more like a peculiar discomfort in the head than true pain. It is always associated with other epileptic symptoms. In a more recent report by Laplante et al. (1983), one of their patients complained of "painful emptiness of the head" and the other one "a painful feeling of pressure or shiver in the temporal regions"; Both patients suffered from long standing epilepsy. Depth electrode studies during ictal "headache" showed this to be associated with paroxysmal activity from the right hippocampus. Headache following a visual aura is difficult to attribute to epilepsy because the diagnosis of migraine is more likely. Epilepsy is not easily accepted as a diagnosis in such cases even if convulsive or other "epileptic" manifestations are present. A chance coincidence of the two diseases, or epileptic phenomena "triggered off" by the migrainous vasoconstriction in a predisposed brain, are the most familiar explanations. In this respect, it is interesting that headache followed after the seizures with visual symptoms in 3 of the 60 patients with traumatic epilepsy reported by Russell and Whitty (1966):

CASE 1 with a midline wound. One type of fit: "Zigzag ring of light in front — gets bigger till ring reaches limit of sight range — clears — headache."

CASE 46 with a left-sided wound. One type of fit: "Right hemianopia, then flashing red light from right spreading to centre and quickening to about one a second, continuing for 30 minutes. Both clear quite suddenly and are followed by left occipital headache."

CASE 48 with right-sided wound. One type of fit: "Feels faint — vision goes black — flashing light on left upper field for a few seconds followed by headache for an hour."

VOMITING AND THE SYNDROME OF BENIGN NOCTURNAL CHILDHOOD OCCIPITAL EPILEPSY

Vomiting is closely related to the headache phase of migraine and also, vomiting attacks are found in the past history of approximately one fourth of migrainous patients (Lance, 1982). In epilepsies, vomiting is accepted only as an after event in the postictal phase of generalized tonic clonic seizures. It has also been reported in the "migrainous headache" phase of "childhood epilepsy with occipital paroxysms" (Camfield et al, 1978; Panayiotopoulos, 1980; see also chapter 3, this volume).

Vomiting has not been reported in association with ictal manifestations of epilepsy except in a new syndrome of "benign nocturnal childhood occipital epilepsy" (Panayiotopoulos, in press). The syndrome has been recently recognized in 8 out of 20 patients with "occipital lobe epilepsy" seen by the author in a 10 year period. The syndrome is characterized by a clinical triad of nocturnal seizures, tonic deviation of the eyes and vomiting. In all eight children, vomiting occurred during the ictal phase of the seizures when the eyes were deviated and always preceded other partial epileptic manifestations and generalized tonic clonic seizures which may have followed. Consciousness is usually, but not always, disturbed. The duration of the seizures varies from a few minutes up to 3 hours. The frequency of the seizures is remarkably low; in all 8 children only 29 seizures were witnessed and two children suffered only solitary ones. Non-nocturnal seizures are extremely rare. The age of onset varies from 2- to 6-years-old with a peak at age 4. The prevalence of this syndrome appeared to be higher than that of "childhood epilepsy with migrainous phenomena and occipital paroxysms;" only two patients were seen with the latter syndrome in the same period. The prognosis is excellent, with all children free of seizures in a 1 to 10 year follow-up. The duration between onset and remission of seizures does not exceed 2 years. Remission occurs before age 7. There is no family history of epilepsy or migraine, both sexes are involved and no definite causative factor has been detected.

Electroencephalography reveals abnormalities identical to those previously reported (Panayiotopoulos, 1980, 1981). In physiological terms they suffer from "fixation-off-sensitive" epilepsy.

DURATION OF THE PRODROME

The duration of the prodrome in migraine is usually longer than 5 minutes, as opposed to the much briefer aura in epilepsy. It is known, however, that particularly in children, the prodrome phase of migraine can be short and therefore impose a differential problem, mainly when, as is not unusual, it occurs with no associated headache. The findings of Bille (1962) regarding visual hallucinations in children are informative: in 16 of 51 children with migraine, the duration of the visual hallucinations was less than 5 minutes (1 minute in 2 children, less than 5 minutes in 14, and approximately 5 minutes in 25 children).

Conversely, long-lasting ictal manifestations are also evident in epilepsy —for example, in complex partial status epilepticus and partial sensory seizures. Relatively long-lasting visual auras in traumatic epilepsy have also been reported (Russell and Whitty, 1955). We have also described cases of young children with tonic lateral deviation of the eyes and vomiting, sometimes lasting over an hour, as a manifestation of mainly nocturnal, occipital lobe epilepsy, terminating abruptly or leading to a generalized tonic-clonic seizure (Panayiotopoulos, 1981; Panayiotopoulos and Siafakas, 1980).

ELEMENTARY AND COMPLEX VISUAL HALLUCINATIONS

Elementary visual hallucinations, which are the most frequent prodromal symptoms of classical migraine, are also a common ictal manifestation of occipital lobe seizures, ranging, in various reports, from 10% to 47%. Their differentiation is usually made possible by coexistent symptomatology, duration, history, and so on. Difficulties are encountered mainly in those cases of juvenile migraine that are isolated and of brief duration. Additionally, EEG abnormalities in the posterior regions should be interpreted with caution, particularly in children with congenital or early-onset ocular or visual defects (Kellaway, 1980).

The morphology of primary visual hallucinations may be similar in the two diseases, although the typical fortification spectra are nearly always indicative of migraine. We have never seen a patient having "epileptic" primary visual hallucinations with fortification spectra; the most common description is of small spots or circular colored lights. Troost and Newton (1975) have also stated that not one of their patients with the visual seizures of symptomatic epilepsy caused by arteriovenous malformations "experienced the 15- to 20-minute episodes that characterize the aura of classic migraine."

More complex hallucinations involving body image as well as illusory changes in the size, distance, or position of objects in the visual field, which often raise the suspicion of epilepsy, have likewise been rarely described as symptoms of migraine (Bille, 1968). The difficulty in differential diagnosis is increased because these hallucinations may occur before, after, or even without the headache. The term "syndrome of Alice in Wonderland" has been coined by Todd (1955) to characterize these symptoms.

BLINDNESS, HEMIANOPIA, BLURRING OF VISION

Blindness, hemianopia, and blurring of vision have been mainly described and are better understood in relation to the vasoconstrictive effect of migraine. There is, however, unequivocal evidence that they also occur in epilepsy. The best example was offered by Russell and Whitty (1955) in their studies of visual seizures in traumatic epilepsy. These "negative phenomena" were found as "a frequent and perhaps best-defined clinical manifestation" of epileptic seizures in wounds of the higher visual cortex, and it was noted that in some cases "complete visual loss seems to occur ab initio." It was suggested that these phenomena emphasize the functional integration of the visual cortices and indicate rapid transmission of impulses between the occipital lobes. Kooi (1970) has also described three cases of young people with brief (less than 1 minute) episodic blindness attributed to a late epileptic effect of head trauma. Troost and Newton (1975), in their study of arteriovenous malformations of the occipital lobes, described sudden dimming of vision in one or both visual fields and regarded these "periodic visual phenomena as manifestations of occipital lobe epilepsy."

Blindness as a manifestation of epilepsy has also been reported by Lennox and Lennox (1960). We too have described such a case, a patient with unequivocal evidence of epilepsy who would awaken with total blindness lasting for approximately 3 minutes; this would be followed by a tonic upward deviation of the eyes and probable loss of consciousness without convulsions as the patient would go into "deep sleep" again (Panayiotopoulos et al., 1978). Case 2 described by Huott et al. (1974), in a study of occipital lobe seizures, is also of much interest. The difficulties in differential diagnosis between migraine and epilepsy are manifested:

CASE 2   A 14-year-old boy. Family history of migraine. A "mild concussion" at age 9 followed by blurred vision for a few hours. Six months later a 30-minute attack of automatic and agitated behaviour. Started on anticonvulsants. Frequent attacks of loss of vision mostly associated with the hallucination of one or more female faces. A 9-minute attack of blurred vision was recorded and showed bilateral-synchronous occipital spike-wave activity.

According to the above authors (Huott et al., 1974): "These attacks might represent a blend of hereditary migrainous elements and acquired traumatic brain damage, but this remains debatable, and the physiopathogenesis of the seizures remain obscure."

Postictal hemianopia and blindness are also well known phenomena in epilepsy, regarded as a form of Todd's paralysis. If the clinical manifestations of the preceding epileptic attack are not striking, the differential problem is again difficult, as illustrated by Case 1 of Kosnik et al. (1976), who studied postictal blindness:

CASE 1   A 10-year-old girl admitted for evaluation of a seizure disorder. She had a history of paroxysmal episodes of abdominal pain and nausea occurring at intervals of 2 weeks to 2 months. In addition, she had had two generalized seizures.

An electroencephalogram done the day of admission showed a right temporal focus. Two days after admission, she complained of headache, dizziness, and abdominal pain with a sensation of twitching of the abdominal muscles on the left. An EEG taken during this episode showed accentuation of the abnormality noted previously and runs of high voltage 4 to 5 Hz and 2 to 3 Hz activity in the right temporal region, with some spread to the parietal and occipital areas. Neurologic examination shortly after the seizure showed a left homonymous hemianopia and hemisensory extinction to double simultaneous stimulation. On repeat examination 24 hours later, the deficit had completely resolved. She was treated with phenobarbital and no additional seizures have occurred.

Symptoms which arise from other than the occipital cortical areas are much less common. Unilateral paraesthesia associated with hemiparesis or dysphasia is encountered in 4% of patients with migraine (Lance, 1972). The differential diagnosis from epilepsy is again difficult, as is illustrated in Case 1 of Hanson and Chodos (1978) reported as epilepsy:

CASE 1   A 12-year-old, right-handed boy had a mild ill-defined illness 2 weeks prior to admission. He was then well until the day before admission when he had an episode of vomiting and headache. The morning of admission, while taking a bath, he found himself unable to move or talk. He was aware, in retrospect, of some left-sided shaking and he may have fallen to the ground. He claimed to have been conscious throughout. He remained paralyzed on the left side. When admitted, approximately 8 hours after onset, he was able to walk unassisted but had a clear left hemiparesis. He was fully oriented but complained of severe headache and mild lethargy. His neck was supple, and there was weakness of the left arm and leg, and mild left central facial palsy with widening of the left palpebral fissure. The visual fields were full and the fundi were normal. There was bilateral hyperreflexia, more on the left, and a left Babinski sign.

VISUAL TRIGGERING FACTORS

Visual stimuli (bright or dimmed light, darkness, television, pattern images) are well-documented triggering factors in both epilepsy and migraine. Photo-, scoto-, and pattern-sensitive epilepsy are varieties in which seizures are evoked by visual stimuli. These disorders affect mainly young adolescents, girls more often than boys. Migraine attacks are also elicited by similar stimuli, the reported frequency ranging from 3% to 84% (see Chapter 23, this volume). The author, who suffers from rare episodes of classical migraine with teichopsia, scintillating scotoma and hemianopia, has observed that most of his attacks are elicited when he walks from bright sunlight to a semi-dark room.

ELECTROENCEPHALOGRAPHY

Electroencephalography has been the subject of much dispute in the study of migraine. An apparent increase in the frequency of abnormalities, although usually nonspecific and not confirmed by all, has been used as the main supportive evidence for a causal relationship between migraine and epilepsy

(Lance, 1982). Moreover, there is no evidence of a progressive EEG deterioration, which would be expected from recurrent migrainous attacks if such a relationship did indeed exist.

Irrespective of the present controversy, EEG abnormalities and particular spikes sometimes present a most difficult puzzle and a very interesting topic for interpretation and investigation, particularly in children.

SUSCEPTIBILITY OF OCCIPITAL REGIONS TO MIGRAINE AND EPILEPSY: THE SYNDROME OF BASILAR MIGRAINE(?) SEIZURES, AND OCCIPITAL SPIKES*

Clinical manifestations common in migraine and epilepsy most often follow a certain pattern that makes the distinction between the two disorders relatively easy. There are cases, however, in which the problem is extremely difficult and any decision is only speculative. One interesting observation that should be emphasized is that it appears that the neuronal networks subserving vision and the posterior brain regions show some particular susceptibility to both epilepsy and migraine at a certain stage of their development, especially in females. Children with congenital ocular or visual disturbances have a high incidence of occipital abnormalities in their EEGs. Blindness and hemianopia as ictal or postictal manifestations of epilepsy are nearly exclusive to children; light-sensitive epilepsy predominantly affects the young female population; basilar artery migraine has mainly been reported in girls. Furthermore, the majority of cases that raise the question of a relationship between migraine and epilepsy are usually associated with visual disturbances.

The susceptibility of the visual cortex and the posterior brain regions might also explain the recently described syndrome of "basilar migraine(?), seizures, and severe epileptiform EEG abnormalities" (Camfield et al., 1978; Panayiotopoulos, 1980). We have placed the question mark on basilar migraine in order to emphasize the difficulties encountered in distinguishing whether these cases represent just another variety of basilar artery migraine or a simple coincidence of epilepsy and migraine. It is most likely that migrainous headache is triggered by epileptic discharges (Epilepsy-Migraine Syndrome).

The syndrome appears mainly in adolescents (too few patients have been described to show sex preponderance), with symptoms of elementary visual

---

*In view of Chapter 3, this volume, by Gastaut & Zifkin, it is felt that this section should remain as originally presented at the Symposium on Migraine and Epilepsy in Bologna. However, it may be unjustifiable to include this interesting syndrome in one clinical entity "childhood epilepsy with occipital paroxysms", with other occipital epilepsies, on the basis of common EEG findings. The latter have also been seen in other forms of epilepsies and their reactivity to fixation, darkness, elimination, or preservation of central vision, etc. needs further documentation.

hallucinations, blindness, headache, and convulsions. In most of them there is a family history of migraine. All patients responded extremely well to anticonvulsant medication, and the prognosis seemed to be good, although the patient described by the author (Panayiotopoulos, 1980) who had been free of symptoms for 3 years experienced, on awakening from sleep, a generalized tonic-clonic seizure preceded by a focal adversive movement.

The EEG show gross abnormalities of posterior spike and slow wave activity inhibited by eye opening (Camfield, et al. 1978; Panayiotopoulos, 1980). The occipital spike and slow wave discharges in our patient showed a similar distribution in the posterior regions and an identical response to eye opening and closing, darkness, and fixation as in definite cases of occipital lobe epilepsy (Panayiotopoulos, 1980, 1981).

The spike and slow wave activity was inhibited with eyes open in the illuminated recording room (Figure 2.1). Darkness induced the abnormal activity (Figure 2.2). Opening and closing the eyes in darkness did not influence

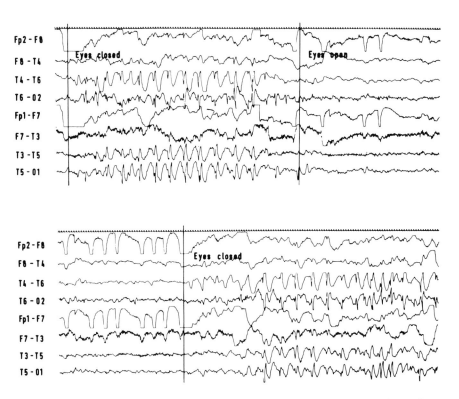

Figure 2.1 EEG recorded in an illuminated room at 120 lux showed continuous high-amplitude spike and slow wave activity confined to the posterior regions. This abnormality occurred only when eyes were closed and was inhibited by eye opening. (From Panayiotopoulos, 1980. By permission of *Neurology.*)

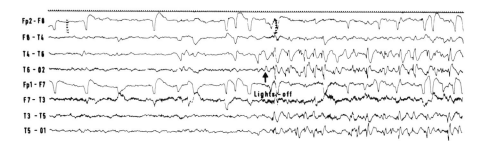

Figure 2.2   Darkness with eyes open evoked the same abnormality as that occurring with eyes closed. (From Panayiotopoulos, 1980. By permission of *Neurology.*)

the continuous posterior discharges (Figure 2.3). A marked inhibition was induced when the child was fixating on a spot of red light in darkness (Figure 2.4). Thus, these cases are indeed "fixation-off-sensitive" epilepsies. Identical results were obtained in patients with occipital lobe seizures (Figure 2.5; Panayiotopoulos, 1981). A similar response to eye opening and darkness has also been described in a case of television epilepsy during the period of conversion to scotosensitive epilepsy, thus indicating the flexibility of the visual cortex in children (Figures 2.6 and 2.7; Panayiotopoulos, 1979). This girl reverted back

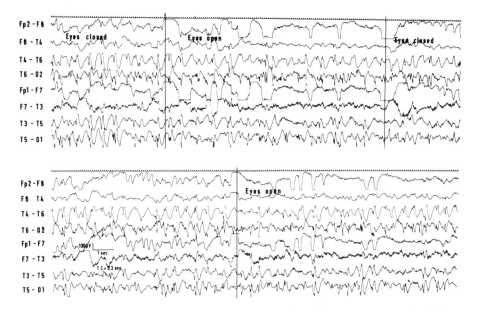

Figure 2.3   Eyes closed and eyes opened in darkness did not bring about any changes; continuous spike and slow wave activity occurred whether eyes were opened or closed. (From Panayiotopoulos, 1980. By permission of *Neurology.*)

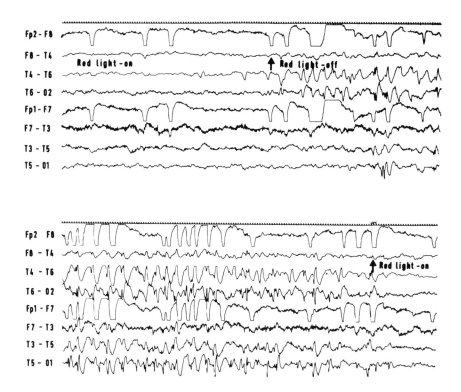

Figure 2.4 EEG abnormalities occurring on eyes open, inhibited in darkness, were attenuated when the patient looked at a red spot of light and reappeared when the red spot was switched off. (From Panayiotopoulos, 1980. By permission of *Neurology.*)

to photosensitivity in a later follow-up. It is interesting that the so-called functional occipital spikes in children with no clinical evidence of epilepsy are more abundant when their eyes are closed. Additionally, Beaumanoir et al. (1981) have shown an inhibitory effect on these spikes by "visual perception." Exaggeration of the "functional" occipital spikes by anticonvulsants, mainly phenobarbital, was not found in other patients, who showed an extremely good clinical and electroencephalographic response to medication (Panayiotopoulos, 1980, 1981).

Whatever the significance of these findings may be, the gross EEG abnormalities distinguish this syndrome from other forms of basilar artery migraine, in which the EEG is usually normal. Regarding the diagnosis, Camfield et al. (1978) have concluded that this is primarily a migrainous syndrome with probable secondary epileptic features "resulting from ischemic changes caused by repeated migraine auras" and related "to the lower epileptic threshold in the young brain." This cannot be easily refuted and is probably correct. It is also in agreement with the consensus that a migraine attack might progress and trigger an epileptic seizure in a susceptible individual who is predisposed to epileptic

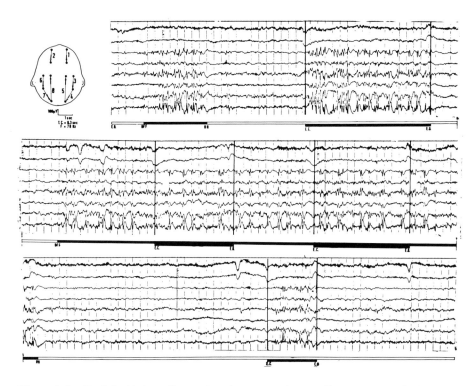

Figure 2.5   Occipital lobe epilepsy. Continuous EEG recording. Darkness (induced by switching off the lights of the recording room) and eyes closed induce posterior "epileptiform" discharges. Eyes closed and eyes opened in darkness do not bring about any changes in the EEG, i.e., continuous spike and slow waves occur whether eyes are opened or closed. Eye opening in an illuminated room completely blocks the EEG abnormalities. EC = eyes closed. EO = eyes open. Off = complete darkness in the recording room. On = room is illuminated at 120 lux near the eyes of the patient. (From Panayiotopoulos, 1981. By permission of *Neurology.*)

disturbances by virtue of heredity. However, Panayiotopoulos (1980) has questioned basilar migraine as a primary disorder in this syndrome.

The arguments in favor of migraine or epilepsy appear to be balanced, although one is impressed by the excellent response to anticonvulsants and the fact that the main clinical features of the syndrome could equally well be attributed to epilepsy in accordance with the data presented. It is also impressive that the vast majority of cases presented as indicative of a possible relationship between migraine and epilepsy are those with visual symptoms (Basser, 1969). Therefore, the subject of the final diagnosis and therefore of the pathogenesis of the syndrome should be left open to further research and evaluation with new methods.

Positron computed tomography, for example, is opening new avenues for investigation of the local cerebral metabolism and cerebral blood flow, and it may provide the data to answer many of the questions raised in this book. Phelps et al. (1981) have already published the results of their investigation of the local cerebral metabolic rate for glucose (LCMRGLc) in the visual cortex. They found a progressive increase in LCMRGLc of the visual cortex from eyes closed control to stimulation with white light, alternating a checkerboard pattern with a complex visual scene. The most interesting findings in relation to the subject of this book were revealed in their study of a patient with seizures originating in the visual cortex. Ictal positron computed tomography showed a

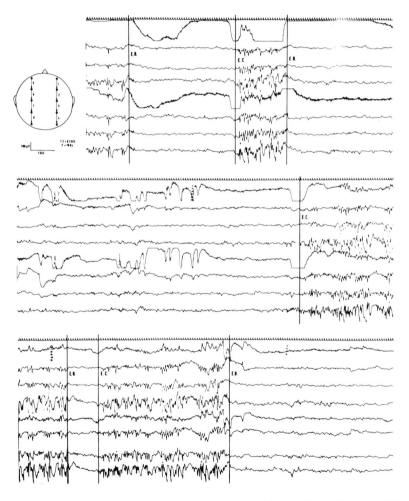

Figure 2.6 Conversion of photosensitive to scotosensitive epilepsy. Scotosensitive period. Room illumination 115 lux. High amplitude continuous spike, polyspike, and slow wave activity appeared only when eyes were closed; it was inhibited on eye opening. (From Panayiotopoulos, 1979. By permission of *Neurology*.)

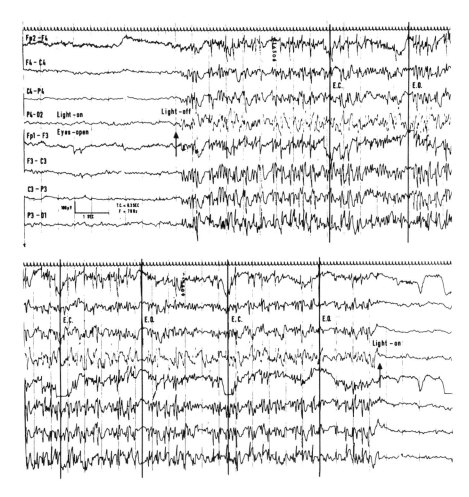

Figure 2.7   Same case as Figure 2.6. Abnormalities were induced by darkness. Eye closure and opening in darkness did not bring about any changes, i.e., continuous epileptiform discharges occur independently of eye opening or closure. (From Panayio-topoulos, 1979. By permission of *Neurology*.)

167% increase of the LCMRGLc in the discharging primary visual cortex in relation to the contralateral one, whereas an 81% decrease relative to the state with eyes closed control was found in the interictal study. This reduction was greater than that found in their hemianopic patients, and was attributed to the functional damage to the visual cortex from the seizure activity. The application of this method to subjects with migrainous or ictal and postictal paralysis, in cases such as those described here and which pose differential and pathogenetic problems, may be of immense help.

MIGRAINE-EPILEPSY SYNDROME?
EPILEPSY-MIGRAINE SYNDROME?
OR A DIFFERENTIAL PROBLEM?

There are many cases, particularly children, where a distinction between migraine and epilepsy is difficult if not impossible to make. Regarding the relationship between them, the prevailing view that an epileptic seizure might be triggered by a migrainous attack in a susceptible subject cannot be easily ruled out (migraine-epilepsy syndrome). However, the reverse (epilepsy-migraine syndrome) is most likely; that is, an epileptic discharge might trigger a vascular sequence of events in an individual susceptible to migraine, particularly since migraine is a neurovascular reaction in which many chemical transmitter agents appear to be involved (Lance, 1981).

Finally, a causal relationship between migraine and a secondary "autonomous" epilepsy should not be accepted without much reservation: There is no evidence that clinical and EEG manifestations of epilepsy deteriorate progressively as would be expected from the frequent "epileptogenic" insults of migrainous attacks to the brain, recurring sometimes throughout life. It is possible that the link suggested between migraine and epilepsy may reflect the differential diagnostic difficulties between the two diseases.

In conclusion I support that: (a) migraine and epilepsy are two entirely different disorders although some symptoms are common for both; (b) most of the cases presented as a migraine-epilepsy syndrome reflect problems in differential diagnosis or pure coincidence; (c) there is no evidence that migraine, secondarily, causes epilepsy, as this would be expected to result in multiple epileptic foci and a bad prognosis and; (d) there is a strong possibility that epileptic discharges may trigger migrainous phenomena, particularly in children, and to describe this disorder the term "childhood epilepsy with migrainous phenomena and occipital paroxysms" is proposed.

REFERENCES

Basser LS. The relation of migraine and epilepsy. Brain 1969; 92:285–300.

Beaumanoir A, Inderwildi B, Zagury S. Paroxysmes EEG "non épileptiques." Med Hyg 1981;39:1911–8.

Bickerstaff ER. Basilar artery migraine. Lancet 1961a;1:15–7.

Bickerstaff ER. Impairment of consciousness in migraine. Lancet 1961b;2:1057–9.

Bickerstaff ER. The basilar artery and the migraine-epilepsy syndrome. Proc R Soc Med 1962;55:167–9.

Bille B. Migraine in school children. Acta Paediatr Scand 1962;51 (Suppl 136):1–151.

Bille B. Headaches in children. In: Vinken PJ, Bruyn GW, eds. Handbook of clinical neurology. Amsterdam: North-Holland, 1968;5:239–46.

Camfield PR, Metrakos K, Andermann F. Basilar migraine, seizures and severe epileptiform EEG abnormalities. Neurology 1978;28:584–8.

Gascon G, Barlow C. Juvenile migraine presenting as an acute confusional state. Pediatrics 1970;45:628–35.

Gowers WR. The borderland of epilepsy. London: J & A Churchill, 1907:6–87.

Hanson PA, Chodos R. Hemiparetic seizures. Neurology 1978;28:920–3.

Heyck H. Headache and facial pain. Stuttgart-New York: Georg Thieme Verlag, 1981.

Huott AD, Madison DS, Niedermeyer E. Occipital lobe epilepsy. Eur Neurol 1974;11:325–39.

Kellaway P. The incidence, significance and natural history of spike foci in children. In: Henry CE, ed. Current clinical neurophysiology. Update on EEG and evoked potentials. Elsevier/North-Holland. 1980;152–75.

Kooi KA. Episodic blindness as a late effect of head trauma. Neurology 1970;20:569–73.

Kosnik E, Paulson GW, Laguna JF. Postictal blindness. Neurology 1976;26:248–50.

Lance JW. Headache. Ann Neurol 1981;10:1–10.

Lance JW. Mechanism and management of headache, 4th ed. London: Butterworth Scientific. 1982;146–147.

Lapkin ML, French JH, Golden GS et al. The electroencephalogram in childhood basilar artery migraine. Neurology 1977;27:580–3.

Laplante P, Saint-Hilaire JM, Bouvier G. Headache as an epileptic manifestation. Neurology 1983;33:1493–5.

Lee CH, Lance JW. Migraine and stupor. Headache 1977;17:32–8.

Lennox GW, Lennox MA. Epilepsy and related disorders. Boston: Little, Brown, 1960.

Manzoni GC, Terzano MG, Mancia D. Possible interference between migrainous and epileptic mechanisms in intercalated attacks. Case report. Eur Neurol 1979;18:124–8.

Panayiotopoulos CP. Conversion of photosensitive to scotosensitive epilepsy. Neurology 1979;29:1550–5.

Panayiotopoulos CP. Basilar migraine? seizures, and severe EEG abnormalities. Neurology 1980;30:1122–5.

Panayiotopoulos CP. Inhibitory effect of central vision on occipital lobe seizures. Neurology 1981;31:1331–3.

Panayiotopoulos CP. Benign nocturnal childhood occipital epilepsy: A new syndrome with nocturnal seizures, tonic deviation of the eyes and vomiting. (in press)

Panayiotopoulos CP, Hatziconstantinou M, Scarpalezos S. Clinical and EEG observations on occipital lobe epilepsy. Arch Med Greek Soc 1978;4:254–6 (in Greek).

Panayiotopoulos CP, Siafakas A. Triggering factors in occipital lobe epilepsy (Abstr). Acta Neurol Scand 1980;62 (Suppl 79).

Penfield W, Kristiansen K. Epileptic seizure patterns. Springfield: Thomas, 1951.

Phelps ME, Mazziotta JC, Kuhl DE et al. Tomographic mapping of human cerebral metabolism: visual stimulation and deprivation. Neurology 1981;31:517–29.

Russell WR, Whitty CWM. Studies in traumatic epilepsy 3. Visual fits. J Neurol Neurosurg Psychiatry 1955;18:79–96.

Slatter KH. Some clinical and EEG findings in patients with migraine. Brain 1968;91:85–98.

Swanson JW, Vick NA. Basilar artery migraine. Neurology 1978;28:782–6.

Todd J. The syndrome of Alice in Wonderland. Can Med Assoc J 1955;73:701–4.

Troost BT, Newton TH. Occipital lobe arteriovenous malformations. Arch Ophthalmol 1975;93:250–6.

3

Benign Epilepsy of Childhood with Occipital Spike and Wave Complexes

Henri Gastaut
Benjamin G. Zifkin

In the course of our investigation of the benign partial epilepsies of childhood with a mainly, if not exclusively, functional focus (Gastaut, 1981, 1982a), also called primary or idiopathic partial epilepsies (Gastaut, 1983; Gastaut and Zifkin, 1985), we had the good fortune to identify a new variety of epilepsy that is characterized by: 1) seizures with elementary visual symptomatology frequently associated with other ictal phenomena and at times followed by postictal headache, and 2) interictal occipital rhythmic paroxysmal electroencephalographic (EEG) activity appearing only after eye closure.

The existence of this benign epilepsy of childhood with occipital paroxysms (BEOP) had been foreseen years ago by many investigators who nevertheless did not recognize it as a distinct clinical and electrographic syndrome. In 1950, Gastaut (1950a) reported several cases of benign childhood epilepsy with visual seizures and occipital spike and wave complexes. Emphasis was placed on the EEG pattern of high-amplitude occipital spike and wave complexes that repeated rhythmically at 2 – 3/sec and appeared with eye closure or intermittent photic stimulation. This pattern was found in the absence of any demonstrable cortical lesion. Gibbs and Gibbs (1952) noted that "Seizure foci in one or both occipital lobes are most commonly found in young children. . . . Occipital foci tend to disappear in adult life, and the subsidence of the electroencephalographic abnormality is usually accompanied by a cessation of seizures." Sorel and Rucquoy-Ponsar (1969) described an occipital epilepsy, along with rolandic epilepsy, as a part of their "age-dependent" idiopathic epilepsy of childhood. Rodin (1972) suggested two types of focal epilepsy, one based on a focal structural lesion and the other possibly genetic. Ludwig and Ajmone-Marsan

(1975) suggested the existence of a benign occipital epilepsy in infants and children. Aicardi and Chevrie (1977) distinguished a form of benign partial epilepsy in which bilaterally synchronous, symmetric, parieto-occipital spike and wave complexes, at times very abundant, were seen in place of the usual rolandic spikes. Beaumanoir et al., (1981) emphasized the possible relationship between a functional occipital focus and a "benign parieto-occipital epilepsy with the same characteristics as benign epilepsy with rolandic spikes." Delwaide et al. (1971) described a benign occipital epilepsy of childhood in which the ictal visual phenomena were at times followed by headaches and even vomiting. That so distinct a form of epilepsy had not previously been described is no doubt explained by the fact that its two fundamental characteristics are not always obvious and must be carefully sought. The typical visual symptoms may be forgotten or poorly described by children, especially younger ones, and they may not be elicited while obtaining the history. Moreover, the attenuation of the occipital spikes with opening of the eyes may not be obvious in a routine EEG recording, during which the eyes may be opened only once or twice for a few seconds at a time.

MATERIALS AND METHODS

We have previously described BEOP in 36 patients selected solely on the basis of occipital paroxysmal activity appearing with eye closure (Gastaut, 1982b, 1982c, 1982d, 1982e). This led us to distinguish two clinical varieties of this disorder depending on the presence or absence of initial visual phenomena. Nevertheless, we did not then rule out the possibility of a third variety in which the typical visual phenomena would occur in the absence of the typical interictal occipital activity.

Since that time we have found 27 more cases and have concluded that these three electroclinical subtypes do indeed exist: the complete syndrome, including seizures with ictal visual symptoms and interictal occipital paroxysmal activity; and the two incomplete syndromes, in which either the ictal visual symptoms or the interictal EEG abnormalities are absent. Furthermore, one can distinguish two other electroclinical varieties of BEOP in which the complete or incomplete electroclinical syndrome is associated with the symptoms of another form of epilepsy, which may be generalized or partial, primary or secondary. Most often, the coexisting disorder is one of the "primary" childhood epilepsies — usually primary generalized epilepsy or benign partial epilepsy with rolandic spikes. Much less frequently, the associated partial or generalized seizure disorder is caused by some lesion or diffuse cerebral disturbance, emphasizing the interaction of these organic factors with the idiopathic predisposition to seizures that may be present in any patient with epilepsy.

The present study is based on 63 observations, of which 33 represent the complete syndrome of BEOP, 17 are examples of an incomplete syndrome, and 13 are associated with other forms of epilepsy. We will summarize illustrative cases of each type.

CASE REPORTS

The Complete Syndrome of BEOP

CASE 1   The patient is a 23-year-old female. Seizures began at age 9, with formed visual hallucinations that occurred when she closed her eyes at night. These hallucinations caused her to hide under her bedclothes; they were sometimes followed by a hemiclonic convulsion of either side of the body. These convulsions occurred before her menses for 9 years, although she was treated with phenobarbital and carbamazepine. The addition of clobazam resulted in complete control of the seizures. Anticonvulsants were stopped at age 19, and there have been no seizures in the last 4 years. Over a 9-year period, 20 EEGs were performed all showing typical bilaterally synchronous and symmetrical occipital 3/sec spike-and-wave complexes (Figure 3.1). With the disappearance of her seizures at age 19, the EEG also returned to normal.

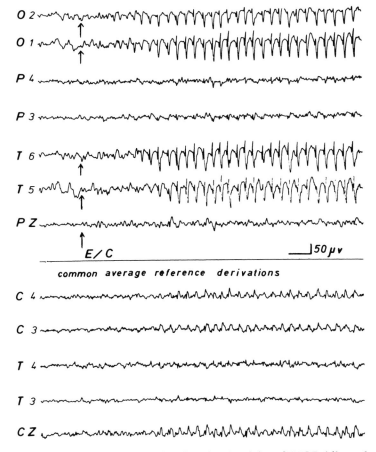

Figure 3.1   Case 1, age 14½. The typical interictal activity of BEOP: bilateral, synchronous, symmetric surface-negative high amplitude spike and wave complexes repeating at 3/sec, localized to the occipital and posterior temporal regions. They appear within only 2 seconds of eye closure.

CASE 2   This patient, a 14-year-old male, had two brothers with epilepsy and one sister with migraine. Seizures began at age 6, with four attacks of complex visual hallucinations over 2 days. During these attacks the patient attempted to play with toys that he imagined were on the kitchen table. These hallucinations were followed by loss of vision lasting for 4 to 5 minutes and headaches with nausea and vomiting. At age 8, he noted sparkling flashes throughout his visual field for several seconds. At age 10, while he was on an ocean cruise, the flashes were followed by a hemiclonic convulsion that continued for 2 hours until stopped by intravenous diazepam. Over a 7-year period, seven EEGs all showed typical occipital spike and wave complexes, either bilaterally synchronous, asynchronous, or with shifting lateralization (Figure 3.2). Several seizures with elementary visual

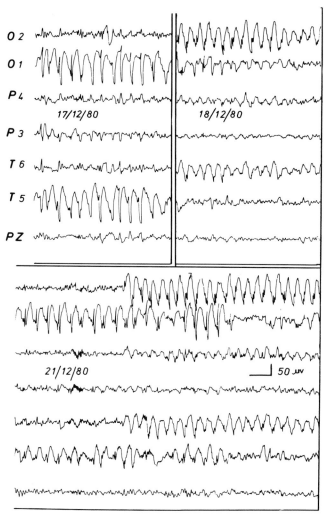

Figure 3.2   Case 2, age 11. Morphology characteristic of the interictal epileptiform activity but seen over each hemisphere or both, independently or synchronously.

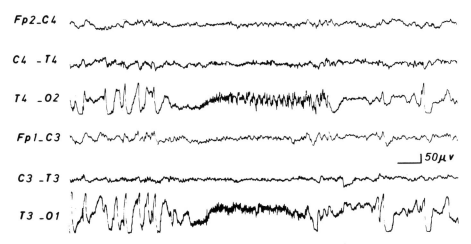

Figure 3.3   Case 2, age 11. Ictal 16–18 Hz activity over both posterior regions. The child describes "seeing stars."

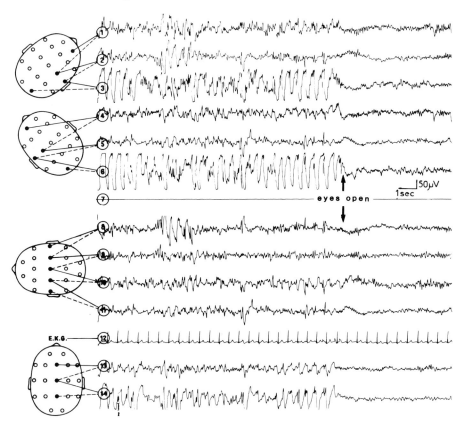

Figure 3.4   Case 3, age 6. Bilateral occipital spike and wave activity with left-sided predominance, suppressed by opening the eyes. Note the occasional centrotemporal spike over each hemisphere.

symptoms were recorded (Figure 3.3). He has been free of seizures and epileptiform activity during the last 4 years, since the time that phenobarbital was prescribed.

Case 3   This patient, a 6½-year-old male, is the brother of the patient in Case 2.
A single seizure occurred at age 6, as it did in his brother's case. Loss of vision
lasting 45 minutes was followed by dysphasia lasting 2 minutes and a major
convulsion. An EEG (Figure 3.4) showed the same typical occipital spike and
wave activity as that of his brother.

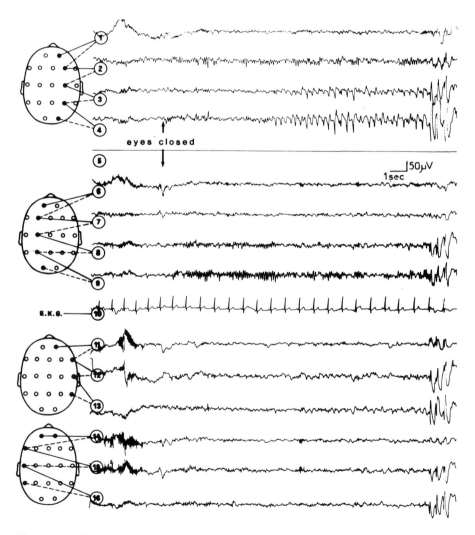

Figure 3.5   Case 4, age 13. Repetitive rhythmic sharp waves over the right posterior
quadrant, beginning 6 seconds after eye closure. Note the spread to homologous areas of
the left side after the sudden increase in amplitude of the right-sided discharge. Alpha
activity is also reduced on the right side.

CASE 4   The patient is a 13-year-old male. A single febrile convulsion occurred at age 3. Seizures began at age 9, heralded by the hallucination throughout the visual field of a glowing yellow sphere that the patient would describe by saying, "Here it comes. I see yellow!" This was followed by a deviation of the head and eyes to the left, with twitching of the left side of the mouth for 30 seconds and sometimes a 2- or 3-minute left-sided hemiclonic convulsion. These attacks occurred usually but not always when he was at the movies or watching television. Three EEGs showed typical posterior sharp-wave activity confined to the right hemisphere (Figure 3.5). A spontaneous seizure was recorded (Figure 3.6),

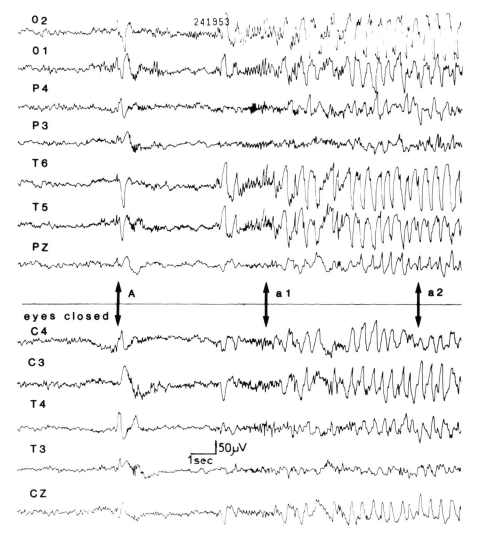

Figure 3.6   Case 4, age 13. Occipital and posterior temporal ictal discharge with right-sided predominance. At (A), the child said, "Here it comes! I see yellow!" At a1 and a2 he was asked what he saw and described "the lights of a car at night." At (B), he returned his head and eyes to the left and did not respond. At (C), he suddenly asked, "Where am I?"

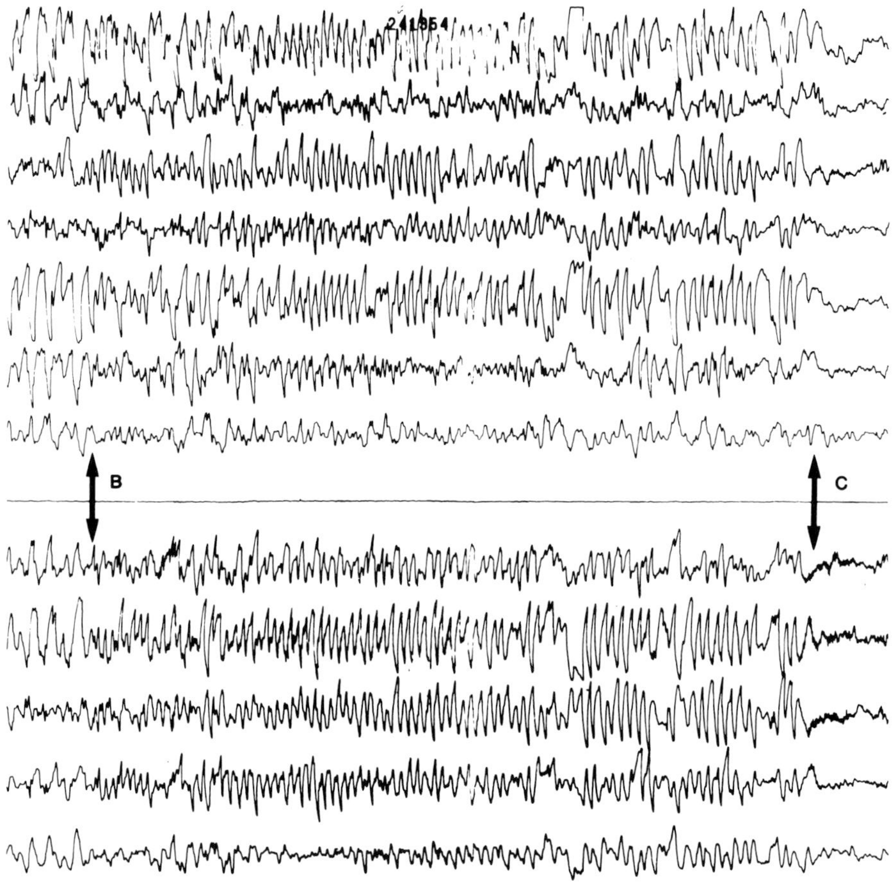

Figure 3.6 *(continued)*

beginning with the hallucination of two yellow lights in blackness like the lights of a car at night. Treated with 150 mg/day of phenobarbital and 250 mg/day of phenytoin, he had no further seizures or EEG abnormalities during 2 years of follow-up.

CASE 5   This patient is a 21-year-old female. At age 8, an episode of metamorphopsia was reported during which the watertaps of the patient's bathtub took on a frightening shape. From ages 9 to 14, adversive and giratory seizures occurred to the right side. If she was hindered in turning around, she would say, "But let me look!", but she could never describe what she saw since the initial phase of the seizure was followed after about 20 seconds by loss of consciousness, automatisms, and amnesia for the event. Postictally, she noted right temporal headache that lasted up to 2 hours. From the age of 14, these attacks were replaced by visual hallucinations consisting of very small and brilliant numerals in the center of her visual field, sometimes followed by a centripetal visual obscuration leading to complete loss of vision. On 5 occasions, a generalized tonic-clonic convulsion followed the attack. A large number of EEGs have invariably shown typical occipital spike and wave activity over the left side alone. One seizure was recorded that consisted of this unusual visual hallucination followed by confusion and automatism (Figure 3.7). No anticonvulsant treatment was successful until clobazam was prescribed, which was followed by the disappearance of seizures and epileptiform EEG activity for the past 2 years.

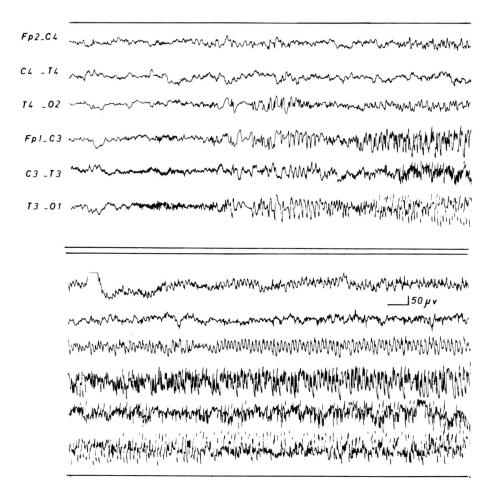

Figure 3.7 Case 5, age 9. Ictal discharge lasting 130 seconds predominantly over the left posterior quadrant. During the first 30 seconds, she saw the figure 57, which gradually faded away and was followed by loss of vision lasting 20 seconds after which she did not respond to questions. During the final 40 seconds (as shown on page 56), she had oral and gestural automatisms.

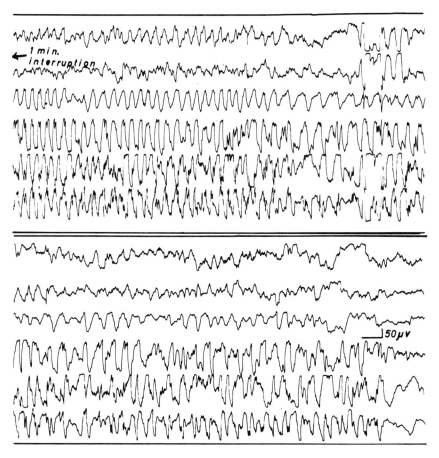

Figure 3.7 *(continued)*

The Incomplete Forms of BEOP

BEOP without Visual Symptoms

In these cases, seizures occur in neurologically normal children whose EEGs show the typical occipital paroxysms but who do not or cannot report any visual symptoms.

CASE 6   The patient is a 9½-year-old female. Seizures began at age 7, with 20- to 30-second psychomotor attacks characterized by gestural and verbal automatisms with no reported visual symptoms. Several EEGs showed typical occipital sharp waves over both hemispheres with clear right-sided predominance, which repeated at about 2/sec (Figure 3.8), as well as independent right-sided rolandic spikes and occasional generalized 3/sec spike and wave complexes. On one occa-

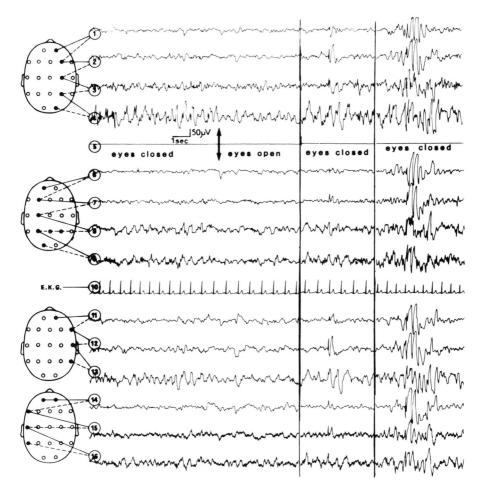

Figure 3.8   Case 6, age 9½. Right occipital and posterior temporal sharp waves suppressed by eye opening. Note the right centrotemporal spike and wave activity and the bursts of generalized spike and wave complexes.

sion, the EEG recorded a psychomotor attack that began during sleep with right occipital discharges and then rapidly generalized (Figure 3.9). Seizures persisted for 2 years despite carbamazepine, 400 mg per day; but she has been free of seizures and interictal EEG abnormalities for 1 year since clobazam, 20 mg daily, was added.

CASE 7   A 14-year-old female has had seven generalized convulsions that have occurred during early sleep over a period of 7 years, each followed by severe headache. The two EEGs obtained have shown typical bilateral occipital spike and wave activity (Figure 3.10). An eighth, most recent seizure that occurred when the patient went to bed before the light was turned out was immediately preceded by a 1 minute loss of vision.

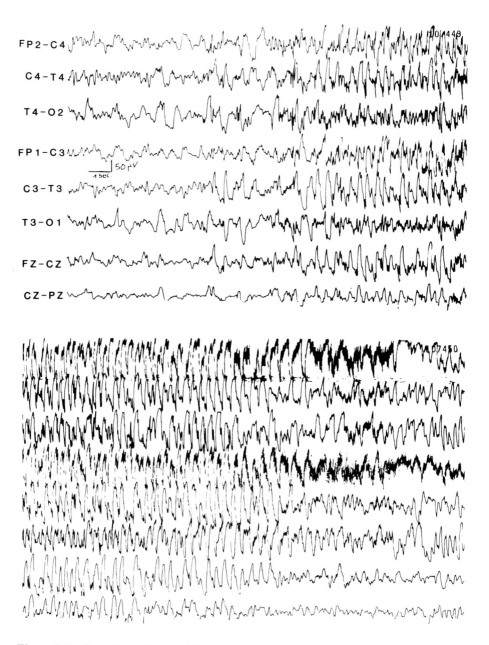

Figure 3.9 Case 6, age 9½. Ictal discharge lasting 20 seconds beginning during sleep. While this was occurring she sat up in bed without awakening and looked to her left side, apparently attentively, before lying down again.

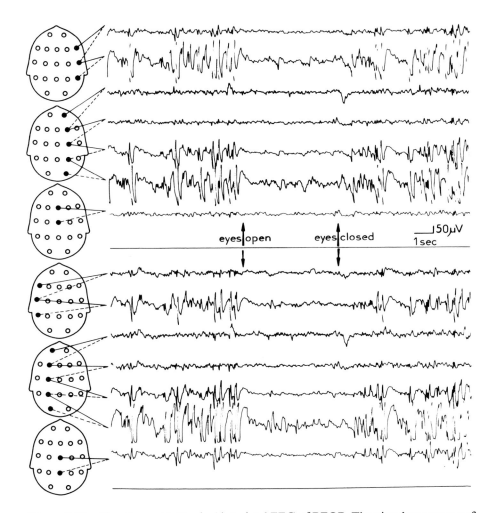

eyes open   eyes closed   50μV
1 sec

Figure 3.10 Case 7, age 14. Typical interictal EEG of BEOP. The visual symptoms of this patient's nocturnal seizures were not apparent for 7 years.

Comment

This case was selected to show that certain instances that seem to be examples of the incomplete syndrome are, in fact, complete cases in which the history of the initial visual symptoms was not obtained because the patient was amnestic for the attacks or because the seizures began during sleep.

BEOP without Occipital Paroxysmal Activity with Eye Closure

In these children, the seizure pattern is that of typical BEOP, but the EEG is normal. These children also have normal neurologic examinations.

CASE 8　This patient is a 10-year-old male. A single seizure occurred at 4 A.M. The child awakened with nausea and vomiting and then fell asleep next to his mother, who was awakened an hour later by her son's generalized convulsion. Several minutes after it ended, nausea and vomiting recurred and were followed by a loss of vision lasting several minutes. An EEG performed the next day and another 1 month later were both normal.

CASE 9　This patient is a 21-year-old female whose seizures began at age 8. She would have progressive loss of vision over a 10-minute period, followed by a lengthy right-sided hemiclonic convulsion and severe headache that lasted several hours. Phenobarbital and phenytoin were given over 13 years; each attempt to taper the medication was followed by a seizure. The two EEGs recorded the day after a right hemiclonic seizure showed the expected left posterior slow activity, but seven further EEGs have all been normal.

CASE 10　A 17-year-old male had a single seizure in which multicolored phosphenes in all visual fields were followed by a left-sided hemiclonic seizure that lasted 45 minutes until intramuscular diazepam was given. An EEG 2 hours later showed the expected right posterior slow activity, which disappeared over 48 hours. Three EEGs obtained since then have all been normal.

Comment

Even in the most typical and complete forms of BEOP, the occipital epileptiform activity may not be seen in some recordings. It is possible, if not probable, that most of the preceding cases are examples of the complete syndrome in which the EEG manifestations have not yet been recorded.

Associated Forms of BEOP

BEOP Associated with Clinical and/or EEG Manifestations of Another Type of "Primary" Childhood Epilepsy

Typical cases of BEOP in which coincidental generalized spike and wave activity and/or rolandic spikes were seen have been excluded here. We are considering only those cases in which BEOP is associated with the seizures and/or the EEG pattern of another type of primary epilepsy. The cases may be classified according to whether the associated primary epilepsy is generalized or partial.

BEOP associated with primary generalized epilepsy.

CASE 11　The patient is a 13-year-old female who has experienced typical absence attacks since age 6. While the patient was changing television channels three other attacks occurred which were heralded by phosphenes in all visual fields, and followed by right-sided hemiclonic seizures with postictal headaches and vomiting that lasted several hours. In seven EEGs bursts of generalized bilaterally synchronous spike and wave activity were seen only during hyperventilation, accompanied by clinical absence (Figure 3.11). The amplitude of visual and

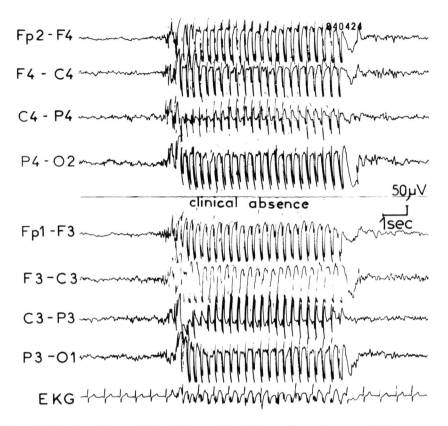

Figure 3.11 Case 11, age 8. Typical generalized 3/sec spike and wave activity accompanied by a clinical absence attack during hyperventilation. The pattern of spontaneous seizures was typical of BEOP but no typical occipital discharge was found.

somatosensory evoked responses was significantly higher over the left hemisphere. She had been initially treated with low doses of barbiturates and, after the substitution of 900 mg of valproate/day, no seizures of any kind have occurred during the past year and no abnormal EEG activity has been seen.

CASE 12 This patient, an 11-year-old female, has one paternal uncle with seizures. After age 7, four identical attacks occurred, each in the evening. Sudden brief losses of vision, which the patient herself described, were followed by loss of consciousness and a tonic seizure lasting about 20 seconds with incontinence of urine, followed by a slow recovery of consciousness with confusion, headache, and vomiting lasting 1 to 2 hours. Of her five EEGs, two were normal and three showed generalized spike and wave and polyspike and wave activity occurring both spontaneously and also with intermittent photic stimulation (IPS) (Figure 3.12). No anticonvulsants have ever been prescribed.

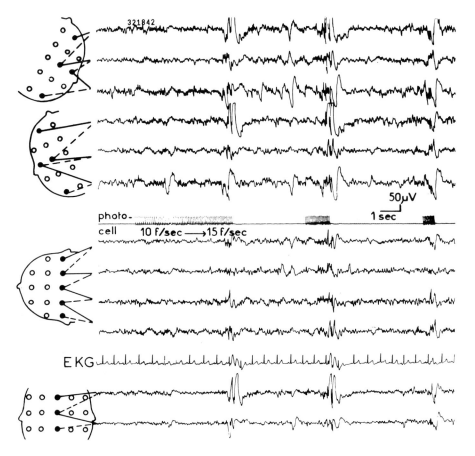

321842

photo-
cell   10 f/sec ——→15 f/sec

50μV

1 sec

EKG

Figure 3.12 Case 12, age 11. Generalized spike and wave and polyspike and wave activity provoked by IPS at 15 Hz in a girl with clinically typical BEOP but without the characteristic occipital spike and wave activity.

CASE 13 The patient is a 20-year-old male whose seizures began at age 13. The seizures were heralded by 30 to 60 seconds of sparkling flashes in all visual fields, followed by adversion to the left, and at times by complete rotation of the body and a subsequent generalized convulsion. All nine EEGs obtained have shown generalized bilaterally synchronous sharp waves with predominance contralateral to the adversion (Figure 3.13), as seen characteristically in "primary generalized versive seizures of adolescents" (Gastaut et al., 1981). Valproate and phenobarbital were prescribed, and no seizures have occurred during the last 6 years.

BEOP associated with benign partial epilepsy of childhood with rolandic spikes.

CASE 14 This patient, a 7-year-old male, has a paternal uncle with primary generalized epilepsy. His seizures first occurred at age 4. The patient awakened around midnight and had an adversive seizure to the right followed by nausea,

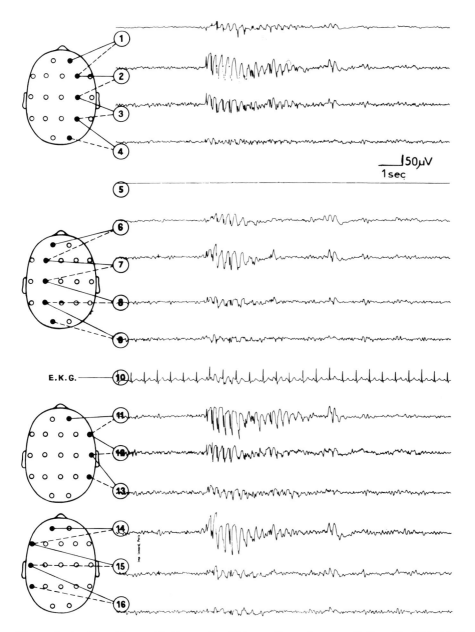

Figure 3.13 Case 13, age 16. Generalized 3/sec spike and wave activity with right-sided predominance in a patient whose turning attacks were preceded by typical phosphenes of BEOP and followed by tonic-clonic seizures.

vomiting, and sudden copious diarrhea before losing consciousness for over an hour. Since then, numerous other attacks of right hemifacial twitching, salivation, and anarthria have occurred. Two EEGs showed typical left occipital spike and wave complexes attenuated by eye opening, and left-sided rolandic spikes (Figure 3.14). He was initially treated with low doses of barbiturates. The addition of 15 mg of clobazam daily has resulted in seizure control and the disappearance of the epileptiform EEG abnormalities for the past 2 years.

CASE 15   The patient is a 10½-year-old male who had two identical seizures at age 8. Both occurred during sleep. He awakened his parents and complained of a sensation of pins-and-needles in the right arm. He then muttered incomprehensibly, turned his eyes and head to the right, and had a right-sided hemiclonic convulsion. This was followed by vomiting and loss of vision lasting 15 minutes,

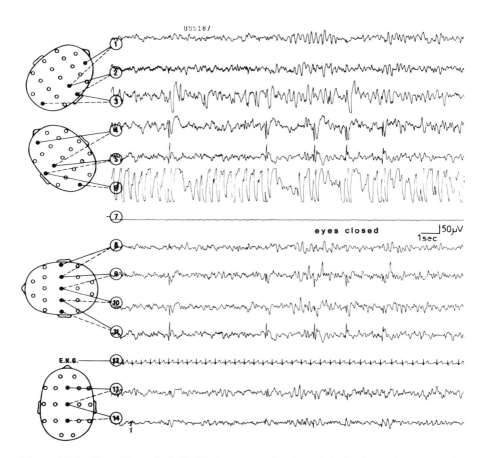

Figure 3.14   Case 14, age 7. Left-sided quasi-rhythmic occipital spike and wave activity with eyes closed. Note the associated left rolandic spikes, seen with the highest-amplitude occipital spikes. In this patient, clinical attacks were typical of epilepsy with rolandic spikes.

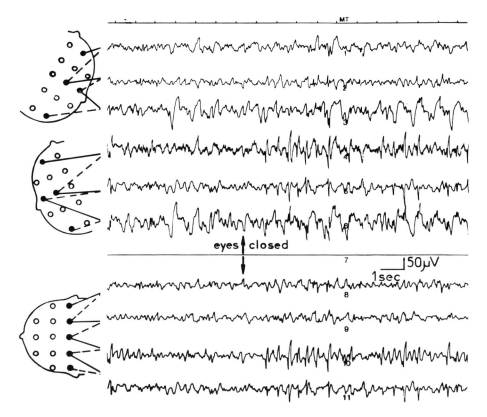

Figure 3.15   Case 15, age 8. Left rolandic spikes seen principally after eye closure in a child with clinical BEOP.

accompanied by right-sided dysesthesiae and subsequent severe headache lasting several hours. An EEG (Professor Montanari) done after his second seizure showed left-sided rolandic spikes only when the eyes were shut (Figure 3.15). Phenobarbital, 100 mg daily, was prescribed. No further seizures have occurred, and the epileptiform activity has not been present during 2 years of follow-up.

BEOP Associated with Clinical and/or EEG Manifestations of Epilepsy Secondary to a Brain Lesion

These forms of BEOP may be classified according to whether the associated secondary epilepsy is generalized or partial.

BEOP associated with secondary or symptomatic generalized epilepsy.

CASE 16   The patient is a 12-year-old female with a mild developmental delay. The first seizure occurred at age 5½, beginning with a loss of vision that occurred while the patient was playing in the sea. An EEG done immediately thereafter showed spike and wave activity seen only at the occipital poles with left-sided predominance, attenuated by eye opening. At age 8, frequent diurnal atonic seizures and nocturnal tonic seizures appeared. The EEG then showed diffuse spike and wave complexes with posterior predominance, unaffected by opening of the eyes (Figure 3.16a). With anticonvulsant treatment, the seizures became less frequent, and the patient is now seizure-free. Four EEGs, recorded at ages 8½, 9, 10, and 10½, respectively (Figure 3.16b), have shown the gradual disappearance of the diffuse spike and wave activity and the appearance of typical left occipital spike and wave complexes with eye closure. A computerized tomography (CT) scan revealed mild diffuse cerebral atrophy.

BEOP associated with secondary or symptomatic partial epilepsy.

CASE 17   This patient, a 19-year-old male, has a twin brother and a father with primary generalized epilepsy. During an attack of scarlet fever at age 2, an episode of left-sided status epilepticus occurred. As a result, there was a residual left hemiparesis. The patient is left-handed and has an IQ of 77. Further seizures were noted at age 5, consisting of the hallucination of a luminous ball followed by deviation of the head and eyes to the left, and dysphasia. Since age 15, psychomotor seizures followed by dysphasia without initial visual phenomena have occurred. The EEG showed sharp and slow wave complexes over both occipital regions with right-sided predominance seen with eye closure and repeating at 1/sec (Figure 3.17). A CT scan revealed right hemisphere atrophy similar to that seen with the hemiconvulsion-hemiplegia-epilepsy (HHE) syndrome.

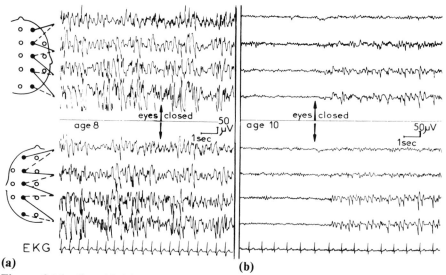

Figures 3.16   Case 16. (a) At age 8, diffuse spike and wave activity is seen, with occipital predominance not reactive to opening of the eyes. (b) At age 10, occipital sharp waves after eye closure are seen.

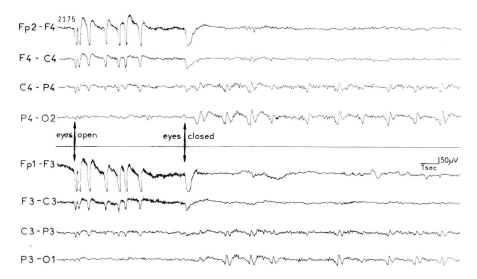

Figure 3.17 Case 17, age 19. Occipital sharp-and-slow waves with eye closure in an adolescent with BEOP in childhood and, subsequently, complex partial seizures.

Comment

In addition to these 17 cases, a retrospective diagnosis of BEOP was made in one other case. This case is of particular interest because the visual seizures of BEOP followed by migraine were succeeded 50 years later by an episode of transient global amnesia, also followed by migraine.

> **CASE 18** This patient is a 60-year-old female who, at age 58, began to experience brief episodes of dizziness, sudden loss of muscle tone, and falling. An EEG was performed the day after an episode of transient global amnesia that lasted 5 hours and was followed by a severe migraine headache. The EEG (Figure 3.18) showed posterior 3-Hz delta activity attenuated by eye opening as previously described in vertebrobasilar insufficiency (Gastaut and Naquet, 1966) and in a case of transient global amnesia (Rowan and Protass, 1979). Further inquiry revealed that when she was of school age, the patient had many episodes of visual illusions associated with severe headache. On several occasions these had been associated with convulsions for which she had been treated with phenobarbital for 10 years.

RESULTS

Our findings on the interictal and ictal symptomatology, the natural history, and the diagnosis of BEOP are based on all 63 cases studied.

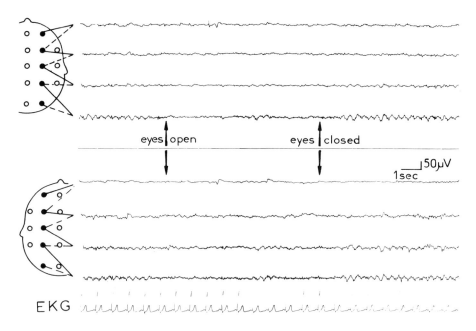

Figure 3.18   Case 18, age 58. Rhythmic 3 Hz occipital delta activity when eyes are closed, the day after an attack of transient global amnesia. Retrospective diagnosis of BEOP in childhood.

Interictal Symptoms of BEOP

There were 33 males (52%) and 30 females (48%). The age at onset was 15 months to 17 years (mean age, 7 years 5 months). Investigation showed that 23 patients had a family history of epilepsy, including febrile convulsions, and 10 cases had a history of migraine. There were 7 cases (11%) of prematurity and/or mild perinatal distress, nine cases (14%) of febrile convulsions, three cases (5%) of breath-holding spells, one case of posttraumatic subdural hematoma, one case of skull fracture, and one case of HHE syndrome.

Neurologic Examination.   Neurologic examination was normal in 57 patients (90%). Of the six patients who had abnormal examinations, all were developmentally delayed, five of them only slightly so; two patients had a hemiparesis, and one a hemiplegia. Of the patients with normal examinations, 11 (17%) seemed to be of above average intelligence, and 9 patients had mild behavioral disturbances.

Ophthalmologic Examination.   Visual acuity was normal in all patients. The visual fields were normal in the 33 patients in whom they were examined interictally.

Neuroradiologic Examination.   CT scans of 39 patients showed 35 cases to be normal. Angiograms, pneumoencephalograms, and isotope brain scans were normal in all patients who underwent these procedures (specifically 11 angiograms, 4 pneumoencephalograms and 7 isotope brain scans).

Visual Evoked Potentials.   Flash-evoked responses were obtained in 11 patients whose ictal symptoms and/or ictal EEGs suggested a unilateral origin for their seizures. In nine patients these responses were asymmetric, with higher-amplitude late responses seen over the involved hemisphere. Somato-sensory evoked responses were obtained in three patients with hemiclonic attacks, and these were similarly of higher amplitude over the involved hemisphere.

Electroencephalography.   Each patient had several EEGs, which were sepa-rated by intervals ranging from several days to 12 years. Background activity was unremarkable for each patient's age, but abundant and unusual interictal epileptiform activity was recorded. There were spike and wave com-plexes in 48 of 63 cases, or 76%; sharp waves in 19%; and rhythmic poste-rior slow waves in 5%. Amplitude sometimes reached $300\,\mu$V. Distribution was over the occipital and posterior temporal regions (standard electrode positions 0_1 and/or 0_2 as well as T_5 and/or T_6) of one hemisphere, most often the left, or over both hemispheres simultaneously or independently. It was usually seen as rhythmically repeated paroxysms from 1 to 3/sec, occurring in bursts or in trains that might continue for virtually the entire recording with eyes closed. On rare occasions, isolated paroxysmal activity was seen at irregular intervals.

Prompt disappearance of the paroxysmal activity with eye opening was seen in 59 of the 63 patients or 94%. The paroxysmal activity was seen almost exclusively after eye closure, usually with a latency of 1 to 10 seconds. Very occasionally, latencies of up to 20 seconds were seen.

Before BEOP had been fully described, Panayiotopoulos (1980, 1981) showed that this interictal activity is not suppressed with the eyes open in darkness but that subsequent fixation on a very small light source abolishes it. He concluded that the loss of macular vision with eye closure was responsible for the appearance of the epileptiform activity.

Intermittent photic stimulation evoked bursts of occipital sharp waves unrelated to eye opening and closing in seven patients who did not display such activity at rest. This effect of IPS is not related to the stimulus frequency and occurs several seconds after the beginning of stimulation, suggesting that the resulting bursts are related to an induced hyperexcitability of the occipital cortex rather than being a response locked to the photic stimuli. In seven other patients with typical occipital paroxysmal activity with eye closure, IPS evoked generalized bursts of spike or polyspike and wave activity, at times with asso-ciated myoclonus.

Hyperventilation had no significant effect on the occipital epileptiform activity. Sleep EEGs were obtained after partial sleep deprivation in 17 patients, whereas spontaneous sleep was recorded in 5 others. In 13 of these 22 patients, the occipital paroxysms disappeared with drowsiness and were not seen during the following slow wave sleep. Conversely, in five patients occipital paroxysmal activity, not seen in wakefulness, was noted; whereas five patients also had apparent electrographic seizures over the occipital regions during slow wave sleep, with no clinical accompaniment. In six patients, bursts of generalized bilaterally synchronous spike and wave complexes were seen.

Generalized bilaterally synchronous spike and wave or polyspike and wave complexes, characteristic of primary generalized epilepsy; and rolandic spikes, typical for benign partial epilepsy of childhood, were recorded in 19 of the 50 children (38%) who had no clinical evidence of either of these forms of epilepsy. The coexistence of rolandic spikes and typical occipital paroxysmal activity was seen principally in patients with hemiclonic seizures. It is noteworthy that a similar association was described by Beaussart (1972) in children with benign partial epilepsy and nocturnal hemiclonic seizures.

Ictal and Postictal Symptoms of BEOP

Clinical Ictal Symptoms

Visual Symptoms.   All patients old enough to answer questions about their attacks reported visual phenomena. In others, behavior during their seizures often suggested visual symptoms that they could not describe or remember. Several different visual experiences might be reported by the same patient as part of one or several seizures.

Partial or complete visual loss was the commonest visual symptom, noted by 33 of 63 patients (52%). It was almost always associated with other phenomena but could occur alone. It might be preceded by simple or complex visual hallucinations and be followed by convulsions, automatic behavior, or headache. The visual loss typically lasted up to several minutes and the entire visual field was eventually affected, although an initial hemianopia sometimes occurred. Laloue (1965), in a study of 158 seizures with visual symptoms, also noted the frequency of visual loss as an epileptic aura in children and its association with convulsions and headache suggestive of migraine.

Elementary visual hallucinations occurred in 29 of 63 subjects (46%). Generally taking the form of moving multicolored flashing spots occupying only one homonymous visual hemifield in one-third of these cases, such hallucinations could begin in the visual field either ipsilateral or contralateral to the discharging focus before filling the entire visual field in the remaining two-thirds. These phenomena could be either isolated or associated with other symptoms. If isolated, they usually occurred in flurries, each hallucination lasting up to 10 seconds. Longer lasting teichopsia might be followed by seizures, visceral sensations such as nausea, or headache.

Complex visual hallucinations were described by nine patients (14%). These too might occur alone or be followed by further symptoms. The most unusual hallucination — a 1- or 2-digit number — was noted by three patients. Since this writing, a further example of a similar occipital ictal hallucination was reported and confirmed by EEG and positron emission tomography (Engel et al., 1983).

Of the 63 patients, nine (14%) reported visual illusions, including micropsia, metamorphopsia, and palinopsia.

Nonvisual Symptoms.   Typically, nonvisual symptoms, either motor or somatosensory, follow one or more of the visual phenomena noted above.

Hemiclonic attacks were seen in 27 patients (43%). Most often, they were preceded by a visual aura and were usually contralateral to the occipital paroxysmal activity when it was unilateral, but this was not always the case, and at times alternating hemiclonic attacks occurred.

Complex partial seizures with automatisms were seen in nine patients (14%). These were indistinguishable from typical attacks arising in the temporal lobe, but were always preceded by visual auras.

Generalized tonic-clonic seizures were seen in eight patients, whereas three had bilateral clonic attacks and two had tonic seizures.

Adversive seizures, including turning of the whole body, were seen in seven subjects. Ocular movements were also seen in seven, but we were unable to determine whether or not these were examples of true epileptic nystagmus (Gastaut and Roger-Beaumanoir, 1954). Fluttering of the eyelids was seen in six patients while their visual auras were occurring.

Ictal dysphasia was described in eight patients.

Unilateral dysesthesia was described by five children. It usually occurred following visual symptoms in the hemifield of vision ipsilateral to the sensation. Elementary auditory hallucinations were described by three patients, always occurring in conjunction with their visual hallucinations.

EEG Ictal Features

Spontaneous seizures were recorded in six patients, four of which are described here. Electrographic seizures during sleep were seen in five others.

CASE 4   A seizure lasting 80 seconds began with phosphenes in all visual fields followed by turning of the head and eyes to the left and was accompanied by right posterior temporal and occipital ictal activity that then spread throughout the right hemisphere (Figure 3.6).

CASE 5   A 3-minute attack began with visual hallucinations followed by mild confusion associated with left occipital ictal activity (Figure 3.7).

CASE 6   An attack lasting 30 seconds occurred in stage 3 sleep and consisted of motor and verbal automatisms. It was associated with ictal activity that began in the right occipital region and rapidly spread over both hemispheres (Figure 3.9).

Note: The attacks in cases 4, 5 and 6 were followed by postictal delta activity lateralized over the hemisphere where the ictal discharge began.

CASE 2   Three elementary visual seizures were recorded, each lasting up to 5 seconds and accompanied by shifting 16-Hz epileptic recruiting rhythms over both occipital regions (Figure 3.3).

In five other cases, similar short-lived activity was seen during sleep. This activity was without any clinical manifestations and probably represented subclinical electrographic seizures.

Postictal Symptoms

The postictal symptoms of BEOP are quite specific and only rarely encountered in any other type of epilepsy. Diffuse headache, only rarely hemicranial, was found in 33% of the cases, whereas nausea and vomiting, at times associated with headache, were seen in 17%. Postictal diarrhea was observed in 3%.

These postictal phenomena became less severe and disappeared over several hours without any disturbance in the level of consciousness. Their postictal quality was further emphasized by the absence of any ictal discharge in the 13 cases in which the EEG was recorded during the postictal headache.

This association of headache, nausea, and vomiting lasting several hours, so characteristic of migraine, is further discussed below.

Frequency and Precipitating Factors

The frequency of BEOP attacks is extremely variable, ranging from a few attacks daily over several months to occasional seizures followed by seizure-free intervals of several years.

Because recognition of this syndrome depends on a characteristic visual aura, it will not be recognized as occurring during sleep. However, we have recorded typical occipital electrographic seizures during sleep without any clinical accompaniment. It is therefore possible that some of the seizures of BEOP may occur during sleep but go unreported as such because the typical history of visual disturbance cannot be obtained.

Although there are no clear precipitating factors, ambient light and the menstrual cycle contribute to their occurrence. Seizures that were apparently precipitated by light were reported by 16 patients. Some occurred on going from a dark area into a brighter one, or, conversely, from a well-lit area into a darkened one, as described by Pazzaglia et al. (1970). Three occurred while on a sunlit beach or at sea, or while watching television. In 5 of 12 pubescent girls with BEOP, seizures began with puberty and continued to occur with menstruation.

Prognosis of BEOP

BEOP generally carries a good prognosis, although it is not as benign as childhood epilepsy with rolandic spikes. In none of our cases have the seizures persisted into middle adulthood, and other types of recurring seizures in adulthood were seen in only three patients. The prognosis, as expected, is poorer in patients with other evidence of cerebral disturbance such as mental retardation or abnormal CT scans, or whose EEGs show an additional secondary epileptiform disturbance. Complete seizure control with anticonvulsant drugs was achieved in 38 patients (60%), and seizures persisted in 3 patients followed beyond age 19. Seizure control may be achieved, although the epileptiform EEG may persist for several months or years after the seizures have ceased.

Almost all available anticonvulsants have been tried without any one being the obvious drug of choice. The rapid response to clobazam (Gastaut and Low, 1979) is noteworthy. In seven of nine patients in whom it was used, both seizures and interictal spikes ceased after only several days of treatment.

Diagnosis of BEOP

In patients with the complete syndrome, diagnosis is not difficult. However, since the presence of occipital interictal discharges increases suspicion and directs the physician in seeking a history of visual disturbance, diagnosis is more difficult in cases in which the syndrome is incomplete, particularly when the characteristic EEG pattern is absent. Thus, many cases of BEOP may be missed if the history of visual phenomena is not carefully sought.

Five conditions must be differentiated from BEOP:

1. Occipital "needle-like" spikes (Gibbs and Gibbs, 1952; Gibbs et al., 1968; Beaumanoir et al., 1981) may be seen with eye closure in nonepileptic children with defective vision. This unusual pattern is not associated with seizures.

2. Very rarely, the EEGs of patients with secondary generalized epilepsy suggesting the Lennox-Gastaut Syndrome show occipital slow spike and wave complexes with eyes open as well as closed, in place of the more usual generalized epileptiform activity.

3. Focal epilepsy caused by occipital lesions is much rarer in childhood than BEOP. It is characterized by a less complex ictal pattern, usually marked by visual seizures followed by tonic deviation but without hemiclonic or psychomotor attacks or postictal headaches. In such patients, the neurologic and neuro-ophthalmologic examinations, as well as the CT scan, will be abnormal. The interictal EEG shows intermittent spikes, which do not react to eye opening, over a single occipital lobe where continuous polymorphous delta activity, or attenuation of background activity, also suggests a focal lesion.

4. Complex partial seizures arising in the temporal lobe are at least as frequent in children as BEOP. The two may be confused in those rare instances where the psychomotor attacks are preceded by visual illusions or hallucina-

tions. The two can be differentiated clinically at times, but the EEG is especially useful in showing the typical anterior sylvian abnormalities associated with epilepsy arising in the temporal lobe.

5. Basilar migraine (Bickerstaff, 1961) is usually seen in adolescent women who subsequently develop common migraine. It is characterized by a prodrome, typically lasting up to 30 minutes, of visual loss or flashing lights together with signs of pontine and midbrain dysfunction such as vertigo, dysarthria, bilateral paresthesiae, or transient loss of consciousness, followed by headache lasting several hours. No paroxysmal EEG activity is seen during or between these attacks, but bilateral posterior slow waves may be seen for hours or days afterwards (Lapkin et al., 1977). The absence of interictal epileptiform occipital activity attenuated by eye opening in patients with basilar migraine (Bickerstaff, 1961; Lees and Watkins, 1963; Slatter, 1968; Hockaday and Whitty, 1969; Watson and Steele, 1974; Golden and French, 1975) is of major importance in differentiating basilar migraine from BEOP.

The diagnosis of BEOP should not be made when seizures first occur in adult life. Although several authors (Naquet et al., 1960; Gastaut et al., 1963; Fischer-Williams et al., 1964; Swanson and Vick, 1978) have described occipital seizures evoked by intermittent photic stimulation in adults without evidence of brain lesions, these cases are extremely rare and are not believed to form a separate type of epilepsy.

DISCUSSION

Etiology of BEOP

Cerebral seizures with visual symptoms and occipital spike and wave complexes that attenuate with eye opening have been reported in the past (Slatter, 1968; Camfield et al., 1978; Panayiotopoulos, 1980). However, because of the prominent headache and postictal visceral symptoms in their few patients, these authors felt that the attacks were a variety of basilar migraine. To account for the epileptiform EEG, Camfield et al. (1978) suggested that initial migrainous vasospasm produced an ischemic cortical lesion in the territory of the basilar artery, giving rise to the occipital spike and wave activity in both hemispheres.

The results reported here suggest, on the contrary, that BEOP does not depend on an initial migrainous lesion but is a primary and independent epileptic disorder.

In our patients, the majority of seizures began with brief unilateral teichopsia or hallucinations that were characteristically epileptic. This was confirmed in six patients who had seizures during EEG monitoring. Headache was seen in only one-third of our patients and, even in these patients, it only followed some, not all, of their attacks. Their headaches were not always typically migrainous and occurred only following a seizure. Visual evoked responses in some patients suggested an occipital hyperexcitability on the side where the typical occipital paroxysmal activity was predominant. The seizures and the headaches that may accompany them respond to antiepileptic drugs rather than to anti-migraine treatment, and the seizures and epileptiform abnormalities disappear spontaneously after several years. In our cases a family history of epilepsy was twice as frequent as one of migraine, whereas almost no patient gave a personal history of common or basilar migraine.

It therefore seems clear that the seizures in our 63 patients were not a variety of basilar migraine and that the attacks were definitely epileptic, although they were followed by a migraine-like headache in one-third of cases. It is, moreover, noteworthy that the only other reported epileptic seizures followed by postictal migrainous symptoms also arose in the occipital lobe, after head trauma. Prior to the well-known report of Ritchie Russell and Whitty (1955), Marchand and Ajuriaguerra (1948) reviewed reports of several authors from 1917 to 1933 who described posttraumatic visual seizures after occipital lesions, with violent hemicranial headaches at times followed by convulsions. However, only 7% of Ritchie Russell and Whitty's cases of posttraumatic seizures with visual symptoms in adults were associated with migraine, compared with one-third of the cases of benign occipital epilepsy in children. It is thus possible that there exists a genetic link between migraine and benign focal epilepsy of childhood as suggested by Kinast et al. (1982), who found that 9% of 100 children with migraine but without epilepsy had benign focal epileptiform discharges in their EEGs.

BEOP is seen almost exclusively in children with no clinical or radiological evidence of brain lesions, and 36% of them have a family history of epilepsy or febrile convulsions. These seizures usually respond well to antiepileptic drugs and cease spontaneously in adulthood, as do the epileptiform EEG paroxysms. From this, it seems clear that BEOP must be grouped with the "primary," "benign," or "functional" partial epilepsies as opposed to the secondary epilepsies related to some focal or more widespread lesion. We have suggested this distinction in the past (Gastaut, 1951) and have also recommended the inclusion of the primary partial epilepsies in the International Classification of the Epilepsies (Gastaut, 1983; Gastaut and Zifkin, 1985). The epileptic focus in such primary partial epilepsies is associated with a constitutional and often inherited predisposition to seizures (Gastaut 1981, 1982a) expressed, when generalized, by 3/sec spike and wave complexes (Gloor et al., 1982). Thus, it is not surprising that more than one-third of our patients also have generalized spike and wave activity or rolandic spikes and that 16% had the typical seizures associated with these abnormalities.

We have thus been led to group all the primary partial epilepsies together and consider them, along with the primary generalized epilepsies, as forming a class of primary epilepsies of childhood carrying a relatively good prognosis. A similar association has been proposed by Bray and Wiser (1965), Beaumanoir

(1974), and Niedermeyer (1981), who classified rolandic epilepsy with primary generalized epilepsy.

Nevertheless, we do not suggest that all cases of primary epilepsy, particularly BEOP, can be attributed exclusively to a basic predisposition to seizures. Although it is possible that certain cases depend on this mechanism alone, as in Cases 2 and 3 reported above, it is probable that many cases arise from the interaction between this tendency and a cerebral lesion that is insufficient to cause spontaneous seizures on its own. It is also possible that in certain cases this secondary factor is at least as important as the primary one. This would explain those patients (Cases 16 and 17) in whom a Lennox-Gastaut Syndrome or an organic partial epilepsy coexists closely with the electroclinical findings of BEOP.

We suggest that, just as for the classic spike and wave discharge (Gloor et al., 1982), the EEG pattern of BEOP may be contributing to epileptogenesis in many patients with evidence of acquired or genetic encephalopathies. This hypothesis is in agreement with the reports of Andermann and Metrakos (1969) and Andermann (1982), who showed a similar multifactorial etiology in patients with focal and generalized epilepsy.

The diagnosis of typical BEOP, like that of primary generalized epilepsy, is based predominantly on negative findings. That is, the history and examination are unremarkable, the EEG shows typical findings without other abnormalities, and there is no radiological evidence of focal lesions or other more diffuse abnormalities. Again in similarity to generalized epilepsy (Gloor, 1977), mixed BEOP syndromes, in which one or more of these conditions is not met, have been encountered and will continue to be seen. Often they will not fit precisely the classical phenotypes of primary or secondary epilepsy, sharing the elements of the typical syndromes to a variable degree. One might predict that patients with such mixed syndromes have a worse prognosis for total control of seizures and their eventual disappearance than do patients with typical BEOP.

Pathophysiology of the Seizures of BEOP

Any discussion of the pathophysiology of BEOP must consider both the genesis of the interictal and ictal neuronal discharge in the absence of any evident lesion and also the pattern of ictal spreading of this discharge that is responsible for the clinical symptoms.

To explain the rhythmic spike and wave complexes seen with eye closure or IPS over an intact occipital lobe, Gastaut (1950a) proposed a thalamocortical mechanism, driven by a thalamic pacemaker. Ludwig and Ajmone-Marsan (1975) suggested that bilateral, rhythmic, synchronous occipital spike and wave complexes in epileptic patients could be the result of an atypical "centrencephalic" disturbance, similar to that responsible for generalized 3/sec spike and wave complexes, which we have seen in 19 of our patients. A subcortical mechanism in the electrogenesis of these occipital spike and wave complexes is also suggested, for two reasons. First, there is the absence of discernible occipital lesions. Second, there is a resemblance between the interictal occipital spike and wave complexes and (1) the normal posterior slow waves of youth (Aird and Gastaut, 1959), and (2) the posterior delta rhythm often found in association with typical spike and wave complexes in classic absence. The response to IPS at 3 Hz in some photosensitive patients, in whom occipital and posterior temporal bilateral spikes are seen prior to generalization (Gastaut, 1950b), also suggests a similar subcortical mechanism.

The spread of occipital epileptiform discharges has been previously studied in adults with secondary occipital epilepsy. Ajmone-Marsan and Ralston (1957), Bancaud (1969), and Bancaud et al. (1961, 1969, 1973) have shown that occipital epileptic discharges may remain localized or spread to either the parietal lobe, the temporal lobe and rhinencephalon, or even to subcortical structures. In addition, Bancaud et al., showed that such discharges could give rise to secondary epileptogenesis at a distance, thus explaining the variability of seizure patterns in which either the primary or the secondary focus may be manifested clinically. These findings, which we had suggested earlier (Gastaut, 1958), and which have been recently confirmed by Olivier et al. (1982), certainly apply to BEOP. They also explain the existence of the four major seizure patterns of BEOP:

1. Purely visual seizures associated with a nonpropagated focal occipital discharge
2. Visual auras followed by hemisensory and/or hemiconvulsive attacks; related to the spreading of the occipital discharge to the parietal and central regions
3. Visual auras followed by psychomotor seizures; related to the spreading of the occipital discharge to the temporal lobe and/or the rhinencephalon
4. Seizures without visual auras; corresponding either to secondary spreading of the occipital discharge in which the visual phenomena were not reported or to the discharge of an independent secondary epileptogenic focus (Bancaud et al., 1969).

The postictal migrainous symptoms of some attacks may be explained by a persistence in the territory of the posterior cerebral and basilar arteries of the initial vasodilation accompanying the occipital ictal activity in children with impaired or labile cerebrovascular autoregulation who are predisposed to migraines. This hypothesis is the converse of the theory of Camfield et al. (1978), since we suggest that the occipital seizure is responsible for the migraine and not vice versa. This agrees with the observations of Caplan et al. (1981), who suggested a similar mechanism to explain the occurrence of migraine symptoms with transient global amnesia. Case 18 in our series is therefore of particular interest, as this patient reported the seizures of BEOP followed by migraine in childhood, whereas in later life there was transient global amnesia followed by migraine and accompanied by posterior slow waves attenuating with eye opening.

CONCLUSIONS

We have described 63 cases of a childhood epilepsy in which seizures are characterized by visual symptoms that are often followed by sensory, motor, or psychomotor symptoms and postictal migrainous and visceral symptoms. The EEG usually shows characteristic repetitive occipital paroxysmal activity attenuated by eye opening. No occipital lesions have been found, and the seizures cease in adult life. It is suggested that this syndrome represents a separate variety of relatively benign primary partial epilepsy that derives at least in part from a constitutional predisposition to such attacks similar to that proposed for primary generalized epilepsy. The migrainous and visceral phenomena may be attributable to a persistence of the initial vasodilation in the posterior cerebral and basilar artery territories, accompanying the occipital ictal activity.

REFERENCES

Aicardi J, Chevrie J. Epilepsies partielles bénignes de l'enfant. In: Congrès de la société de neurologie infantile, Diffusion générale de librairie. Marseille, 1977;233–42.

Aird R, Gastaut Y. Occipital and posterior electroencephalographic rhythms. Electroencephalogr Clin Neurophysiol 1959;11:637–56.

Ajmone-Marsan C, Ralston B. The epileptic seizure: its functional morphology. Springfield, Ill.: Charles C Thomas, 1957:211–5.

Andermann E, Metrakos J. EEG studies of relatives of probands with focal epilepsy who have been treated surgically (Abst). Epilepsia 1969;10:45.

Andermann E. Multifactorial inheritance of generalized and focal epilepsy. In: Anderson VE, Hauser WA, Penry JK, Sing CF, eds. Genetic basis of the epilepsies. New York: Raven Press, 1982:355–74.

Bancaud J, Bonis A, Morel P, Talairach J, Szikla G, Tournoux P. Epilepsie occipitale à éxpression "rhinencéphalique" prévalente. Rev Neurol 1961;105:219.

Bancaud J. Les crises épileptiques d'origine occipitale. Rev Oto Neuro Ophtalmol 1969;41:229–311.

Bancaud J, Talairach J, Bonis A, Bernoulli C, Bordas-Ferrer N. Constitution chez l'homme des foyers épileptogènes secondaires. Rev Neurol 1969;121:297–305.

Bancaud J, Talairach J, Geier S, Scarabin J. EEG et SEEG dans les tumeurs cérébrales et l'épilepsie. Paris: Edifor, 1973:320–32.

Beaumanoir A, Ballis T, Varfis G, Ansari K. Benign epilepsy of childhood with Rolandic spikes. A clinical, electroencephalographic, and telencephalographic study. Epilepsia 1974;15:301–15.

Beaumanoir A, Inderwildi B, Zaguri S. Paroxysmes EEG "non-épileptiques." Med Hyg Genève 1981;39:1911–8.

Beaussart M. Benign epilepsy of children with rolandic foci. Epilepsia 1972;13:795–811.

Bickerstaff E. Basilar artery migraine. Lancet 1961;1:15.

Bray P, Wiser W. The relation of focal to diffuse epileptiform EEG discharges in genetic epilepsy. Arch Neurol 1965;13:223–37.

Camfield P, Metrakos K, Andermann F. Basilar migraine, seizures and severe epileptiform EEG abnormalities. Neurology 1978;20:584–8.

Caplan L, Chedru F, Lhermitte F, Mayman C. Transient global amnesia and migraine. Neurology 1981;31:1167–70.

Delwaide PJ, Barragan M, Gastaut H. Remarques sur l'épilepsie partielle occipitale. Acta Neurol Belg 1971;71:383–91.

Engel J, Kuhl DE, Phelps ME, Rausch R, Nuwer M. Local cerebral metabolism during partial seizures. Neurology 1983;33:400–13.

Fischer-Williams M, Bickford RG, Whisnant JP. Occipito-parieto-temporal seizure discharge with visual hallucinations and aphasia. Epilepsia 1964;5:279–92.

Gastaut H. Evidence électrographique d'un mécanisme sous-cortical dans certaines épilepsies partielles — la signification clinique des "secteurs aréo-thalamiques." Rev Neurol 1950a;83:396–401.

Gastaut H. Combined photic and Metrazol activation of the brain. Electroencephalogr Clin Neurophysiol 1950b;2:249–61.

Gastaut H. Etiologie des épilepsies. In: Les épilepsies. Encyclopédie médico-chirurgicale, tome Système Nerveux. Paris, 1951.

Gastaut H. A propos des décharges neuroniques développées à distance d'une lésion épileptogène. In: Alajouanine T, ed. Bases physiologiques de l'épilepsie. Paris: Masson, 1958:163–83.

Gastaut H. Individualisation des épilepsies dites "bénignes" ou "fonctionnelles" aux différents âges de la vie. Rev EEG Neurophysiol Clin 1981;11:346–66.

Gastaut H. "Benign" or "functional" (versus "organic") epilepsies in different stages of life. In: Broughton R, ed. Henri Gastaut and the Marseille school's contribution to the neurosciences. Electroencephalogr Clin Neurophysiol 1982a; (Suppl)35:17–44.

Gastaut H. L'épilepsie bénigne de l'enfant à pointe-ondes occipitales. Rev EEG Neurophysiol Clin 1982b;12:179–201.

Gastaut H. Die benigne Epilepsie des Kindesalters mit okzipitalen Spike-wave. EEG EMG 1982c;13:3–8.

Gastaut H. A new type of epilepsy: benign partial epilepsy of childhood with occipital spike-waves. Clin Electroencephalogr 1982d;13:13–22.

Gastaut H. A new type of epilepsy: benign partial epilepsy of childhood with occipital spike-waves. In: Advances in epileptology, XIIIth Epilepsy International Symposium. New York: Raven Press, 1982e;19–25.

Gastaut H. A proposed completion of the current international classification of the epilepsies. In: Rose FC, ed. Research progress in epilepsy. London; Pitman, 1983;8–13.

Gastaut H, Franck G, Krolikowska W, Naquet R, Regis H, Roger J. Etude des potentiels évoqués visuels chez les hémianopsiques présentant des crises épileptiques visuelles dans leur champ aveugle. Rev Neurol 1963;108:316–22.

Gastaut H, Iemolo F, Menendez-Gonzalez P. L'épilepsie versive à pointe-ondes généralisées de l'adolescent. In: Epilepsies de l'adolescent et adolescents épileptiques. Paris: Documentation médicale Labaz, 1981:25–30.

Gastaut H, Low M. Antiepileptic properties of clobazam. Epilepsia 1979;20:437–46.

Gastaut H, Naquet R. Etude électroencéphalographique de l'insuffisance circulatoire cérébrale chronique. Symposium internationale sur la circulation cérébrale. Paris: Sandoz, 1966:163–91.

Gastaut H, Roger-Beaumanoir A. Les formes inhabituelles de l'épilepsie: le nystagmus épileptique. Rev Neurol 1954;90:130–2.

Gastaut H, Zifkin BG. Classification of the epilepsies. J Clin Neurophysiol 1985; 2:313–26.

Gibbs F, Gibbs E. Atlas of electroencephalography. Vol. 2. Cambridge, Mass.: Addison-Wesley Press, 1952:222–4.

Gibbs F, Gibbs E, Gibbs E, Gibbs T. Relation between specific types of occipital dysrythmia and visual defects. Johns Hopkins Med J 1968;122:343–9.

Gloor P, Metrakos J, Metrakos K, van Gelder N. Neurophysiological, genetic, and van Huffelen AC, eds. Current concepts in clinical neurophysiology. The Hague: Trio, 1977:9–21.

Gloor P, Metrakos J, Metrakos K, van Gelder N. Neurophysiological, genetic, and biochemical nature of the epileptic diathesis. In: Broughton R, ed. Henri Gastaut and the Marseille school's contribution to the neurosciences. Electroencephalogr Clin Neurophysiol 1982;(Suppl)35:45–56.

Golden GS, French JH. Basilar artery migraine in young children. Pediatrics 1975;56:722–6.

Hockaday JM, Whitty CWM. Factors determining the electroencephalogram in migraine: a study of 560 patients according to clinical type of migraine. Brain 1969;92:769–88.

Kinast M, Lueders H, Rothner A, Erenberg G. Benign focal epileptiform discharges in childhood migraine. Neurology 1982;32:1309–11.

Laloue R. Crises épileptiques comportant des phénomènes visuels. Bordeaux: Thèse, 1965.

Lapkin ML, French JH, Golden GS, Rowan AJ. The EEG in childhood basilar artery migraine. Neurology 1977;27:580–3.

Lees F, Watkins SM. Loss of consciousness in migraine. Lancet 1963;2:647–9.

Ludwig B, Ajmone-Marsan C. Clinical ictal patterns with occipital EEG foci. Neurology 1975;25:463–71.

Marchand L, Ajuriaguerra J. Epilepsies. Paris: Desclée de Brower, 1948:389–90.

Naquet R, Fegerstein L, Bert J. Seizure discharges localized to the posterior cerebral regions in man provoked by intermittent photic stimulation. Electroencephalogr Clin Neurophysiol 1960;12:305–16.

Niedermeyer E. Complexities of primary generalized epilepsies. Clin Electroencephalogr 1981;12:177–91.

Olivier A, Gloor P, Andermann F, Ives J. Occipito-temporal epilepsy studied with stereotaxically implanted depth electrodes and successfully treated by temporal resection. Ann Neurol 1982;11:428–32.

Panayiotopoulos CP. Basilar migraine? Seizure and severe epileptic EEG abnormalities. Neurology 1980;30:1122–5.

Panayiotopoulos CP. Inhibitory effect of central vision on occipital lobe seizures. Neurology 1981;31:1330–3.

Pazzaglia P, Sabattini L, Lugaresi E. Crisi occipitali precipitate dal buio. Riv Neurol 1970;40:184–92.

Ritchie Russell W, Whitty CWM. Studies in traumatic epilepsy III. J Neurol Neurosurg Psychiatry 1955;18:79–96.

Rodin E. Discussion in: Alter M, Hauser WA, eds. The epidemiology of epilepsy. Bethesda: US Department of Health, Education, and Welfare Publication No. NIH 73–390, 1972:110.

Rowan AJ, Protass LM. Transient global amnesia: clinical and EEG findings in 10 cases. Neurology 29;1979:869–72.

Slatter K. Some clinical and EEG findings in patients with migraine. Brain 1968;91: 85–98.

Sorel L, Rucquoy-Ponsar M. L'épilepsie fonctionnelle de maturation. Rev Neurol 1969;121:288–97.

Swanson JW, Vick NA. Basilar artery migraine. Twelve patients with an attack recorded electroencephalographically. Neurology 1978;28:782–6.

Watson P, Steele JC. Paroxysmal dysequilibrium in the migraine syndrome of childhood. Arch Otolaryngol 1974;99:177–9.

4

Benign Epilepsy with Occipital Paroxysms and Migraine: The Question of Intercalated Attacks

Mario Giovanni Terzano
Gian Camillo Manzoni
Liborio Parrino

There are some forms of epilepsy that may be described as benign syndromes because the suppression of seizures continues even after administration of drugs has been suspended. Indeed, in some forms of epilepsy not only generalized but also focal seizures are known to disappear, perhaps spontaneously, with age (Terzano et al., 1980a; Gastaut, 1981). Among the clinical and electroencephalographic (EEG) features most suggestive of benign syndromes are the absence of obvious lesions to account for the seizures; the decreased frequency of seizures following drug therapy; the absence of accompanying neuropsychiatric symptoms that might interfere with a normal social life; and, finally, the complete remission of seizures at a certain age, even after drug therapy has been discontinued. Early detection of these features in an increasing number of epileptic disorders is especially important because patients and their families can then be adequately informed about the benign nature of the syndrome and the good prognosis that might be expected, whatever the therapeutic approach.

Traditionally remission has been considered to be more likely in those forms of epilepsy that manifest with generalized seizures (primary generalized epilepsies) induced by genetically inherited factors. The concept of benign focal epilepsies has been less widely accepted, because these have generally been assumed to have an "organic" rather than a "functional" cause, even when no lesion was found.

In the last 10 years, several benign focal epileptic syndromes have been identified. In addition to centrotemporal epilepsy with rolandic spikes (Beaussart, 1972), which has for some time been recognized as a benign epilepsy, benign epilepsy with affective seizures and temporal lobe spikes (Dalla Bernardina et al., 1980) and benign epilepsy with parietal lobe spikes (De Marco, 1980) have also been defined. More recently, a form of benign epilepsy with visual seizures and occipital lobe spikes has been reported by a number of authors (Camfield et al., 1978; Manzoni et al., 1979; Terzano et al., 1980b, 1980c; Panayiotopoulos, 1980; Terzano et al., 1981; Gastaut, 1982a, 1982b; Beaumanoir, 1983).

Our patients, during late childhood and adolescence, had epilepsy with occipital spikes and seizures that were closely associated with classical migraine attacks. In this form of epilepsy, some of the epileptic and migrainous symptoms originate in the occipital lobe, which is involved with both the epileptic neuronal discharge and the vascular phenomena characteristic of the migraine attacks.

MATERIALS AND METHODS

Among 450 patients with classical or common migraine treated at the Headache Center of the University of Parma, 16 (6 males and 10 females), or 3.6%, also had epileptic seizures. At the time of this study, headache was regarded by the patients as their main clinical problem. Headache was diagnosed according to the Ad Hoc Committee classification (1962) and seizures according to the classification suggested by the International League against Epilepsy (Gastaut 1969).

Data concerning both migraine and epilepsy were obtained from a 34-section questionnaire, which was regularly updated at follow-up visits. For both disorders, the questionnaire recorded the personal and family history, age at onset of the first migraine attack or seizure, their frequency, triggering circumstances, prodromes, accompanying clinical manifestations, and transient sequelae. For headache, the location and type of pain were also determined. Additionally, the patient's general medical condition was investigated, and a behavioral profile was obtained by testing each subject on an outpatient basis.

All patients who had epilepsy in addition to headache were screened by at least one neuroradiologic examination (computerized tomography [CT] scan, angiography, or cerebral scintiscan). Serial EEG records were obtained over a period of time in order to determine the interictal and, when possible, ictal correlates of both phenomena. Polygraphic recordings were carried out during nocturnal sleep in six patients in an attempt to more accurately assess the location and activation of paroxysmal abnormalities.

For both disorders, the temporal relationships between migraine attacks and epileptic seizures were studied and inquiries were made as to possible interactions between the two types of attack.

RESULTS

In none of the 16 patients with migraine and epilepsy were brain lesions found on neuroradiologic examination. We identified three groups of patients according to the interval between the onset of migraine and that of epilepsy.

Patients with Associated Attacks

This group included four subjects (three females and a male) in whom onset of migraine and epilepsy were not simultaneous (Table 4.1). Onset of the seizures either preceded or followed that of the migraine attacks by 5 to 19 years. Migraine attacks and epileptic seizures occurred independently of each other, and their frequencies were in no way related.

In this group the two disorders appeared to be quite distinct conditions and their association a purely coincidental one.

Patients with Combined Attacks

This group included five subjects (four females and a male) in whom the onset of epilepsy and migraine was almost simultaneous, occurring during late childhood or the early teens (Table 4.2).

In these patients, the two types of attack were still quite distinct from each other but were often, if not always, closely related, so that an epileptic seizure was often followed by a migraine attack and vice versa. The migraine that followed the seizures was different from postictal headache, since it lasted longer, was associated with photophobia, nausea, and vomiting, and was responsive to ergotamine preparations.

In these cases, migraine and epilepsy appeared to act as stress stimuli that could mutually trigger each other. Their clinical courses turned out to be closely related as well.

Patients with Intercalated Attacks

This association between migraine and epilepsy was found in seven subjects who were also in late childhood or in their teens.

The seizures started at an occipital focus and were almost always closely related to attacks of classical migraine in which the headache was usually preceded by a visual aura. The chronological sequence of events revealed that the seizures were intercalated between the migrainous aura and the headache (Manzoni et al., 1979).

Table 4.1   Associated Attacks: Independent Occurrence of Migraine Attacks and Epileptic Seizures

Case Number	Sex	Age at Onset		Family History		Type of Migraine	Type of Seizure	EEG Abnormalities
		Migraine	*Epilepsy*	*Headache*	*Epilepsy*			
1	M	12	1	yes	no	Classical	Convulsive generalized	Generalized
2	F	17	22	yes	yes	Common	Complex partial	Left temporal
3	F	30	15	yes	no	Common	Complex partial	Left temporal
4	F	20	39	yes	no	Common	Complex partial	Left and right temporal

Table 4.2 Combined Attacks: Migraine Attack → Epileptic Seizure or Epileptic Seizure → Migraine Attack

Case Number	Sex	Age at Onset		Family History		Type of Migraine	Type of Seizure	EEG Abnormalities
		Migraine	Epilepsy	Headache	Epilepsy			
5	M	12	11	no	no	Common	Generalized convulsive Non-convulsive	Generalized
6	F	9	11	no	no	Classical	Convulsive generalized	Generalized
7	F	12	9	yes	no	Common	Complex partial	Left temporal
8	F	10	10	yes	no	Classical	Convulsive generalized	Generalized
9	F	8	8	yes	no	Common	Complex partial	Left temporal

This group included four males and three females who had (Table 4.3) suffered from classic migraine for 8 to 15 years. All had a family history of headache, and two also had a family history of epilepsy. The first seizure appeared as late as 2 years after the onset of migraine in six patients. In one case, epilepsy preceded the first migraine attack by 7 years.

Clinical Manifestations

Clinically, the epileptic seizures always started in the occipital region. They consisted initially of positive visual images — highly stylized contours of plain figures, or single or multiple colored spots that often rotated.

These visual seizures lasted 1 or 2 minutes and came out of a scintillating scotoma slowly developing in the visual field and evolving into unilateral or bilateral hemianopia. The change of visual perception from negative back to the positive visual images usually corresponded to the beginning of the epileptic seizure, which was later followed by migraine headache.

Visual seizures became secondarily generalized in three cases. In three other cases, illusions and psychomotor automatisms occurred, suggesting spread to the temporal lobe. In one patient the seizures remained confined to the occipital lobe.

The migraine attacks were usually much more frequent than the epileptic seizures. In three subjects visual seizures sometimes occurred independently of the migraine attacks.

EEG Features

All of these patients had at least one EEG showing an epileptogenic focus in the posterior head regions (occipital, parieto-occipital, or temporo-occipital). Some patients had bilateral independent foci; in such cases one of these foci showed consistent predominance. When the patient's eyes were closed, the EEG recorded high-amplitude, almost continuous discharges that ceased as soon as the eyes were opened (Figure 4.1). Over the years these abnormalities continued to appear from time to time, especially after eye closure.

The EEGs of three subjects revealed diffuse as well as focal abnormalities. There were four other patients who exhibited marked photosensitivity.

During nocturnal sleep, a decreased activation of the occipital EEG abnormalities was observed during slow wave sleep (SWS).

The EEG abnormalities tended to disappear before the third decade.

Clinical Course

Six of the seven patients ceased having seizures before age 20. Antiepileptic therapy varied considerably, with frequent changes in type and dosage of drugs; in some cases, medication was discontinued for some time. Drugs used were phenytoin, phenobarbital, benzodiazepines, and carbamazepine. In these six patients the mean period of time during which they had seizures was 4 years.

Table 4.3　Intercalated Attacks: Prodromes → Epileptic Seizure → Migraine Attack

Case Number	Sex	Age at Onset		Family History		Type of Migraine	Type of Seizure	EEG Abnormalities
		Migraine	Epilepsy	Headache	Epilepsy			
10	M	15	16	yes	no	Classical	Partial & generalized	Left occipital
11	M	7	8	no	no	Classical	Partial	Right temporo-occipital
12	M	11	4	yes	yes	Classical	Partial	Right temporo-occipital
13	M	7	8	yes	yes	Classical	Partial & generalized	Occipital
14	F	7	16	yes	no	Classical	Partial	Occipital & generalized
15	F	14	16	no	no	Classical	Partial & generalized	Occipital & generalized
16	F	11	12	yes	no	Classical	Partial	Occipital

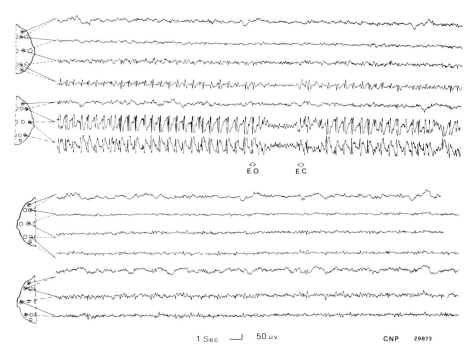

E.O. E.C.

1 Sec ⊔ 50 μv   CNP 29873

Figure 4.1 Focus of rhythmic spike and slow wave discharges in the right temporo-occipital region in an 8-year-old child. Opening of the eyes (EO) suppresses the abnormalities, which reappear as eyes are closed (EC).

Migraine continued, but their attacks became increasingly less frequent, and the patients proved responsive to antimigraine prophylaxis with ergotamine and pizotifen.

The seventh patient, a woman still under 20, continues to have migraine attacks and both isolated and intercalated occipital lobe seizures. After the frequency of migraine attacks and seizures was determined over a 6-month drug-free period, she was treated with 600 mg of sodium valproate, plus placebo, daily for 6 months and a combination of 600 mg of sodium valproate and 1.0 mg of pizotifen over the following 6 months (Figure 4.2). The combination of these two drugs was more effective in reducing the number of both migraine attacks and seizures.

DISCUSSION

The existence of a special relationship between migraine attacks and epileptic seizures has often been suggested. Both epilepsy and migraine are characterized by a chronic course with recurring, paroxysmal clinical manifestations.

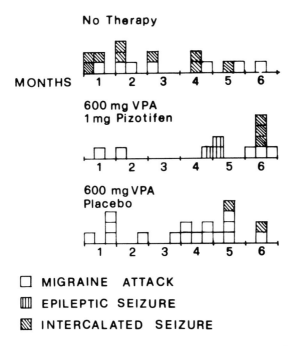

Figure 4.2 Results of pharmacologic trials in a young woman with migraine and intercalated seizures. The number of migraine attacks, isolated occipital lobe seizures, and intercalated seizures occurring in three 6 month periods, during which the patient received (1) no treatment, (2) 600 mg of valproic acid (VPA) plus 1.0-mg of pizotifen, and (3) VPA plus placebo. The combination of the antiepileptic drug (VPA) and the antimigraine drug (pizotifen) appeared to be the most effective therapy in controlling both migraine attacks and intercalated seizures.

Common Features of Epilepsy and Migraine

1. Epilepsy and migraine are fairly widespread among the general population. The prevalence of epilepsy is 0.5% to 2%, whereas that of migraine is 5% to 10%. A significant family history of migraine in epileptics (28%) (Alvarez, 1959) and of epilepsy in migraine sufferers (2%–3%) (Selby and Lance, 1960) suggests that these subjects may share some genetic traits. Moreover, 6% to 8% of migraine sufferers have seizures (Slatter, 1968; Basser, 1969), which is a higher frequency than that found in control subjects.
2. Signs of brain involvement, which may differ depending on the structures involved, are always present during epileptic seizures. Focal signs characterize the aura of classical migraine.
3. Interictal EEG abnormalities can be observed in both syndromes. Paroxysmal abnormalities, that is, spikes and spike and wave complexes, predominate during seizures. These abnormalities can also be found in migraine

(Terzano et al., 1981), but slow discharges, generally focal, are more frequently found in the EEG during a migraine attack.
4. Both epileptic seizures and migraine attacks can be prevented by appropriate regular medication.

Differences between Epilepsy and Migraine

1. The pathophysiologic mechanisms of epilepsy and migraine are entirely different. Epilepsy is a neuronal disorder, since the symptoms of epileptic seizures result from the pathologic activation of neuronal aggregates. On the other hand, migraine is a vascular condition; its accompanying neurologic symptoms are merely concomitant or secondary. Several types of mechanism are known to play a role, among them for example, genetic, humoral, hormonal, and neurotransmitter abnormalities. Involvement of the arterial tree of the head is constantly present, with vasoconstriction occurring in the prodromal phase and vasodilation in the painful phase.
2. The classification of different types of generalized and focal seizures is based on clinical and EEG features. Pain is a rare occurrence in seizures, and it tends to appear during the preictal or postictal phases. Most migraine attacks, by contrast, are characterized by headache in which the pain is generally unilateral and the premonitory or accompanying symptoms of the aura are usually minor.
3. The EEG during epileptic seizures is characterized by features that are described as "ictal" and consist of a sequence of spikes or spike and wave complexes that often clearly signal the moment when the seizures begin or cease. In focal seizures the ictal discharges, if appropriately recorded, indicate the area where the paroxysm started and those areas to which it subsequently spread. The EEG during migraine attacks may be unchanged or may show a slowed background rhythm but no ictal paroxysmal abnormalities.
4. Although attacks in both disorders can be prevented by drug therapy, the types of medication are different. Drugs commonly used in seizures are aimed at controlling abnormal neuronal discharges. Drugs used in migraine attacks often block neurohumoral or vasomotor mechanisms that are responsible for pain. Treatment must be continuous for epilepsy, whereas separate courses of therapy are possible for migraine.

Clinically, the early symptoms of an attack of classical migraine may resemble the conscious sensations reported by epileptic patients during focal seizures or seizures that later develop into generalized convulsions (Giovanardi-Rossi et al., 1982; Mancia et al., 1982). Misdiagnosis can also result from the fact that loss of consciousness may occur during a migraine attack and, conversely, a seizure may be characterized by the appearance of marked autonomic reactions (Barolin, 1966).

Finally, when migraine and epilepsy are known to coexist, as in our patients, the clinical pictures of the two syndromes overlap to the point that a causal relationship may be suspected (Basser, 1969).

In patients with associated attacks, the two types of event appear at different times, probably because of the different nature of the genetic factors involved. In patients with combined attacks, migraine and epilepsy appeared almost simultaneously before puberty. In these cases, there does not seem to be definite direct interaction between the two types of pathophysiologic mechanisms. However, the chronological sequence in which migraine attacks and epileptic seizures occurred suggests some process of mutual activation.

The patients with intercalated attacks all had classical migraine with visual prodromes and benign occipital lobe seizures that subsided in adulthood.

The location of the scotomata of migraine and the lateralization of hemianopia suggest that the aura always starts in the occipital lobe, where the epileptogenic EEG foci are also localized. Clinically, the seizures begin with a change in the nature of the visual symptoms that characterize the scotomata of migraine and evolve into an elementary visual seizure of occipital origin.

Visual symptoms that are part of the epileptic seizure starting in the occipital lobe are described by the patients themselves as being different from those that are part of the visual prodrome preceding an attack of classical migraine. The visual aura in seizures consists of rotating, colored balls of light in which red predominates, or of unformed contours or images that are not precisely localized in the visual field (Ludwig and Ajmone-Marsan, 1975).

The visual aura of migraine consists of scintillating scotomata that give rise to blind areas that are localized in the visual field. Milner (1958), when commenting on the observation made by Lashley (1941) on his own scotoma of migraine, pointed out that this clinical phenomenon may correspond to the spreading depression reported by Leão (1944). Lashley assumed that an intense wave of excitation travels across the visual cortex at a speed of 3 mm/min; this excitatory process might be followed by total inhibition of cortical activity, which slowly dies away.

The phenomenon of spreading depression, induced experimentally in animals through different types of chemical or mechanical stimuli, consists of a slowly spreading wave that inhibits electrical activity in the brain. This wave is preceded by a phase of intense neuronal excitation accompanied by a massive, outflow of potassium ions. The excitatory wave travels at a speed of 2 to 3 mm/min (Grafstein, 1956). Normal neuronal activity of the cortex is completely restored within 10 to 20 minutes, corresponding to the average duration of the migraine aura. Until recently, the spreading depression reported by Leão had been considered little more than an artificial phenomenon; the analogy to the aura of migraine has been the only attempt to implicate this mechanism in the explanation of a clinical phenomenon. Basser (1969) suggested that vasoconstriction in the posterior cerebral artery is the specific stimulus responsible for the development of spreading depression and the appearance of the migraine aura.

This mechanism has been confirmed in clinical and experimental studies conducted recently on the brains of rats by using estimates of the cerebral blood flow (Olesen et al., 1981, 1982; Lauritzen et al., 1982). The identity of the classical migraine aura with spreading depression is again suggested. The initial phenomena characterizing the migraine aura and spreading depression consist of focal hyperemia that leads to intense neuronal activation; this is soon followed by reduced cerebral blood flow corresponding to the inhibitory phase characterizing both the scotomata of migraine and spreading depression. During the excitatory phase, spreading depression activates and increases the frequency of the discharge recorded intracellularly from experimentally induced epileptic foci. A decrease in the frequency of the discharge until all spikes are suppressed is recorded only during the phase in which neuronal activity is depressed, and lasts a few minutes (Goldensohn, 1975).

Thus, an interaction is possible between the pathophysiologic mechanisms responsible for the migrainous aura and the visual epileptic aura, even though they are quite distinct from a clinical point of view.

The scotoma that precedes the migrainous headache results from slow, "extrasynaptic" cortical mechanisms. By contrast, the visual epileptic aura or the elementary visual seizure originating from an occipital focus is a paroxysmal phenomenon that depends on massive synaptic activation of certain groups of neurons. The epileptic paroxysm may not be confined to the cortex but can spread along the corticofugal pathways to activate other structures in motor centers or the temporal lobe, which in turn lead to more elaborate clinical manifestations of the seizure.

We believe that in intercalated occipital lobe seizures the phase of massive cellular excitation giving rise to the migrainous aura may trigger the epileptic discharge, which then continues autonomously. The visual migraine aura turns into an elementary occipital lobe seizure; this may remain restricted or may lead to paroxysmal activation of other brain structures or secondary generalization.

The seizures are manifested much more rapidly than the classical migraine process, owing to the characteristics of the neuronal mechanisms involved; they may therefore be intercalated between the visual aura of the migraine attack and the headache that follows.

REFERENCES

Ad Hoc Committee on Classification of Headache. JAMA 1962;179:717–8.
Alvarez G. Migraine plus epilepsy. Neurology 1959;9:487–91.
Barolin GS. Migraines and epilepsies. A relationship? Epilepsia 1966;7:53–66.
Basser LS. The relation of migraine and epilepsy. Brain 1969;92:285–300.
Beaumanoir A. Infantile epilepsy with occipital focus and good prognosis. Eur Neurol 1983;22:43–52.
Beaussart M. Benign epilepsy of children with Rolandic (centro-temporal) paroxysmal foci. A clinical entity. Study of 221 cases. Epilepsia 1972;13:795–811.

Camfield P, Metrakos K, Andermann F. Basilar migraine, seizures and severe epileptiform EEG abnormalities. Neurology 1978;28:584–8.

Dalla Bernardina B, Colamaria V, Bondavalli S et al. Epilepsie partielle bénigne de l'enfant à sémiologie affective. In: Angeleri F, Canger R, eds. Progressi in epilettologia. Boll Lega It Epil 1980;29/30:183–8.

De Marco P. Evoked parietal spikes and childhood epilepsy. Arch Neurol 1980;37: 291–2.

Gastaut H. Classification of the epilepsies: proposal for an international classification. Epilepsia 1969;10(Suppl):514–21.

Gastaut H. Individualisation des épilepsies dites "bénignes" ou "fonctionnelles" aux différents âges de la vie. Appréciation des variations correspondantes de la prédisposition épileptique à ces âges. Rev EEG Neurophysiol 1981;11:346–66.

Gastaut H. A new type of epilepsy: benign partial epilepsy of childhood with occipital spike and waves. Clin Electroencephalogr 1982a;13:13–22.

Gastaut H. L'épilepsie bénigne de l'enfant à pointe-ondes occipitales. Rev EEG Neurophysiol 1982b;12:179–201.

Giovanardi-Rossi P, Santucci M, Gobbi G, Sacquegna T. Diagnosi differenziale fra emicrania ed epilessia nell 'età evolutiva. Boll Lega It Epil 1982;37/38:77–81.

Goldensohn ES. Initiation and propagation of epileptogenic foci. In: Penry JF, Daly DD, eds. Complex partial seizures and their treatment. Advances in neurology, Vol 14. New York: Raven Press, 1975:141–62.

Grafstein B. Mechanism of spreading cortical depression. J Neurophysiol 1956;19: 154–71.

Lashley KS. Patterns of cerebral integration indicated by the scotoma of migraine. Arch Neurol Psychiatry 1941;46:331–6.

Lauritzen M, Jørgensen MB, Diemer NH, Gjedde A, Hansen AJ. Persistent oligemia of rat cerebral cortex in the wake of spreading depression. Ann Neurol 1982;12:469–74.

Leão AAP. Spreading depression of activity in cerebral cortex. J Neurophysiol 1944;7:359–90.

Ludwig BJ, Ajmone-Marsan G. Clinical ictal patterns in epileptic patients with occipital electroencephalographic foci. Neurology 1975;25:463–71.

Mancia D, Manzoni GC, Terzano MG, Lechi A. Criteri differenziali tra fenomeni accessuali emicranici ed epilettici. Società Italiana di Neurologia. Atti del VI Corso di Aggiornamento 1982;209–15.

Manzoni GC, Terzano MG, Mancia D. Possible interference between migrainous and epileptic mechanisms in intercalated attacks. Eur Neurol 1979;18:124–8.

Milner PM. Note on a possible correspondence between the scotoma of migraine and spreading depression of Leão. Electroencephalogr Clin Neurophysiol 1958;10:705.

Olesen J, Larsen B, Lauritzen M. Focal hyperemia followed by spreading oligemia and impaired activation of rCBF in classic migraine. Ann Neurol 1981;9:344–52.

Olesen J, Lauritzen M, Tfelt-Hansen P, Henriksen L, Larsen B. Spreading cerebral oligemia in classical and normal cerebral bloodflow in common migraine. Headache 1982;22:242–8.

Panayiotopoulos CP. Basilar migraine, seizures and severe epileptiform EEG abnormalities. Neurology 1980;30:1122–5.

Selby G, Lance JW. Observation of 500 cases of migraine and allied vascular headache. J Neurol Neurosurg Psychiatry 1960;23:23–32.

Slatter KH. Some clinical and EEG findings in patients with migraine. Brain 1968;91:85–98.

Terzano MG, Mancia D, Zacchetti O, Manzoni GC. L'epilessia nella terza età: persistenza delle crisi dopo i 60 anni. Riv Pat Nerv Ment 1980a;101:185–201.

Terzano MG, Manzoni GC, Maione R, Mancia D. Epilessia benigna con parossismi occipitali ed emicrania: problema delle crisi intercalate. Atti del IX Congresso Nazionale della Società Italiana di Neuropsichiatria Infantile, Repubblica di San Marino, 17–19 Ottobre 1980c;827–32.

Terzano MG, Manzoni GC, Maione R, Moretti G, Mancia D. Case study of association patterns between epileptic and migraine attacks: In: Abstract Book, International Congress on Headache 1980, Florence, 1980b:79.

Terzano MG, Manzoni GC, Maione R, Moretti G, Mancia D. Association patterns between epileptic and migraine attacks. Acta Neurol (Napoli) 1981;36:587–98.

5

Occipital Spikes, Migraine, and Epilepsy

Anne Beaumanoir
Eduna Grandjean

The occasional coexistence of basilar migraine and occipital lobe epilepsy has raised the question of a causal relationship. We have studied a group of patients with this combination of disorders in an attempt to identify any correlations that might suggest a common pathologic mechanism. Relationships between epilepsy and migraine were considered, as in most other studies, by examining interictal electroencephalograms (EEG) and clinical aspects of the two syndromes. The present study concentrated on migrainous attacks with visual symptoms and on occipital epilepsies with posterior spike and wave activity.

MATERIALS AND METHODS

We selected 41 patients, 23 males and 18 females, aged 17 to 27 at the time of their last EEG, for the following EEG criteria: (1) the most recent EEG showing no spike discharges and obtained at least 6 years after the first recording; (2) background activity normal for their age; and (3) presence in at least one EEG of a unilateral or bilateral parieto-occipital focus of pseudorhythmic spikes and/or spike and wave complexes. The characteristic paroxysmal discharges were inhibited by visual perception (Figure 5.1). They generally increased during slow-wave sleep and disappeared during rapid-eye movement (REM) sleep. They did not correlate with ocular movements (Beaumanoir et al., 1981).

This EEG pattern is thus identical to the one first identified in 1951 by Levinson et al. in children with strabismus and later by Kellaway et al. (1955) in amblyopic children. This pattern has been extensively studied by Enge et al. (1973), Lairy et al. (1964), Beaumanoir (1983), and Beaumanoir et al. (1981) in epileptic and nonepileptic children with or without amblyopia; by Camfield et al. (1978) in young patients who had epilepsy associated with basilar migraine; by Panayiotopoulos (1981) in his so-called scotosensitive epilepsy which has

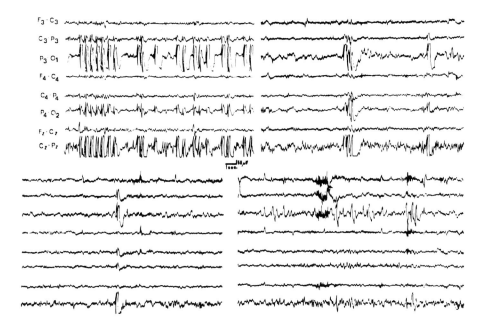

$F_3 \cdot C_3$
$C_3 \, P_3$
$P_3 \, O_1$
$F_4 \cdot C_4$
$C_4 \, P_4$
$P_4 \, O_2$
$F_z \cdot C_z$
$C_z \cdot P_z$

Figure 5.1   Telemetered EEG record of a child with amblyopia. Visual acuity: 1/10 in the left eye, 3.5/10 in the right eye. This child had a normal neurologic and psychological examination. Note characteristic paroxysmal discharges. See text for description.

also been reported on by Herranz-Tanaro et al. (1984) and Lugaresi et al. (1984); and, finally, by Gastaut (1981, 1982) in benign occipital epilepsy of childhood.

RESULTS

Electroencephalographic Data

The interictal EEG necessarily shows a posterior focus of spikes and/or spike and wave complexes.

The mean age at discovery of this pattern is 6½ years, with extremes ranging from 3½ years to 11 years. The age at which this activity first appears cannot be inferred from these data. In most cases it is discovered in the first EEG, recorded at a time when clinical findings already suggest some functional or structural disturbance of the central nervous system.

The mean age at disappearance of this pattern is 12½ years, with extremes ranging from 8 to 19 years. This was determined by follow-up EEGs every 6 to 12 months.

Clinical Data

Distribution of Patients According to Clinical Data

The first EEG was usually performed for one of four indications: (1) behavioral disturbances or learning disability; (2) disturbances of visual function; (3) migraine; or (4) epileptic seizures. In many cases these symptoms were combined, defining 12 different clinical categories correlated with similar occipital foci (Table 5.1). In this study, 26 patients (63.4% of cases) had epilepsy, which was associated in 12 cases with a deficit in visual function, in five with migraine, and in five with a behavioral or learning disorder. In addition, 8 patients (19.5% of cases) had migraine, which was associated in 5 with epilepsy, in 5 with visual function deficit, and in 1 with behavioral problems. Finally, 12 patients (29.3% of cases) were free of both seizures and migraine; 6 of these children had behavioral disturbances, associated in 2 cases with a deficit in visual function, and 6 had disturbances of visual function alone.

Thus, 22 patients (53.6%) had disturbances arising from congenital deficit of visual function and 11 (26.8%) had behavioral or learning problems; 21 (51.2%) had epilepsy but no migraine, and only 5 (12.2%) suffered from both migraine and epilepsy.

Table 5.1 Clinical Characteristics of the Patients

Clinical Categories*	Number of Cases (Total = 41 Cases)	Sex	
		M(23 Cases)	F(18 Cases)
1	4	2	2
2	6	3	3
3	1	0	1
4	9	5	4
1 + 2	2	1	1
1 + 4	3	3	0
1 + 2 + 4	1	0	1
2 + 3	2	1	1
2 + 4	8	5	3
2 + 3 + 4	3	2	1
3 + 4	1	0	1
1 + 3 + 4	1	1	0

*Categories: 1 Behavior disturbance or learning disability
2 Disturbances of visual function
3 Migraine
4 Epileptic seizures

Epilepsy

In the cases studied, 26 patients had seizures. These were of variable frequency but usually occurred rarely. Of those patients over age 15, 10 had not had a seizure since age 13. When the seizures ceased, the EEG abnormalities also disappeared, with one exception. The EEG abnormality was still present after age 13 in only 2 patients.

Seizures were diurnal in 5 patients, diurnal and nocturnal in 14, and exclusively nocturnal in 7. The diurnal attacks always presented sensory and visual symptoms, and oculoclonic twitching was often associated with these attacks. One patient described episodes of left orbital pain either alone or followed by brief palinopsia. Nocturnal seizures were characterized by partial motor seizures involving the eye and face in all but one case. Sometimes the arm was also involved. One patient seemed to have additional alternating hemiconvulsions, and a generalized seizure was noted in another.

Migraine

Migraine occurred in eight patients, five of whom also had epilepsy (Table 5.2); a sixth suffered an episode of febrile convulsions at age 18 months. EEGs showed a rolandic focus in addition to the occipital discharges in two cases. Of these two patients, one had nocturnal seizures typical of benign rolandic epilepsy that were independent of his diurnal visual seizures and migraine (Case 4). The other had typical absences as well as diurnal visual seizures and episodes of basilar migraine (Case 8).

Migrainous attacks were always characteristic of either classical or basilar migraine.

Table 5.2   Clinical Details on Eight Patients with Migraine and Abnormal Occipital EEG Activity

| | | | | | Family History | |
| | | | | Visual | | |
Case	Sex	Epilepsy	Migraine	Disorder	Epilepsy	Migraine
1	F		+		+	+
2	F		+	+		
3	M		+	+		
4	F	+	+	+	+	+
5	M	+	+	+		+
6	M	+	+	+		
7	F	+	+			+
8	M	+	+			+

CASE REPORTS

CASE 1   A female born in 1967 had a family history of one aunt with childhood febrile convulsions, and migraine until her first pregnancy. Her personal history was normal.

Migraine.   The first migrainous episode occurred at age 9. It consisted of a feeling of general discomfort, perspiration, and blurred vision lasting 5 hours. A second attack, 10 months later, started with a right visual field scotoma followed by diffuse headache and marked photophobia, and lasted about 10 hours.

EEG.   An EEG recorded in October 1977 showed bilateral continuous posterior spike and wave activity which was most prominent on the left and ceased with eye opening. A year later, skull films and a computerized tomography (CT) scan were normal and the EEG unchanged. In 1981, an EEG done because of minor head trauma after a fall from a bicycle was again normal.

CASE 2   A female, born in 1967 had a normal family history. She was born 3 weeks prematurely and suffered one benign febrile convulsion.

Migraine.   Her attacks started at age 5, lasting a couple of hours each and consisting of violent posterior headaches associated with abdominal discomfort, vomiting, vertigo, and perhaps also diplopia.

Visual Function.   The child was markedly myopic and attended a special school for amblyopic children.

EEG.   The record showed a bilateral posterior paroxysmal focus. On follow-up in February 1981, migraine attacks still occurred, and the EEG still showed left occipital spikes activated by eye closure that persisted during drowsiness (Figure 5.2).

CASE 3   A male, born in 1966 had an unremarkable family history. His personal history included a 10-day postmature birth, normal psychomotor development, and dyslexia first noted at age 6.

Migraine.   The child recounted that since he was little, bright lights had bothered him and sunlight would provoke violent retro-orbital headache, especially on the right. His mother recalled transient ophthalmoplegia. In 1974 and 1975, he had two migrainous episodes with occipital headaches lasting 7 and 12 hours. These were preceded by brilliant flashes in the entire visual field, followed by blindness and then by retro-orbital pain, both lasting a few minutes.

EEG.   A record in 1973 showed a continuous bilateral posterior paroxysmal focus (Figure 5.3). At a follow-up in 1976 while the child was hospitalized, the record was unchanged. All other examinations were normal.

Visual Function.   An ophthalmologic examination showed a macular deficit of degenerative type with normal visual acuity. The electroretinogram was abnormal, with a decrease of the a-wave on both sides and abnormal response to red, most prominent on the right. Visual evoked potentials were abnormal on both sides.

CASE 4   A female, born in 1965 had a family history of one brother with benign rolandic epilepsy; both her father and another brother had migraine.

Visual Function.   A congenital strabismus was treated surgically at age 5. The patient had significant myopia and wore glasses.

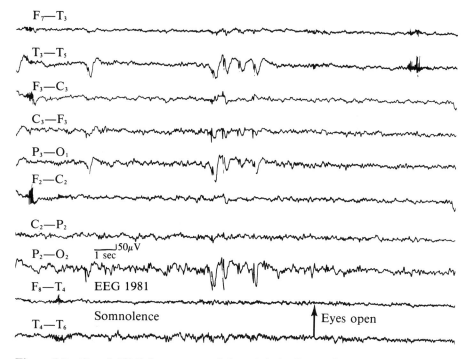

Figure 5.2   Case 2. EEG demonstrates left occipital spikes activated by eye closure that persisted during drowsiness.

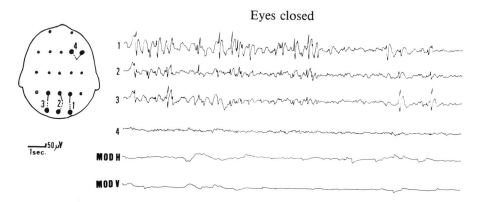

Figure 5.3   Case 3. Polygraphic recording demonstrates a continuous bilateral posterior paroxysmal focus. MOD = ocular movement, right eye; H = horizontal; V = vertical.

Epilepsy.   Her first nocturnal epileptic seizure occurred in January 1973 after a day spent skiing; it consisted of jerking of the left side of the face and hypersalivation. A second attack lasting 1 minute occurred later that night with, in addition to the previous symptoms, spasms of the left arm and tonic deviation of the head to the left. The parents thought the seizures were the same as those of her brother, but they occurred on the opposite side.

EEG.   An EEG tracing in February 1973 (Figure 5.4) showed right parietal spikes and bilateral occipital spikes most prominent on the left. Treatment with phenytoin was then started.

Migraine.   Her first migrainous episode occurred during a hot day in July 1973. It started with dazzling light flashes, followed by blindness lasting about 20 minutes. The child was agitated and anxious, and she vomited. She complained of paresthesiae in both hands, vertigo, nausea, a feeling of coldness, numbness of the back of her head, and diffuse headaches most prominent over posterior head regions.

Her last seizure occurred in 1974. The parietal focus had disappeared by 1979. On follow-up in 1981, migraine attacks were still present but the occipital foci had disappeared.

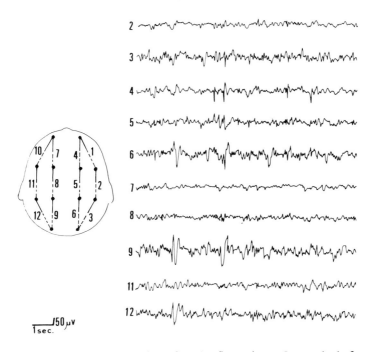

Figure 5.4   Case 4. Initial recording after the first seizure 5 months before the first attack of migraine. Right parietal spikes and bilateral occipital spikes are most prominent on the left.

CASE 5   A male, born in December 1966 had a family history that included his father and one uncle having migraine. The patient was born 1 week premature and was delivered by forceps but without obstetrical trauma.

Visual Function.   The child had marked amblyopia. His psychomotor development was normal despite very low visual acuity. He showed no behavioral problems.

Epilepsy.   Febrile convulsions started at age 3 with a single episode followed 2 months later by a diurnal febrile, probably hemiclonic, seizure. In April 1973, while playing, the child suddenly pointed at a tree and shouted, "I see, I see . . . it's all red!" A seizure occurred a few minutes later with left tonic deviation of the eyes and head, and clonic jerking of the eyes to the left. It lasted about 3 minutes; there was no loss of consciousness. A little later, in the school infirmary, a second seizure occurred. It started with a scream and was generalized. All investigations except the EEG were normal.

EEG.   The EEG tracing showed continuous occipital spike and wave activity reactive to eye opening and most prominent on the left (Figure 5.5).

Migraine.   Migrainous attacks started in October 1974, characterized by occipital headaches and vomiting after a prodromal phase of 15 minutes. Dazzling lights

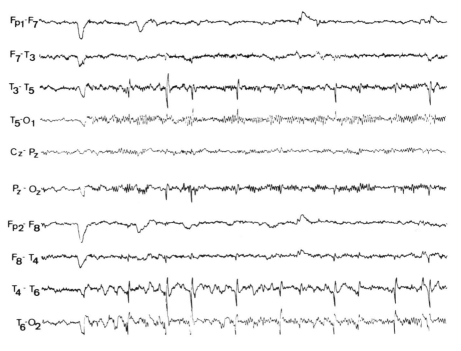

Figure 5.5   Case 5. Recording 2 weeks after the first epileptic seizure. Tracing shows continuous occipital spike and wave activity reactive to eye opening. Abnormal activity is most prominent on the left.

evolved to a red spot in front of both eyes or hemianopia, soon followed by complete blindness and paresthesiae of both arms and the tongue. Awareness was reduced during these attacks and continued to fluctuate for some hours after the headaches stopped.

Migrainous episodes were frequent in 1978 and 1979 and are still present. Seizures have been rare, and the last one occurred in 1982. The EEG focus in the waking state disappeared in 1977, as it also did in the sleeping state in 1981.

CASE 6 A male, born in 1964, had an unremarkable family and personal history.

Visual Function. In 1971 there was an operation for congenital divergent strabismus of the left eye.

Epilepsy. His epileptic seizures started 2 weeks after the surgery for strabismus. The first seizure began with micropsia, followed by blindness lasting less than 1 minute, according to his father. A few hours later, the child refused to go on reading because "pages are dancing and the letters are becoming smaller." In March 1972 his schoolteacher noticed brief episodes of deviation and jerking of the eyes to the left, which occurred in bursts of three to four jerks. The child remained conscious and could describe his eyes "dancing." In January 1973 his father observed that the patient showed the same critical phenomenon during night sleep.

Migraine. Migrainous attacks started around the same time as the epilepsy. An altitudinal hemianopia was followed by diffuse headaches lasting 5 to 24 hours and was associated with marked photophobia, abdominal discomfort, and intermittent vomiting. A marked confusional state with agitation and ataxia twice led to hospitalization. All investigations, including a CT scan, were normal.

EEG. The EEG record showed bilateral posterior spike and wave complexes that were most prominent on the right. Primidone was prescribed. In January 1974, a 24-hour EEG recording still showed the occipital epileptogenic discharges. A seizure starting with oculoclonic jerks followed by tonic spasm of the left arm was recorded. There was suppression of the occipital discharges during the seizure. No postictal abnormalities were seen, and the posterior spike and wave complexes resumed shortly after the ictal discharge was over (Figure 5.6).

Between January 1973 and January 1974, he had at least six diurnal and nocturnal oculoclonic seizures, one visual seizure with micropsia, a short episode of palinopsia, and three migraine attacks each lasting more than 10 hours. On a follow-up examination in January 1982, the patient had been seizure-free for 5 years and had had one migraine attack in 1981. His EEG was normal.

CASE 7 A female, born in 1958, had a family history in which her mother had had ophthalmic migraine from menarche through her second pregnancy.

Migraine. Her first migrainous attack occurred at age 7. She became agitated while showering, complaining of a feeling of heat in the back of her head lasting for 3/4 hour, and then of headache over the calvarium lasting a few more hours. Three hours after onset she lost consciousness while standing. Her face was very pale. There were no abnormal movements. She was hospitalized. Examinations were normal except for the EEG, the result of which is unknown. On the basis of the EEG, phenytoin was prescribed. After November 1964, migrainous episodes recurred every two months, usually starting with a glittering scotoma in the right visual field, sometimes followed by hemianopia or complete blindness. Bilateral occipital headaches, abdominal discomfort, diarrhea, vomiting, and anxious agi-

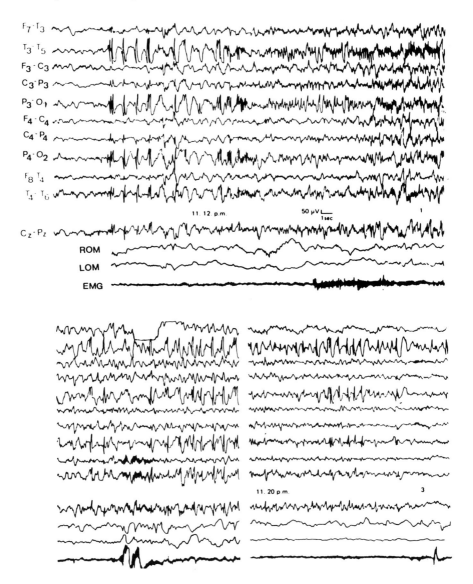

Figure 5.6 Case 6. Seizure recorded during nocturnal sleep, January 1974. Bilateral posterior spike and wave complexes were most prominent on the right. Oculoclonic jerks were followed by tonic spasm of the left arm. Occipital discharges were suppressed during seizure. ROM = Right ocular movement; LOM = Left ocular movement; EMG = Electromyogram.

tation were constant features of her attacks. Anxiety was also thought to be linked to her reading disability.

EEG. In 1966 an EEG showed continuous spike and wave complexes over both parieto-occipital regions (Figure 5.7). Barbiturates were added to the phenytoin without improvement.

Epilepsy. Epilepsy started at age 15 with a nocturnal motor seizure involving the right arm that probably became generalized. Investigations, including carotid and vertebral arteriography, were normal, but the EEG was unchanged.

In February 1977, she had a prolonged migraine attack. The EEG was again unchanged, and antiepileptic treatment was tapered and stopped. In August 1978, a follow-up tracing obtained after the patient had delivered a normal baby showed disappearance of the focus. In 1982, an EEG during a second pregnancy remained normal, although another prolonged migrainous episode with blindness lasting 15 minutes had occurred in 1980.

CASE 8   A male, born in 1965, had a family history that included his father having migraine. At 2 weeks of age the patient was hospitalized for 3 days because of acute dehydration related to gastroenteritis. Febrile convulsions occurred during gastroenteritis when he was 17 months old.

Epilepsy. Epileptic seizures began about age 2 with eyes rolling upward, pallor, and hypotonia lasting 1 minute, followed by jerking of the left side of the mouth. At age 5½, a focal nocturnal seizure occurred with recurrence on awakening a few hours later.

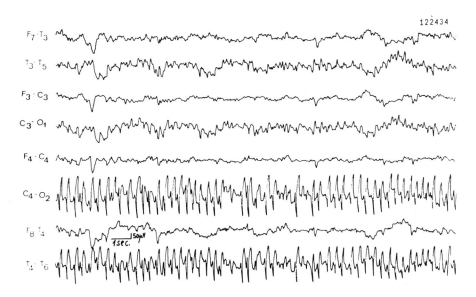

Figure 5.7   Case 6. EEG record at 8 years of age. The patient was receiving phenytoin. Continuous spike and wave complexes are seen over both parieto-occipital regions.

EEG.   The first record at age 2 was normal. After the seizure at age 5½, the EEG showed left midtemporal spikes. A record 4 months later showed, in addition, bilateral posterior spike and wave activity. Treatment with phenytoin was started.

In 1971 psychotherapy was started because of behavioral disturbances. Focal seizures did not recur, but typical absences with generalized 3 Hz spike and wave discharges occurred and were controlled by sodium valproate.

Migraine.   The first migrainous episode occurred in 1972. He suddenly saw the landscape becoming very bright and appearing as though he was looking at it "through a broken mirror." Blindness followed after a few seconds, lasting 15 minutes. The child was ataxic and felt paresthesiae in both hands. He was agitated, and talked continuously, but his father could not understand what he was saying. Occipital headache, lasting several hours, started once vision had returned. Vomiting was present in a few similar episodes.

In 1979 a follow-up EEG was normal. The patient was still taking sodium valproate. He had been seizure-free since 1974. His migraine continued with the last attack occurring in 1982.

DISCUSSION

In this study, the nonspecificity of the clinical findings linked to characteristic epileptogenic EEG abnormalities was confirmed, although the statistics might be slightly biased. Indeed, some categories, such as amblyopia, were over-represented because of our special interest in EEG-neuro-ophthalmologic correlations. Others, such as behavioral or learning disturbances, were underrepresented as compared with other studies (Lairy et al., 1964) because of the makeup of our referral base. However, there would hardly be a bias with regard to the relative frequency of epilepsy and migraine. Most cases were examined at a neuropediatric outpatient facility to which children suffering from epilepsy and migraine had been referred.

Thus, the triad of basilar migraine, epilepsy, and functional occipital epileptogenic discharges is highly unspecific and does not point to a particular pathology. Moreover, most of the authors who have studied basilar migraine, among them Bickerstaff (1961, 1962), do not describe interictal EEG abnormalities. Only Camfield et al. (1978), Panayiotopoulos (1981), Suter et al. (1959), and Manzoni et al. (1979) noted epileptogenic abnormalities (Interestingly, these were always occipital spikes and waves).

CONCLUSIONS

In our small group of five patients who had basilar migraine and epilepsy with interictal EEG occipital epileptogenic abnormalities, migraine always started (except in Case 7) many months or years after the first epileptic attack. On the other hand, in four patients the EEG focus was already present before the first migrainous attack and disappeared before migraine stopped (Table 5.3). These

Table 5.3 Age at Onset and Disappearance of EEG Foci, Epilepsy, and Migraine in Eight Patients with Migraine and Abnormal Occipital EEG Activity

Case Number	EEG Foci		Epilepsy		Migraine	
	First	Last	Onset	End	Onset	End
1	9 yr	14 yr			9 yr	?
2	5 yr	?			5 yr	?
3	7 yr	?			7 yr	?
4	8 yr	15 yr	8 yr	9 yr	8½ yr	?
5	6 yr	11 yr awake, 15 yr asleep	6 yr	?	8 yr	?
6	7 yr	12 yr	7 yr	12 yr	7 yr	?
7	8 yr	19 yr	15 yr	15 yr	7 yr	?
8	6 yr	14 yr	2 yr	9 yr	7 yr	?

facts speak against the hypothesis of Camfield et al. (1978) in which the occipital spike focus would be secondary to transient ischemia accompanying the prodromal phase of migraine.

REFERENCES

Beaumanoir A. Infantile epilepsy with occipital focus and good prognosis. Eur Neurol 1983;22:43–52.

Beaumanoir A, Inderwildi B, Zagury S. Paroxysmes EEG "non épileptiques." Med Hyg 1981;1425:1911–8.

Bickerstaff E. Basilar artery migraine. Lancet 1961;1:15–7.

Bickerstaff E. The basilar artery and migraine-epilepsy syndrome. Proc R Soc Med 1962;55:167–9.

Camfield PR, Metrakos K, Andermann F. Basilar migraine, seizures, and severe epileptiform EEG abnormalities; a relatively benign syndrome in adolescents. Neurology 1978;28:584–8.

Enge S, Kaloud H, Lechner H. EEG investigations in totally and almost blind children. Paediat Paedol 1973;8:175–80.

Gastaut H. Individualisation des épilepsies dites "bénignes" ou "fonctionnelles" aux différents âges de la vie. Rev EEG Neurophysiol 1981;11:346–66.

Gastaut H. L'épilepsie bénigne de l'enfant à pointes-ondes occipitales. Rev EEG Neurophysiol 1982;12:179–201.

Herranz-Tanaro FJ, Lope ES, Sassot SC. La pointe onde occipitale avec et sans epilepsie bénigne chez l'enfant. Rev EEG Neurophysiol 1984;14:1–7.

Kellaway P, Bloxsom A, Mac Gregor M. Occipital spike foci associated with retrolental fibroplasia and other forms of retinal loss in children. Electroencephalogr Clin Neurophysiol 1955;7:469–70.

Lairy GC, Harrison A, Leyer EM. Foyers EEG bioccipitaux asynchrones de pointes chez l'enfant mal voyant et aveugle d'âge scolaire. Rev Neurol 1964;3:351–3.

Lairy GC, Harrison A. Functional aspects of EEG foci in children. In: Kellaway P, Petersen I, eds. Clinical electroencephalography in children. Stockholm: Alm-l'enfant mal voyant et aveugle d'âge scolaire. Rev Neurol 1964;3:351–3.

Levinson JD, Gibbs EL, Stillermann ML, Perlstein MA. Electroencephalogram in eye disorders. Pediatrics 1951;7:422–7.

Lugaresi J, Cirignotta S, Montagna P. Occipital lobe epilepsy with scotosensitive seizures: The role of central vision. Epilepsia 1984;25:115–20.

Manzoni GC, Terzano MG, Mancia D. Possible interference between migrainous and epileptic mechanism in intercalated attacks. Case report. Eur Neurol 1979;18:124–8.

Panayiotopoulos CP. Inhibitory effect of central vision on occipital lobe seizures. Neurology 1981;31:1331–3.

Suter C, Klingman WO, Austin H, Lacy OW. Migraine and seizure states in children. Dis Nerv Syst 1959;20:9–16.

6

Clinical Findings in Children with Occipital Spike Wave Complexes Suppressed by Eye Opening

Jean Aicardi
Richard Newton

Continuous, rhythmic, high-voltage slow-and-sharp-wave activity seen over one or both occipital lobes, completely or significantly suppressed by eye opening and augmented by hyperventilation, is an uncommon electroencephalographic (EEG) abnormality in children (Figures 6.1 and 6.2). This abnormality has been reported in association with two clinical syndromes: (1) that of basilar artery migraine with infrequent generalized or focal seizures heralded by a visual aura (Slatter, 1968; Camfield et al., 1978; Panayiotopoulos, 1980; Andermann, 1983); and (2) that of "benign occipital epilepsy," in which seizures usually begin with visual symptoms that are either isolated or followed by hemisensory, motor, or psychomotor phenomena (Gastaut, 1982a, 1982b).

The four adolescent patients with the syndrome of basilar artery migraine described by Camfield et al. (1978), and the single patient described by Panayiotopoulos (1980), responded well to treatment and presented no behavioral or educational difficulties. The outcome of Slatter's (1968) 8-year-old male patient is not described.

Gastaut's cases included 21 girls and 15 boys whose seizures first appeared between ages 15 months and 11 years. Visual symptoms were said to accompany the seizures in 26 of these. In addition, two had a mild mental handicap and five had behavioral problems. The visual symptoms experienced by both this group and those with basilar artery migraine included transient blindness, complex visual hallucinations, distorted vision, and brightly colored balls or spectra seen on the side contralateral to that of the interictal EEG abnormality.

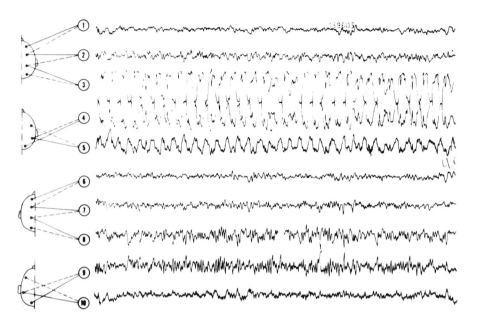

Figure 6.1   Case 12. EEG record with eyes closed. Continuous high-voltage spike wave complexes over the posterior part of the right hemisphere.

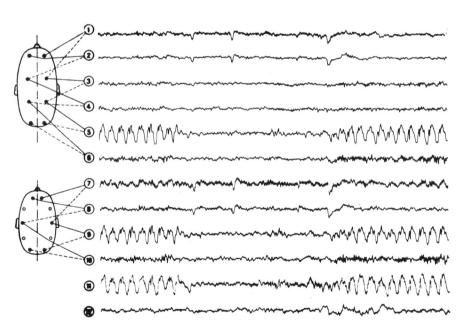

Figure 6.2   Case 12. Interruption of the continuous spike wave activity upon eye opening. The complexes reappear immediately upon eye closure.

Hemiclonic seizures were additionally seen in 16 patients and hemisensory or psychomotor phenomena in 7. Beaumanoir (1983) reported on 10 boys and 8 girls with epileptic seizures and a similar EEG pattern. Her patients had visual phenomena (10) and other seizures including partial complex and motor ones, the latter occurring especially during sleep. Panayiotopoulos (1981) described three such cases with visual seizures. We describe here the wider range of clinical features that was observed in 21 young patients with the same characteristic EEG abnormality.

METHODS AND RESULTS

This characteristic EEG abnormality was present in 21 children who attended two seizure clinics (Hôpital des Enfants Malades, Paris, and Booth Hall Hospital, Manchester) between 1975 and 1980. Of these cases, 16 have been briefly described elsewhere (Newton and Aicardi, 1983). There were 11 girls (52%) and 10 boys (48%).

EEG Abnormality

The background activity was normal in all patients. Sharp waves or spikes of high amplitude usually associated with slow waves occurred over one or both occipital lobes. The appearance varied: in most patients, the abnormal activity was rhythmic, with regular succession of spike wave complexes at 2 to 3 Hz (Figures 6.1 and 6.2). In some, the spikes were less regular (Figure 6.3). The amplitude varied from 75 to 250 μV. The abnormality was bilateral in 12 patients (asymmetrical in 8) but usually asynchronous. It was unilateral in the remaining nine. The paroxysms were augmented by hyperventilation and, in several patients, by drowsiness and the first stage of slow wave sleep. Suppression of the abnormality by eye opening was complete in 11 cases. In the remaining patients, the suppression was striking though not quite complete. Reappearance of the paroxysmal complexes with eye opening was either instantaneous or delayed by 2 to 4 seconds. Ictal records in three patients comprised a rhythmic discharge of spikes at about 10 Hz, starting on the side of the maximal abnormality, spreading to the opposite hemisphere while becoming progressively slower. In a fourth case, very little paroxysmal EEG activity was seen during seizures, although the interictal complexes disappeared several seconds before the onset of the attacks.

Pattern Of the Seizures

Migrainous Features

Transient loss of consciousness was regularly preceded by headache in five patients. In four of these the headache was bilateral, usually frontal, and in the

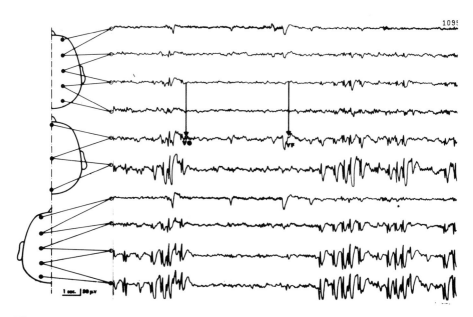

Figure 6.3 Case 5. Continuous spike wave activity arrested on eye opening (first arrow). The complexes reappear 2 seconds after eye closure (second arrow).

fifth it was unilateral, on the same side as the EEG abnormality. The headache was associated with nausea in four patients, and two others experienced nausea and vomiting before a seizure but had no headache.

Visual Phenomena

Of the 21 children 9 experienced visual symptoms at the onset of their seizures. In addition, four patients experienced a transient loss of vision, four saw brightly colored discs in the visual field contralateral to the side of the EEG abnormality, and another described distortion of the visual image.

Nonvisual Phenomena

All but one of the children had transient loss of consciousness with maintenance of posture, often accompanied by fluttering of the eyelids. In three of the children, these bouts were at times prolonged, lasting up to 45 minutes. Two children had only generalized tonic-clonic seizures. One was only 13 months old at presentation: the other had a single seizure at age 9 years 10 months. In two patients, this transient loss of consciousness was not accompanied by other seizure phenomena.

Unilateral tonic-clonic movements, contralateral to the EEG abnormality, sometimes accompanied the transient loss of consciousness in five cases. Of these children, four had transient paresis of the affected limb or face contralateral to the side of the EEG abnormality on at least one occasion. Adversive movement of the head away from the side of the EEG abnormality accompanied the seizures in three patients. Psychomotor phenomena were also seen in five children: two experienced fear during attacks, one in conjunction with auditory hallucinations; one child frequently laughed aloud; and another experienced a feeling of "derealization" prior to attacks. In eight cases, bilateral tonic-clonic movements sometimes accompanied the seizures, and in 1 child the tonic-clonic movements were either unilateral or bilateral.

There were two patients who frequently experienced myoclonic movements of all four limbs shortly after waking each morning; one child developed myoclonic-atonic seizures at age 10, 8 years after the start of the seizure disorder. In five of the children seizures occurred predominantly at night, though in one case this lasted for only a few weeks at the beginning of the seizure disorder.

Other Clinical Data

Age of Onset. The onset of the seizure disorder occurred between the ages of 4 months and 12 years (mean: 6 years 1 month).

Past Medical and Family History. Birth asphyxia was described in one case, severe neonatal respiratory illness in another, and neonatal subarachnoid hemorrhage in a third. Case 5, described in detail later, had "bouts of trembling" at age 2, for which phenobarbitone was subsequently prescribed, prior to a severe encephalopathic illness that appeared 8 months later. One child had had three febrile seizures between ages 18 months and 2½ years; and in seven patients, there was a history of periodic headache and vomiting prior to the onset of the seizure disorder, consistent with a diagnosis of migraine.

In only two cases was there a family history of convulsive disorder and that was in second-degree relatives. Another child had a father with migraine.

Physical Examination. Physical examination did not reveal hard neurologic signs in any of the children, although four of them, on single occasions, had transient postictal paresis of limbs contralateral to the EEG abnormality.

Psychological Assessment. In an effort to explain their learning difficulties, two patients in this series had a psychological assessment. The results of these assessments are summarized in Table 6.1. A brief outline of these patients' histories is given here. Case 18 was a mildly mentally handicapped girl of 11 years whose first seizures began at the age of 4 months. These initial seizures occurred as very brief "absences" associated with bursts of diffuse spike waves up to age 2 and were later replaced by partial complex seizures and occasional tonic-clonic seizures. By age 7 her EEG had changed to match the characteristic abnormality in this study. Her computerized tomography (CT) scan was normal. Case 19 was a boy of 10 years who had a single tonic-clonic seizure at age 9 years, 10 months. His EEG was typical until he was prescribed valproate. Subsequently, he had three complex partial seizures, all of which were heralded by bright colors in the right visual field.

Table 6.1   Summary of Psychological Assessments of Cases 18 and 19

CASE 18: GRIFFITHS MENTAL DEVELOPMENT SCALE

	Quotients (Mental Age in Months)		
Subscales	Aged 59 mo	Aged 62 mo	Aged 77 mo
Locomotor	66 (26)	45 (24)	44 (34)
Personal-social	62 (24)	68 (36)	62 (48)
Hearing-speech	67 (26)	68 (36)	44 (34)
Eye-hand	56 (22)	64 (34)	62 (48)
Performance	44 (17+)	75 (40)	65 (50)
Practical reasoning	—	53 (28)	36 (28)

CASE 18: FROSTIG DEVELOPMENTAL TEST OF VISUAL PERCEPTION AT 77 MONTHS

	Age Equivalent	Scaled Scores
Eye-motor coordination	3 yr 3 mo	5
Figure-ground	3 yr 6 mo	6
Form constancy	2 yr 6 mo	4
Position in space	4 yr 0 mo	6
Spatial relations	4 yr 0 mo	6
Perceptual Quotient — 70		

CASE 19: WISC AT 10 YEARS

	Verbal Tests			Performance Tests	
	Raw Score	Scaled Score		Raw Score	Scaled Score
Information	9	6	Picture completion	9	8
Comprehension	9	7	Block design	18	10
Arithmetic	9	11	Object assembly	12	5
Similarities	9	10	Coding	38	11
Vocabulary	27	8			

	Scaled score	IQ
Verbal scale	42	90
Performance scale	43	90
Full scale		89

CT Scan Appearance.   Scans were performed on nine of the patients, and abnormalities were present in three. There was asymmetric dilatation of the ventricles in 2 patients; in one this was accompanied by some cortical atrophy. In both cases, the side on which the EEG abnormality predominated corresponded to the side of the ventricular dilatation.

Duration of the Seizure Disorder.   In 7 of the 20 patients treated, treatment was stopped after the seizures had abated. In these seven the seizure disorder lasted from 1 month to 11 years (mean: 3½ years). In 3 patients, the response to medication had always been poor before the eventual remission of the seizure disorder. These 3 cases experienced learning difficulties at school that required remedial education.

Despite being medically treated for periods of 6 months to 13 years (mean: 5 years 4 months), the seizure disorder persisted in the other 14 children. Of these, six required remedial education; four others were mildly mentally handicapped.

Details on all 21 patients are summarized in Table 6.2. The following five case histories are illustrative of the wide range of disabilities that accompanied the characteristic EEG abnormality of this study.

CASE REPORTS

CASE 1   At the age of 2 years, 5 months, this boy presented with a poorly defined episode of trembling and was treated with phenobarbitone. He had a respiratory infection in the neonatal period that rendered him oxygen dependent for 4 weeks, and he remained hypotonic for the first 6 months of life. He subsequently showed an expressive language delay in association with a developmental motor dyspraxia and literacy problems for which he received remedial education. At age 7, he had two nocturnal complex partial seizures. Each began with a cry of distress followed by a short period of unconsciousness and tonic-clonic movements of the right side of his body except for the face. A year later the attacks became diurnal and more frequent, each heralded by temporary blindness. A CT scan showed dilatation of the left ventricular system corresponding to the side of the EEG abnormality. When seen, at age 12, his attacks persisted despite treatment with several anticonvulsants. At times he had simple partial motor seizures preceded by transient loss of vision.

CASE 3   At 8 years, this girl presented with bouts of loss of consciousness lasting from a few minutes to 2 hours, the majority being about 30 minutes long. These episodes were heralded by the appearance of red, blue, yellow, and green circles in the left visual field. These were accompanied by an unsteady gait and deviation of the eyes to the left. Her face, initially pale, would become flushed; nausea and vomiting would ensue, but there was no headache. The bouts continued intermittently until she was 13, when she had a left-sided tonic-clonic seizure. The seizure pattern persisted despite medication, and a transient postictal hemiplegia was observed on one occasion. At 14 she was receiving remedial help for her reading difficulty.

Table 6.2   Summary of Cases Showing Characteristic EEG Abnormalities

Case Number	Sex	Age at Onset of Seizures	Type of Seizure	Response to Treatment	Duration of Seizure Disorder
1	M	7 yr 3 mo	CPS Bilateral or right TCS SPS	Poor	4 yr 3 mo+
2	F	6 yr 1 mo	CPS Bilateral TCS Morning myoclonus	Poor	9 yr+
3	F	8 yr 1 mo	CPS (at times prolonged) Left TCS	Initially good, then poor	6 yr+
4	F	12 yr	CPS Morning myoclonus Fear	Poor	6 yr+
5	M	11 yr 3 mo	CPS Fear with auditory hallucinations	Good	6 mo+
6	M	2 yr 6 mo	CPS Monoclonic astatic seizures "Laughter"	Poor	10 yr+
7	F	7 yr	CPS Left TCS	Initially good, then poor	4 yr 6 mo+
8	M	8 yr 3 mo	CPS "Derealization" Head movement Bilateral TCS	Poor	1 yr 6 mo+
9	F	3 yr	CPS (at times prolonged) Bilateral TCS	Poor	13 yr+
10	M	1 yr 1 mo	Bilateral TCS	Poor	3 yr
11	M	5 yr 7 mo	CPS Left TCS	Good	1 mo
12	F	5 yr 3 mo	CPS	Good	3 mo*
13	F	4 yr 10 mo	CPS Left TCS Adversive head movement	Fair	3 yr+
14	F	7 yr	CPS (at times prolonged)	Poor	8 yr
15	F	7 yr 7 mo	CPS	Good	2 mo

CPS: complex partial seizures.
TCS: tonic-clonic seizures.
SPS: simple partial seizures.
+denotes continuation of the seizure disorders.
*Had only two short CPS during this period.

Table 6.2 *(continued)*

Migrainous Phenomena

Headache & Vomiting	Visual Symptoms	Predominance in Sleep	Learning Difficulties	CT Scan Appearance	Medical History
—	Loss of vision	Initially	Yes	Left ventricular dilatation	Neonatal respiratory illness
—	Visual distortion	No	Yes	—	Neonatal subarachnoid hemorrhage
Vomiting	Colored circles	No	Yes	Normal	—
—	Loss of vision	No	Mentally handicapped	Bilateral ventricular dilatation	"Trembling" then encephalopathy
—	—	No	None	—	—
—	—	Yes	Yes	Normal	—
Bilateral headache and vomiting	—	No	Yes		3 febrile convulsions before 30 mo
Headache and vomiting	Vertigo Flashing lights	No	No	Normal	Long history of headache & vomiting
—	—	No	Mentally handicapped	—	—
—	—	No	Yes	Right ventricular dilatation with cortical atrophy	—
Headache and vomiting	Loss of vision	Yes	No	—	—
—	—	No	No	—	—
Headache	—	Yes	No	—	—
Headache and vomiting	Loss of vision	Yes	Yes	—	—
Vomiting	—	No	No	Normal	—

(Continued on pgs 120–121)

Table 6.2   Summary of Cases Showing Characteristic EEG Abnormalities *(continued)*

Case Number	Sex	Age at Onset of Seizures	Type of Seizure	Response to Treatment	Duration of Seizure Disorder
16	M	5 yr 6 mo	CPS Bilateral TCS	Poor	11 yr
17	M	7 yr 3 mo	SPS CPS	Poor	2 yr 8 mo+
18	F	4 mo	"Absence", then CPS and TCS	Poor	10 yr 6 mo+
19	M	9 yr 10 mo	Single TCS	Good	Had one generalized seizure 3 CPS
20	M	4 yr 11 mo	CPS with tonic phase	Good	2 mo
21	F	4 yr 1 mo	Single CPS	No treatment	Had only single seizure

CASE 5   At age 2, this girl presented with bouts of trembling for which phenobarbitone was prescribed. At age 2 years, 10 months, she became ill with an encephalopathic illness of uncertain etiology, and she was unconscious for 48 hours. After this illness she had complex partial seizures that proved to be resistant to medication. At age 18, she had three types of seizure: short-lived lapses of consciousness, lapses of consciousness heralded by a period of temporary blindness, and myoclonic jerks mainly seen soon after waking. After the encephalopathic illness, her CT scan showed moderate ventricular dilatation, and she was mildly mentally handicapped.

CASE 8   Beginning at age 3, this boy had intermittent bouts of headache and vomiting. There was no family history of migraine. At age 8, he had two episodes, 8 days apart, in which a severe frontal headache lasting for ½ an hour was followed by loss of consciousness, staring, clenching of his teeth, and shortly thereafter by vomiting. A year later, after a period of "derealization" lasting for 2 to 3 hours, he went to bed with a frontal headache. He vomited and had an adversive seizure with his head turned to the left. He attempted to speak but his "mouth felt full." Similar seizures continued for the next 11 months, showing no response to valproate, although some improvement was seen with carbamazepine. At age 10 he had his first generalized tonic-clonic seizure. It lasted for 30 minutes and was preceded by a frontal headache and vomiting. He continued to experience many simple and complex partial seizures accompanied by vertigo and brightly flashing lights. The characteristic EEG abnormality persisted in the left posterior head area. He had no problems at school.

Table 6.2 *(continued)*

Migrainous Phenomena

Headache & Vomiting	Visual Symptoms	Predominance in Sleep	Learning Difficulties	CT Scan Appearance	Medical History
—	—	No	Yes	—	Birth asphyxia
—	Bright colors Distortion	No	No	Normal	—
—	—	No	Mild mental handicap	Normal	—
—	Bright colors in right visual field	Single generalized seizure presented in sleep	Visual perceptual problems	—	—
—	—	No	Global developmental delay	—	—
—	—	No	—	—	—

CASE 12   At 5 years, 3 months, this girl had two episodes of loss of consciousness lasting less than 5 minutes with no accompanying abnormal movements. She was treated with phenobarbitone for 5 years, 6 months and had no more seizures. However, the EEG showed the same abnormality until she was 12; thereafter it was normal. Off treatment for 2 years, she remained seizure-free and her development and school performance were normal.

DISCUSSION

This series confirms the association of the interictal EEG pattern of continuous spike-waves over one or both occipital lobes arrested by eye opening, with vertebrobasilar migraine in some patients, and the "benign occipital epilepsy syndrome" in others, as previously reported (Camfield et al., 1978; Panayiotopoulos, 1980, 1981; Gastaut, 1982a, 1982b; Andermann, 1983; Beaumanoir, 1983).

However, visual phenomena that are regarded as the hallmark of "benign occipital epilepsy" were reported by only nine patients. Age or lack of intellectual ability, may have prevented some patients from reporting visual phenomena, but symptoms were specifically excluded in several competent patients.

Other epileptic manifestations were observed in our patients as well as in other studies (Gastaut, 1982a, 1982b; Beaumanoir, 1983). In 13 of our children, epileptic manifestations were not associated with any visual phenomenon. This is similar to the experience of Beaumanoir (1983), who reported that 8 of her 18 patients had only partial complex or partial motor seizures, the latter occurring especially during sleep.

Migrainous symptoms were present in 11 patients, confirming that there is a relationship between posterior spike waves arrested by eye opening and migraine — the migraine-epilepsy syndrome. This relationship is a complex one, since this syndrome may also occur in the absence of EEG abnormality (Andermann, 1983). Migrainous symptoms, however, were absent in 10 of our children.

The benign course emphasized by Gastaut (1982a, 1982b) and Beaumanoir (1983) was by no means always found in our series. Seizures were difficult to control in 14 patients, and 13 had educational problems. A longer follow-up might show that seizures remit in more patients but, as of this writing, this was observed in only 10 and the outlook or prognosis for those patients was certainly not as good as in benign epilepsy of childhood with rolandic spikes (Beaussart and Faou, 1978). The difference in outcome between the present series and those of Gastaut and Beaumanoir may result, in part, from a different selection of patients. The more severe cases were probably overrepresented in our series, which was collected in a referral center dedicated mainly to the care of severe neurologic disorders. Conversely, Beaumanoir's patients were selected *a posteriori* among patients whose epilepsy had remitted, and the original population of patients presenting with similar EEG and clinical data was not described. Our experience indicates that the EEG pattern studied in this chapter does not necessarily indicate a benign prognosis. The history of our Case 12 shows that the EEG abnormality itself cannot be taken as the sole indication to start treatment, nor should it necessarily delay a decision to stop it.

No single etiological factor was evident. The low incidence of a family history of migraine in our patients might well have been spurious, since parents were not specifically questioned about this, and the reliability of such histories in retrospective studies is notoriously limited. The low incidence of a family history of epilepsy is at variance with the experience of Gastaut and that of Beaumanoir, who found such a history in 6 of her 18 patients. This discrepancy is difficult to explain since parents in our study were specifically questioned about a family history of convulsive disorders.

Structural brain damage was present or probable in four patients but, in most, no etiological agent was found. CT scanning showed abnormalities in three of our cases. The CT findings did not alter subsequent management. There was no clear difference in ictal phenomena or EEG signs between patients with or without structural brain damage. Thus, the syndrome studied in this chapter might belong to "lesional" as well as to "nonlesional" epilepsies, and the prognosis might vary accordingly. However, even cases without demonstrable structural abnormality did not necessarily follow a benign course.

Although considerable attention has been given to the association of occipital EEG paroxysms with visual disturbances (Kellaway et al., 1955; Lairy et al., 1964; Lairy and Harrison, 1968), psychological studies of patients with "occipital epilepsy" have not been reported. The psychological testing of Case 18, summarized in Table 6.1, showed that her problems were global, probably representing the underlying etiology of her condition rather than any specific dysfunction related to the EEG abnormality. Testing of Case 19, however, done shortly after he was started on valproate at a time when his EEG had returned to normal, illustrated some residual perceptual difficulties. He scored lowest on the Object Assembly tests, which rely on two-dimensional perception of three-dimensional objects. Other tests of visual perception, such as coding, where one can use verbal reasoning to attack the problem, were completed satisfactorily. Further evidence of problems with visual perception was obtained from his performance on the Bender Motor Gestalt Test. His copying of designs revealed profound problems in orienting the shapes, and his drawing was very primitive. These effects have not been reported with valproate. The observed perceptual difficulties seem to be related to the dysfunction of neurons in visual association pathways rather than to the seizure discharge itself.

The cases described indicate that rhythmic occipital slow-and-sharp-waves suppressed by eye opening are not representative of any clinical entity, but rather of a wide spectrum of symptomatology, neurologic and intellectual deficit, and response to treatment. Perceptual problems that might lead to learning difficulties should be suspected and tested for, even in those children who show good responses to treatment.

Subsequent to the original writing of this chapter, Herranz Tanarro et al. have reported the same EEG pattern in 14 children without clinical epilepsy (Rev EEG Neurophysiol Clin 1984;14:1–7).

REFERENCES

Andermann F. The migraine-epilepsy syndrome. In: Program of the XIVth Epilepsy International Symposium. London, 1982.

Beaumanoir A. Infantile epilepsy with occipital focus and good prognosis. Eur Neurol 1983;22:43–52.

Beaussart M, and Faou R. Evolution of epilepsy with Rolandic paroxysmal foci: a study of 324 cases. Epilepsia 1978;19:337–42.

Camfield PR, Metrakos K, Andermann F. Basilar migraine, seizures and severe epileptiform EEG abnormalities. Neurology 1978;28:584–8.

Gastaut H. Die benigne Epilepsie des Kindesalters mit okzipitalen Spike-wave Komplexen. Z EEG EMG 1982a;13:3–8.

Gastaut H. A new type of epilepsy: benign partial epilepsy of childhood with occipital spike-waves. In: Akimoto H, Kazamatsuri H, Seino M, Ward A, eds. Advances in epileptology: XIIIth Epilepsy International Symposium. New York: Raven Press, 1982b:19–24.

Kellaway P, Bloxsom A, McGregor M. Occipital spike foci associated with retrolental fibroplasia and other forms of retinal sight loss in children. Electroencephalogr Clin Neurophysiol 1955;7:469–70.

Lairy GC, Harrison A, Léger EM. Foyers EEG bi-occipitaux de pointes chez l'enfant mal voyant et aveugle d'âge scolaire. Rev Neurol 1964;3:351–3.

Lairy GC, Harrison A. Functional aspects of EEG foci in children. In: Kellaway P, Petersen, I eds. Clinical electroencephalography in children. Stockholm. Almquist and Wiksell, 1968;179–212.

Newton R, Aicardi J. Clinical findings in children with occipital spike-wave complexes suppressed by eye-opening. Neurology 1983;33:1526–1529.

Panayiotopoulos CP. Basilar migraine(?), seizures and severe epileptic EEG abnormalities. Neurology 1980;30:1122–5.

Panayiotopoulos CP. Basilar migraine(?), seizures and severe epileptic EEG abnormalities. Neurology 1980;30:1122–5.

Slatter KM. Some clinical and EEG findings in patients with migraine. Brain 1968;91:85.

7

Electroclinical Delineation of Occipital Lobe Epilepsy in Childhood

Tomoyuki Terasaki
Yasuko Yamatogi
Shunsuke Ohtahara

Epileptic seizures with focal symptomatology are generally considered to be caused by localized organic brain lesions and to differ from idiopathic epilepsies. Recently, however, a group of benign focal epilepsies based on a genetic predisposition have been identified (Heijbel, 1975). Benign epilepsy of childhood with centrotemporal spike foci (BECCT) (Blom et al., 1972; Heijbel, 1975) is well known, and autosomal dominant inheritance with age-dependent penetrance (Heijbel, 1975) is suspected. Benign occipital foci had been noticed in the 1950s by Gibbs et al. (1954). Gastaut (1982a, 1982b, 1982c) described the electroclinical entity of benign partial epilepsy of childhood with occipital spike waves (BEOSW). This is considered to be a specific form of occipital lobe epilepsy, namely, a partial epilepsy with favorable prognosis and age-dependent manifestation. This type of epilepsy is also frequently accompanied by headache.

To clarify the existence and characteristics of functional occipital foci, 32 cases of occipital lobe epilepsy were studied clinically and electroencephalographically. They were classified into "organic" and "nonorganic" groups. The relationship of the epilepsy to the accompanying headaches was also considered.

SUBJECTS AND METHODS

The subjects consisted of 32 patients, 15 boys and 17 girls, with occipital lobe epilepsy who were seen at the neuropediatric clinic of the Okayama University

125

Hospital during the 16 years from 1967 to 1983. Ages at the initial visit ranged from 10 months to 13 years.

In our study, occipital lobe epilepsy was defined as partial epilepsy with localized epileptic foci in the occipital region and with clinical epileptic seizure phenomena peculiar to the occipital cortex such as visual seizures and oculoclonic seizures.

According to the presence or absence of exogenous causative factors, neurologic and neuro-ophthalmologic abnormalities, low intelligence (IQ less than 85), and computerized tomography (CT) abnormalities, the 32 patients were classified into two groups, i.e., 23 cases without organic brain lesions (Group 1) and 9 cases with findings strongly suggestive of organic brain damage (Group 2). Six cases in Group 2 had more than one acquired etiological factor. None of the patients had visual disturbances.

RESULTS

Age of Onset

The ages of onset of epilepsy and occipital lobe epilepsy were within the first year of life in 3 and 1 cases respectively, from 1 to 3 years in 7 and 1 cases, from 3 to 5 years in 4 and 5 cases, from 5 to 7 years in 3 and 5 cases, from 7 to 9 years in 7 and 9 cases, from 9 to 11 years in 5 and 6 cases, from 11 to 13 years in 3 and 4 cases, and from 13 to 15 years in 0 and 1 case, with a peak age of from 7 to 9 years.

An apparent difference was noted in the age of onset of occipital lobe epilepsy between Groups 1 and 2; Group 1 showed a remarkable age-dependent mode of onset with a peak at 7 to 9 years of age, whereas no age characteristic was observed in Group 2, as shown in Figure 7.1.

As to the sex difference, girls exceeded boys by 1.6 to 1 in Group 1 but boys exceeded girls by 2 to 1 in Group 2.

Presumptive Causes and Neurologic Abnormalities

A family history of convulsive disorders among second-degree relatives was noted in 11 cases (34.4%). The convulsive predisposition was striking in Group 1, i.e., 10 cases (43.5%), but there was only 1 case (11.1%) in Group 2. Predisposition to headache among second-degree relatives was noted in 31.3% of all cases. It was high in Group 1, 39.1%, but only 11.1% in Group 2. All five cases (15.6%) with familial predisposition to both convulsions and headaches were in Group 1.

Exogenous causative factors observed in Group 2 were neonatal asphyxia in two cases, abnormal delivery in four, and acute encephalopathy in one case.

Neurologic abnormalities in Group 2 were: mental defect in four cases; one case each of tetraplegia, hemiplegia, and marked behavioral disorder; and

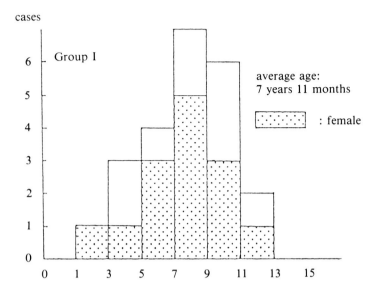

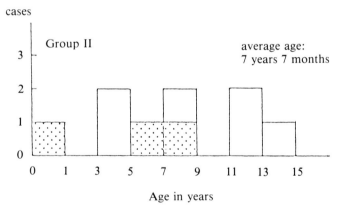

Figure 7.1   Age at onset of occipital lobe epilepsy.

four cases with oculomotor disturbance, including one case of divergent strabismus. CT scans revealed one case with diffuse brain atrophy and another case with moderate unilateral ventricular dilatation.

Clinical Seizure Manifestations

As shown in Table 7.1, which describes ictal manifestations, oculoclonic seizures were observed in 3 cases (9.4%) and visual seizures in 29 cases (90.6%). Visual seizures consisted of blurred vision and/or blindness in 23 cases (71.9%);

Table 7.1   Seizure Symptomatology in Occipital Lobe Epilepsy

Clinical Seizure Patterns	Group 1 (23 Cases)		Group 2 (9 Cases)		Total (32 Cases)	
Visual seizures	21 cases	(91.3%)	8 cases	(88.9%)	29 cases	(90.6%)
Blurred vision, blindness	17	(73.9)	6	(66.7)	23	(71.9)
Phosphenes	8	(34.8)	3	(33.3)	11	(34.4)
Visual hallucinations	5	(21.7)	1	(11.1)	6	(18.8)
Visual illusions	3	(13.0)	2	(22.2)	5	(15.6)
Oculoclonic seizures	2 cases	(9.4%)	1 case	(11.1%)	3 cases	(9.4%)
Seizures evolving to:	11 cases	(47.8%)	6 cases	(66.7%)	17 cases	(53.1%)
Simple partial motor seizures	4	(17.4)			4	(12.5)
Complex partial motor seizures	3	(13.0)	1	(11.1)	4	(12.5)
Complex partial seizures with automatism	1	(4.3)	3	(33.3)	4	(12.5)
Partial seizures evolving to generalized tonic-clonic seizures	3	(13.0)	2	(22.2)	5	(15.6)
Seizures evolving to impairment of consciousness	7/11 cases	(63.6%)	6/6 cases	(100.0%)	13/17 cases	(76.5%)
Autonomic symptoms	18 cases	(78.3%)	6 cases	(66.7%)	24 cases	(75.0%)
Headache	12	(52.2)	4	(44.4)	16	(50.0)
Nausea, vomiting	11	(47.8)	4	(44.4)	15	(46.9)
Vertigo	4	(17.4)	1	(11.1)	5	(15.6)
Preceding seizures	7 cases	(30.4%)	2 cases	(22.2%)	9 cases	(28.1%)
Presence of other types of seizures	3 cases	(13.0%)	6 cases	(66.7%)	9 cases	(28.1%)
Generalized tonic-clonic seizures	2	(8.7)	2	(22.2)	4	(12.5)
Simple partial motor seizures	1	(4.3)			1	(3.1)
Complex partial seizures with automatism			2	(22.2)	2	(6.3)
Tonic seizure, myoclonic absence			2	(22.2)	2	(6.3)

phosphenes described as round, colored, flickering luminous shapes in 11 cases (34.4%); visual hallucinations with images such as human faces, eyes, square patterns, and figures in 6 cases (18.8%); and visual illusions such as distortion of ceilings or floormats in 5 cases (15.6%).

All of the children were able to respond accurately during visual seizures, whereas three patients had impaired consciousness during oculoclonic seizures.

No difference was observed between Groups 1 and 2 in the incidence of visual seizures and oculoclonic attacks, which presumably originate in the occipital cortex.

Visual seizures and oculoclonic attacks were followed by partial seizures with hemifacial involvement and/or hemiconvulsions in eight cases (25.0%), generalized tonic-clonic convulsions in five cases (13.6%), and automatism in four cases (12.5%). It was found that 17 patients (53.1%) went on to another seizure pattern, and this was slightly more frequent in Group 2. Among these patients, alteration of consciousness was recognized in 13 cases (76.5%); complete loss of consciousness was noted in only 5 patients (29.4%) who developed secondarily generalized tonic-clonic convulsions. The seizures evolved predominantly into partial motor seizures in Group 1, whereas complex partial seizures with automatism or generalized tonic-clonic convulsions were frequently observed in Group 2. Thus, alteration of consciousness late in a seizure occurred less frequently (p < 0.02) in Group 1: it was found in 7 of 11 cases (63.6%) and in 6 of 6 cases (100%) in Group 2.

In 24 cases (75.0%) there were autonomic symptoms such as headache, nausea, vomiting, and vertigo during and/or after visual seizures. As many as 16 patients (50.0%) had headaches; these were described mainly as a heavy feeling in 11 cases (68.8%). Pulsatile migraine-like headache was noted in only four cases (25.0%) and occipital pain in only one. In two cases every visual seizure was accompanied by headache. The duration of headache was rather short; it lasted 10 minutes or less in 10 cases (62.5%) and 1 to 2 hours in only 2 cases. Four children (25.0%) fell asleep after every headache. There was no difference in the incidence and features of the headache between Groups 1 and 2.

Occipital lobe epilepsy was preceded by febrile and/or afebrile generalized tonic-clonic convulsions before its onset in nine cases (28.1%), and it was combined with generalized tonic-clonic convulsions and complex partial seizures in nine cases (28.1%). Combination with other types of seizures was significantly more frequent (p < 0.005) in Group 2, which included a patient with the Lennox-Gastaut syndrome.

EEG Findings

Electroencephalographic (EEG) background activity was dysrhythmic in all cases. However, dysrhythmia was slight in 22 (95.7%) of 23 cases in Group 1. On the other hand, moderate or marked dysrhythmia was noted significantly

Table 7.2　Electroencephalographic Features of Occipital Epilepsy

EEG Findings	Group 1 (23 Cases)		Group 2 (9 Cases)		Total (32 Cases)	
Localization of seizure discharges						
Localized occipital focus	**12 cases**	(52.2%)	**1 case**	(11.1%)	**13 cases**	(40.6%)
Occipital focus with generalization	2	(8.7)	2	(22.2)	4	(12.5)
Multiple foci	3	(13.0)	1	(11.1)	4	(12.5)
Occipital and rolandic foci	2	(8.7)			2	(6.3)
Multiple foci with generalization	6	(26.1)	5	(55.6)	11	(34.4)
Occipital and rolandic foci	4	(17.4)	1	(11.1)	5	(15.6)
Effect of activation procedures						
Suppressed by eye opening	**7/7 cases**	(100.0%)	**0/3 cases**	(0%)	**7/10 cases**	(70.0%)
Activated by hyperventilation	9/15	(60.0)	2/7	(28.6)	11/22	(50.0)
Activated by sleep	4/17	(23.5)	5/7	(71.4)	9/24	(37.5)
Suppressed by sleep	6/17	(35.3)	1/7	(14.3)	7/24	(29.2)
Photosensitivity	8/23	(34.8)	2/9	(22.2)	10/32	(31.1)

(p < 0.005) more frequently in Group 2 than in Group 1: four cases (44.4%) versus one case (4.3%), as shown in Table 7.2.

As for epileptic discharges, a single localized occipital spike focus was detected in 13 cases (40.6%); an occipital spike focus with generalization in 4 cases (12.5%); multiple foci, including an occipital focus or foci, in 4 cases (12.5%); and multiple foci with generalization in 11 cases (34.4%). Localized occipital spikes were more frequently (p < 0.02) noted in Group 1 than in Group 2: 12 cases (52.2%) versus 1 case (11.1%). On the other hand, multiple foci, including occipital discharges, with and without generalization, were more frequently observed in Group 2: six cases (66.7%) as compared with nine cases (39.1%) in Group 1. When multiple foci were present, they consisted of rolandic foci in as many as six children of Group 1.

A significant difference between Groups 1 and 2 was noted in the response of occipital discharges to various activation procedures. In Group 1, occipital discharges were suppressed by eye opening in all 7 cases tested and were increased by hyperventilation in as many as 9 (60.0%) of 15 cases examined. Occipital discharges were activated by sleep in only 4 cases (23.5%) but were suppressed in six cases (35.3%). In Group 2, occipital spikes were suppressed by eye opening in none of the three cases and were activated by hyperventilation in two cases (28.6%); they were easily induced by sleep. Photosensitivity was noted in 31.3% of the cases without significant difference between Groups 1 and 2.

Ictal EEGs recorded in five cases showed repetitive occipital spikes or bursts of fast activity from occipital regions, occasionally with gradual generalization followed by irregular spike wave discharges. One patient who had a visual seizure during photic stimulation showed a diffuse spike wave burst with occipital predominance.

Prognosis

For more than 2 years, 21 patients were followed. Prognosis was favorable in Group 1, in which 10 cases (71.4%) were seizure-free for over two years and no case was uncontrolled. On the other hand, patients in Group 2 showed a poor prognosis: only one case (14.3%) was seizure-free for over two years and four cases (57.1%) showed no change or only a slight decrease in seizure frequency (Table 7.3). All four cases that were free of epileptic discharge for over 1 year were in Group 1.

DISCUSSION

Occipital epileptic foci have been studied since the 1950s. Gibbs et al. (1954) considered occipital spike foci to be the most common focal discharges in children around 4 years of age; after this age, the discharges either disappeared or "moved forward" to temporal, diencephalic, or hypothalamic regions. Kel-

Table 7.3 Prognosis of Occipital Lobe Epilepsy

Prognosis	Group 1 (14 Cases)	Group 2 (7 Cases)	Total (21 Cases)
Free of seizures*	10 cases (71.4%)	1 case (14.3%)	11 cases (52.4%)
Medication effective†	4 cases (28.6)	2 cases (28.6)	6 cases (28.6)
Medication poorly effective or ineffective‡		4 cases (57.1)	4 cases (19.0)

*Seizure-free for over 2 years.
†Seizures decreased to less than 1/4 of the frequency at the initial visit.
‡Seizures still occur more frequently than 1/4 of the frequency at the initial visit.

laway et al. (1955) and Smith and Kellaway (1963) noted the relationship between occipital foci and congenital blindness. More recently, Gastaut (1982a, 1982b, 1982c) proposed the reclassification of benign functional epilepsies under broad concepts according to genetic predisposition and age factors. He designated a group of cases who presumably had functional occipital foci with genetic predisposition and with visual seizures as benign partial epilepsy of childhood with occipital spike waves (BEOSW).

As many as 90.6% of our cases had visual seizures; these consisted of loss of vision in 71.9%, elementary visual hallucinations in 34.4%, psychic visual hallucinations in 18.8%, and visual illusions in 15.6%. Oculoclonic seizures, which were observed in only 9.4% of our cases, seem to occur only rarely. The main ictal symptoms in five cases with occipital lobe epilepsy reported by Huott et al. (1974) were blindness, phosphenes, and visual hallucinations, but oculoclonic seizures were experienced in one case. Among 36 cases reported by Gastaut (1982a, 1982c), blindness was noted in 65%, phosphenes in 58%, figurative visual psychic hallucinations in 23%, and visual illusions in 12%— almost the same frequency of incidence as in our series but no case with oculoclonic seizures was mentioned. The similarity in incidence of various visual symptoms among our Groups 1 and 2 and the BEOSW of Gastaut (1982a, 1982c) indicated no difference in the ictal symptoms peculiar to the occipital lobes due to either "functional" or "organic" epileptic foci.

Seizure discharges from occipital foci were considered to propagate preferentially to suprasylvian or infrasylvian structures (amygdala and hippocampus) and also to subcortical systems (Collins and Caston, 1979). According to Bancaud (1969) and Takeda et al. (1969, 1970), seizure discharges originating below the calcarine fissure are likely to transmit to temporal areas and those from supracalcarine regions to parietal areas. Of our cases who initially had occipital seizures, 53.1% showed evidence of spread to other areas. Evolution to partial motor seizures (25.0%), generalized tonic-clonic seizures (15.6%), and complex partial seizures with automatisms (12.5%), indicated that seizure discharges from occipital foci propagate easily to other brain regions. Gastaut (1982a, 1982c) observed secondary spread of seizures in as many as 71% of his cases, namely, hemiclonic seizures in 44%, psychomotor seizures in 19%, and generalized tonic-clonic seizures in 8%. The level of consciousness during the secondary spread of seizures may also indicate the mode of propagation for the seizure discharges. In Group 1, compared with Group 2, secondary spread led more frequently to partial motor seizures and less frequently to complex partial seizures with automatisms and alteration of consciousness, suggesting that in these patients, propagation of occipital spike discharges to the limbic system may be limited. In 72% of Gastaut's series (1982a, 1982c), consciousness was preserved more frequently during seizures in which visual symptoms were succeeded by hemiclonic attacks without loss of consciousness compared to those seizures that evolved into complex partial seizures, as in our series.

As many as 75% of our cases had accompanying autonomic symptoms such as headache, nausea, vomiting, and vertigo during and/or after visual seizures. Headaches were noted in 50%. These autonomic symptoms were frequently noted in Group 1. Autonomic symptoms were observed in 3 (60%) of 5 cases by Huott et al. (1974); headache was seen in 36% and vomiting and/or vertigo in 14% of 36 cases by Gastaut (1982a, 1982c); these autonomic symptoms seem to accompany preferentially occipital lobe epilepsy.

Basilar artery migraine with visual symptoms (Bickerstaff, 1961) must be differentiated from this type of epilepsy. As a rule, basilar artery migraine is not accompanied by convulsions or epileptic EEG abnormalities except when epilepsy or epileptic foci occur as the sequelae of ischemia during migrainous attacks (Parain and Samson-Dollfus, 1984). Cases reported as basilar artery migraine by Slatter (1968), Camfield et al. (1978), Swanson and Vick (1978), and Panayiotopoulos (1980) very likely have occipital lobe epilepsy with migrainous headache for the following reasons: occurrence of visual symptoms followed by headache and hemifacial, lateralized, or generalized convulsions with onset from 4 to 11 years of age; frequent epileptic discharges from occipital areas; and favorable prognosis with good response to anticonvulsants. The headaches observed in our cases were different from migraine, especially basilar artery migraine, because of their characteristics: the headaches were rarely pulsatile and considered primarily of a heavy feeling (68.8%); localization was mainly diffuse and rarely localized to the occipital region; duration was generally short; and they were rarely followed by sleep. They were also different from the long-lasting headache observed in Gastaut's series (1982a, 1982c). However, as Gastaut (1982a) indicated, dysfunction of the subcortical autonomic nervous system may be caused by occipital epileptic discharges (Collins and Caston, 1979); also, these patients may have a genetic predisposition to headaches.

Regarding the etiology, Huott et al. (1974) stressed the importance of acute or subacute brain damage from their experience with patients who had onset of seizures shortly after toxemia or an encephalitic-like state. However, Gastaut (1982a, 1982c) stressed genetic or functional factors because a predisposition to epilepsy was noted in 17 (47.2%) of his 36 cases. Our Group 1 had a significantly higher incidence of predisposition to convulsions, namely 10 (43.5%) of 23 cases, compared with an overall figure of 20.5% in childhood epilepsy (Ohtahara et al., 1981). Genetic predisposition is likely to be one of the major contributing factors to the epilepsy in Group 1. A remarkable difference was noted between Groups 1 and 2 in the mode of onset of occipital lobe epilepsy. The age-dependent mode of onset with a peak at 7 to 9 years of age and a predominance in girls in Group 1 was the same as in Gastaut's series (1982a, 1982c) but differed from the cases with occipital spikes reported by Gibbs et al. (1954) and by Smith and Kellaway (1963).

As to EEG findings, patients with BEOSW described by Gastaut (1982a, 1982c) and benign epilepsy with occipital foci of Beaumanoir (1983) showed normal background activity. Our patients in Group 1 also showed only slight dysrhythmia, suggesting the functional nature of these foci.

Epileptic discharges showed a different response to various activation procedures in Groups 1 and 2. In Group 1, seizure discharges were suppressed by eye opening and activated by eye closure, increased by hyperventilation and suppressed by sleep. These responses to eye opening, eye closure, and sleep were the same as in the BEOSW of Gastaut (1982a, 1982b, 1982c) but different from those in the occipital seizures of Beaumanoir (1983), which were activated by slow-wave sleep like BECTS (Blom et al., 1972). Accordingly, Group 1 is probably a specific group among patients with occipital foci. In Group 1, activation of occipital spikes by hyperventilation and suppression by eye opening are characteristics that they share with those affected by subcortical discharges.

There was a significant difference in the prognosis for Groups 1 and 2: Group 1 had a very good prognosis. These findings suggest that our Group 1, apparently different from Group 2, represents benign occipital lobe epilepsy with functional foci closely related to subcortical dysfunction, genetic predisposition, and age.

SUMMARY

A detailed electroclinical study of 32 children with occipital lobe epilepsy was carried out. Ictal symptoms were specific to the occipital cortex, consisting of visual seizures and oculoclonic seizures. The cases were divided into two groups: 23 cases in a "nonorganic" group (1) and 9 cases in an "organic" group (2), according to presumed etiologies, as well as neurologic and neuroradiologic findings.

1. Group 1 showed a remarkably age-dependent mode of onset, with a peak at 7 to 9 years of age, and there was a predominance in girls.
2. A predisposition to convulsions and headaches was noted in 34.4% and 31.5% of the total and in as many as 43.5% and 39.1%, respectively, of Group 1.
3. Visual seizures such as blindness, blurred vision, phosphenes, visual illusions, and hallucinations were noted in 29 cases (90.6%) and oculoclonic seizures in 3 cases (9.4%). Occipital lobe seizure manifestations led to hemiconvulsions, partial motor seizures, or complex partial seizures with automatisms in 17 cases (53.1%) and autonomic symptoms such as headache were present in 24 cases (75.0%).

   There was no difference in the seizure manifestations peculiar to the occipital lobe in the two groups, but simple partial seizures without alteration of consciousness were significantly more common in Group 1 than in Group 2.
4. Headaches followed in 16 cases (50.0%); these were described as a heavy feeling in 11 cases (68.8%) and as a pulsatile migraine-like headache in 4 cases (25.0%).

5. Other types of seizures were significantly more common in Group 2.
6. Dysrhythmic EEG background activity was more marked in Group 2 than in Group 1. Occipital spike foci in Group 2 were often associated with other spike foci and with secondary generalization, whereas those in Group 1 were easily suppressed by eye opening and sleep.
7. The prognosis for Group 1 was better than that for Group 2.
8. This study suggests the existence of functional or benign occipital epilepsy occurring predominantly in children without "organic" brain lesions.

REFERENCES

Bancaud J. Les crises épileptiques d'origine occipitale: étude stéréo-électroencéphalographique. Rev Oto Neuro Ophtalmol 1969;41:299–311.

Beaumanoir A. Infantile epilepsy with occipital focus and good prognosis. Eur Neurol 1983;22:43–52.

Bickerstaff ER. Basilar artery migraine. Lancet 1961;1:15–7.

Blom S, Heijbel J, Bergtors PG. Benign epilepsy of children with centro-temporal EEG foci: prevalence and follow-up study of 40 patients. Epilepsia 1972;13:609–19.

Camfield PR, Metrakos K, Andermann F. Basilar migraine, seizures and severe epileptiform EEG abnormalities. Neurology 1978;28:584–8.

Collins RC, Caston TV. Functional anatomy of occipital lobe seizures: an experimental study in rats. Neurology 1979;29:705–16.

Gastaut H. Die benigne epilepsie des kindesalters mit okzipitalen spike wave-komplexen. Z EEG EMG 1982a;13:3–8.

Gastaut H. "Benign" or "functional" (versus "organic") epilepsies in different stages of life: an analysis of the corresponding age-related variations in the predisposition to epilepsy, In Broughton RJ, ed. Henri Gastaut and the Marseille school's contribution to the neurosciences. Electroencephalogr Clin Neurophysiol Suppl. No. 35. Amsterdam: Elsevier, 1982b:17–44.

Gastaut H. A new type of epilepsy: benign partial epilepsy of childhood with occipital spike-waves. Clin Electroencephalogr 1982c;13:13–22.

Gibbs EL, Gillen HW, Gibbs FA. Disappearance and migration of epileptic foci in childhood. Am J Dis Child 1954;88:596–603.

Heijbel J. Benign epilepsy of childhood with centrotemporal EEG foci: a genetic study. Epilepsia 1975;16:285–93.

Huott AD, Madison DS, Niedermeyer E. Occipital lobe epilepsy: a clinical and electroencephalographic study. Eur Neurol 1974;11:325–39.

Kellaway P, Bloxsom A, MacGregor M. Occipital foci associated with retrolental fibroplasia and other forms of retinal loss in children. Electroencephalogr Clin Neurophysiol 1955;7:469–70.

Ohtahara S, Ishida S, Oka et al. Epilepsy and febrile convulsions in Okayama Prefecture: a neuroepidemiologic study. In: Fukuyama Y et al., eds. Child Neurology, Proceedings of the IYDP Commemorative International Symposium on Developmental Disabilities. Amsterdam: Excerpta Medica, 1981:376–82.

Panayiotopoulos CP. Basilar migraine? Seizures and severe epileptic EEG abnormalities. Neurology 1980;30:1122–5.

Parain D, Samson-Dollfus D. Electroencephalograms in basilar artery migraine. Electroencephalogr Clin Neurophysiol, 1984;53:392-9.

Slatter KH. Some clinical and EEG findings in patients with migraine. Brain 1968;91:85–98.

Smith MB, Kellaway P. The natural history and correlates of occipital foci in children. In: Kellaway P, Petersén I, eds. Neurological and electroencephalographic correlative studies in infancy. New York: Grune & Stratton, 1963:230–49.

Swanson JW, Vick NA. Basilar artery migraine: 12 patients, with an attack recorded electroencephalographically. Neurology 1978;28:782–6.

Takeda A, Bancaud J, Talairach J, Bonis A, Bordas-Ferrer M. A propos des accès épileptiques d'origine occipitale. Rev Neurol 1969;121:306–15.

Takeda A, Bancaud J, Talairach J, Bonis A, Bordas-Ferrer M. Concerning epileptic attacks of occipital origin. Electroencephalogr Clin Neurophysiol 1970;28: 647–8.

8

Occipital EEG Activity Induced by Darkness: The Critical Role of Central Vision

Fabio Cirignotta
Elio Lugaresi
Pasquale Montagna

Calling it "benign partial epilepsy of childhood with occipital spike-wave," Gastaut, in 1982, described a syndrome that is electroencephalographically characterized by interictal occipital and posterior temporal spikes and spike and wave activity, occurring only when eyes are closed or in darkness, and by ictal discharges over an occipital lobe. Similar cases had previously been reported by Pazzaglia et al. (1970) as scotosensitive epilepsy, by Camfield et al. (1978), and by Panayiotopoulos (1980). Panayiotopoulos (1981) demonstrated that retention of central vision in darkness, by fixation on a small spot of light, inhibited the occipital spike and wave discharges.

We have confirmed that central vision represents the critical factor in the activation and inhibition of the occipital discharges (Lugaresi et al., 1984). However, central vision could also represent the critical stimulus for all synchronizing mechanisms of occipital EEG activities induced by eye closure and darkness. As a result, we have now investigated the effects of central vision on physiological occipital EEG rhythms such as the alpha rhythm and the slow alpha variant rhythm.

PATIENTS AND METHODS

Our investigations were performed on nine patients with benign occipital lobe epilepsy and typical posterior EEG discharges provoked by darkness and by eye closure. Three normal subjects were investigated for the alpha rhythm and one subject for the slow alpha variant rhythm. None of the subjects was photosensitive. EEGs were recorded both in normal lighting conditions (daytime in the EEG laboratory) and in total darkness.

In normal lighting conditions, recordings were made with eyes open and with eyes kept open behind a translucent tape and/or Frenzel glasses, in order to block fixation without changing environmental lighting conditions. The recordings were then continued in total darkness, with eyes kept open for about 10 minutes. Afterwards the patient was asked to fix on an imaginary point about one meter away; the recordings were run for another 10 minutes with eyes closed, and at the end of this period the patient was asked to fix on a small light-emitting diode (LED), 2 mcd in intensity, at a distance of about 3 meters. After this was completed, the subject was asked to avert his gaze so that light from the small LED would fall at the periphery of the visual field. Completing our investigations, the effects of intense bright stimuli were studied in one patient who was asked to close his eyes after being dazzled by a photographic flash unit.

RESULTS

In a lit environment, both eye closure and gazing through a translucent tape and/or Frenzel glasses induced the appearance of the alpha rhythm, the slow alpha variant, and the occipital spikes. The slow alpha variant and the spike and wave discharges had a latency of 2 to 6 seconds.

The alpha rhythm, the slow alpha variant, and the occipital spikes also appeared whenever the subjects held their eyes open in total darkness. The slow alpha variant and the spike and wave discharges started after 2 to 18 seconds. Each of these occipital activities was always blocked, without delay, whenever the subject looked at the LED (Figures 8.1 and 8.2). Fixing the patients' eyes on an imaginary point in total darkness did not block the alpha rhythm, the slow alpha variant, or the occipital spikes.

Eye closure, darkening of the room, and application of a semitransparent tape over the open eyes induced spike discharges in the right parieto-occipital region in one of the nine patients with benign occipital lobe epilepsy. Such discharges appeared with a 20-second to 4-minute delay and lasted between 7 and 120 seconds. Only some of these discharges were perceived by the patient as "confusion"; they were immediately blocked by opening the eyes or by fixation on the small LED in total darkness (Figure 8.3).

Finally, in one patient, the occipital discharges were delayed for a few minutes after he was dazzled by a flash (Figure 8.4).

CONCLUSION

We have shown that central vision represents the critical factor, not only in the appearance of the spike and wave discharges of benign occipital epilepsy, as

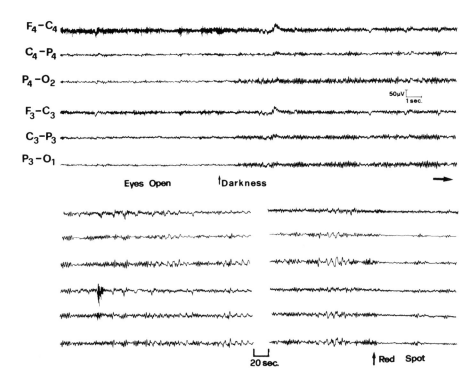

Figure 8.1 Appearance of the occipital alpha rhythm and of the slow alpha variant after total darkening of the environment in a subject with eyes kept open. Looking at a small red spot (light emitting diode, 2 mcd) in total darkness promptly blocks the occipital rhythms.

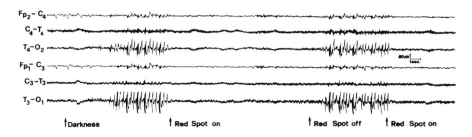

Figure 8.2 Occipital spike and wave discharges induced, after a 4-second delay, by darkness in a patient with benign occipital lobe epilepsy. Looking at a small red spot (light emitting diode, 2 mcd) in total darkness promptly blocks the discharges.

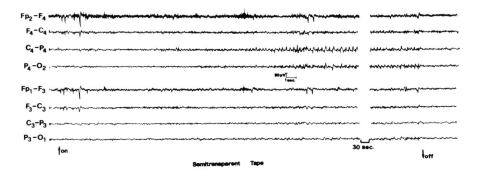

Figure 8.3   Patient with benign occipital lobe epilepsy. A semilucent tape applied over the open eyes in a lighted room induces right parieto-occipital spikes after a delay of about 20 seconds.

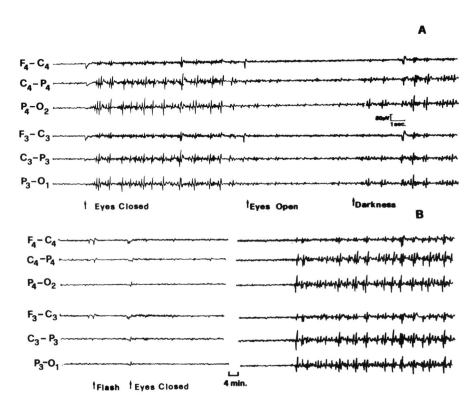

Figure 8.4   Eye closure and darkness with eyes open induce, after 1 second, spikes in a patient with scotosensitive epilepsy. After a dazzling flash, eye closure induces similar spike discharges after a much longer interval (4 minutes 12 seconds).

previously demonstrated by Panayiotopoulos (1981) and later confirmed by us (Lugaresi et al., 1984), but also in the triggering of the alpha and slow alpha variant rhythms and of the ictal occipital discharges provoked by darkness.

The greater influence upon cortical excitability of impulses originating from the macular receptors can be easily understood in the light of some physiological data: macular receptors (cones) have a 1:1 relationship with ganglionic cells, whereas extramacular receptors, mainly rods, converge in a ratio of up to 250:1 upon a single ganglionic cell. Furthermore, the area of the occipital lobe subserving central vision is much larger than the area receiving only peripheral retinal projections (Lugaresi et al., 1984).

The 2- to 4-second delay shown by the interictal occipital spike and wave discharges, and the still longer latency of the ictal scotosensitive discharges, cannot be accounted for, in our opinion, by simple reverberating electric loops, as proposed by Gastaut (1982). It is likely that suppression of central vision exerts longer-lasting metabolic effects upon the occipital cortex, probably mediated by neurotransmitters. Retinal visual mechanisms show lasting adaptation, on the order of minutes; they could conceivably play a role in the long onset delays after dazzling stimuli (Mountcastle, 1980). In conclusion, similar reactivity to eye closure and darkness is displayed by both normal and pathologic occipital lobe EEG activities and is not, as such, a phenomenon restricted to cases of scotosensitive epilepsy. Indeed it represents a basic feature of the visual system.

REFERENCES

Camfield PR, Metrakos K, Andermann F. Basilar migraine, seizures and severe epileptiform EEG abnormalities. Neurology 1978;28:584–8.

Gastaut H. A new type of epilepsy: benign partial epilepsy of childhood with occipital spike-wave. Clin Electroencephalogr 1982;13:13–22.

Lugaresi E, Cirignotta F, Montagna P. Occipital lobe epilepsy with scotosensitive seizures: the role of central vision. Epilepsia 1984;25:115–20.

Mountcastle VB. Medical Physiology. 14th ed., vol. 1. St. Louis: CV Mosby, 1980: 504–43.

Panayiotopoulos CP. Basilar migraine? Seizures and severe epileptic EEG abnormalities. Neurology 1980;30:1122–5.

Panayiotopoulos CP. Inhibitory effect of central vision on occipital lobe seizures. Neurology 1981;31:1330–3.

Pazzaglia P, Sabattini L, Lugaresi E. Crisi occipitali precipitate dal buio. Riv Neurol 1970;40:184–92.

9

The Association of Benign Rolandic Epilepsy with Migraine

Peter F. Bladin

Of all the pediatric entities contained in that group of disorders labeled "the epilepsies," the entity of benign rolandic epilepsy has assumed outstanding diagnostic importance in recent years. Not only has its unsuspected frequency in the juvenile population created great interest, but as has become obvious, it has an almost uniformly good outlook (Blom and Heijbel, 1982). In addition, its prompt response to anticonvulsant therapy and its natural history of regression over the years give great comfort to the clinician and parent alike. In fact, it is one of the few entities in that group of disorders of which the clinician can say with some confidence that the patient will eventually "grow out of it."

Some years ago, in an earlier communication on the subject, I noted that in a small series of children with benign rolandic epilepsy (sylvian spike epilepsy) there seemed to be an unusually high incidence of migraine in both the patient's personal and family histories. During the intervening years, my continued follow-up of these patients has shown that the prognosis for the epileptic seizures was indeed benign, but that they continued to suffer from migraine. In some of these patients, I have even seen the emergence of migraine after the cessation of their seizures.

This study deals with a series of patients, the majority of whom I have personally managed since their first presentation and all of whom I have personally reviewed. The aim of this study was to assess the outcome of seizure tendency and migrainous symptoms.

SELECTION AND REVIEW DATA

This series consisted of 30 patients who were reviewed 5 to 8 years after their first presentation and diagnosis. The appearance of a typical sylvian spike (Lombroso, 1967) was the prime prerequisite for inclusion. As pointed out previously, all patients tended to present a typical clinical profile (Bladin and Papworth, 1974), but it should be noted that almost twice as many clinically suitable patients were excluded from this series as were included because of the lack of evidence of a sylvian spike on their first or subsequent electroencephalographic (EEG) record—a matter to be discussed later.

In light of earlier observations, the historical data obtained for almost all of these patients included thorough documentation of the nature, occurrence, and frequency of seizures and also specific details regarding the presence or absence of possible migrainous symptoms. In particular, information was sought regarding recurrent headache with possible lateralization, "classical" migraine with teichopsia, and migraine equivalents of childhood: recurrent abdominal ache, vomiting, and pallor. All patients were followed-up with regard to their response to anticonvulsant therapy; further EEGs were performed to document continuation or disappearance of the EEG spikes; and all patients were periodically clinically reviewed for 5 to 8 years. This period was regarded as long enough to document with certainty the disappearance of seizures and yet short enough to assure reasonable accuracy in the historical data obtained pertaining to their juvenile years—clinical experience has shown that at later follow-up this data is often forgotten or inaccurate.

Four patients had been followed up over the years, primarily in a hospital pediatric outpatient clinic, but detailed clinical records were available for study, and all review assessments included an interview with at least one parent as well as the patient.

All patients had been followed up at regular intervals with repeated clinical assessments and EEGs. The review assessment was undertaken with the main aim of confirming previously noted epileptic and headache symptomatology and if necessary, questioning the patient and parent regarding the possibility of the presence of headache symptoms at the time of first presentation, if this was not already noted in the clinical history. In addition, a complete and detailed assessment of the present seizure and headache status of the patient was undertaken in the review examination.

RESULTS

Rolandic Seizures (Table 9.1)

The seizures of this group of patients followed the pattern described in the literature. All patients were in the juvenile or prepubertal age group; seizures in each patient were nocturnal or occurred when drowsing, and, except in one instance, presentation resulted from the occurrence of a major tonic-clonic seizure. However, focal seizures were observed in 18 of 30 patients, and in one case a perceptive mother observed a focal seizure and sought medical aid before a generalized seizure occurred.

Table 9.1 Benign Rolandic Epilepsy—Seizures. A Summary of 30 Cases Including 19 Males and 11 Females Between Ages Six and Ten.

Presentation	
Seizure pattern	
Major tonic-clonic seizures	12
Partial and tonic-clonic seizures	17
Partial only (presentation)	1
Drowsing and sleeping seizures only	30
Clinical findings normal	30
Investigations	
EEG: Sylvian spike	30
Left-sided spike	14
Right-sided spike	16
Course	
Duration of seizure tendency	2–3 years
Response to anticonvulsant therapy	100% success

In no instance was gross clinical neurologic deficit detected on clinical examination, and in no patient was organic focal neuropathology discovered as a basis for the seizures. In every case the effect of anticonvulsant medication was to halt the seizures immediately. Most patients had been withdrawn from drugs when examined at follow-up; in one or two patients the family physician had maintained medication for too long, and as a result of our inquiry during this study the patients were weaned from all such medication. This series of patients resembled all other such series reported in the literature (Beaussart and Faou, 1978; Blom et al., 1972; Beaumanoir et al., 1974; Lerman and Kivity, 1975).

EEG Findings

The typical EEG features of this condition have been well described by Lombroso (1967), with the characteristic sylvian spikes best seen in the centrotemporal region but sometimes in the midtemporal region. The spike was always much better seen over one or the other cerebral hemisphere. Change in spike dominance has been reported in the literature, although in this series this was not observed.

    Bilaterally synchronous delta and theta waves mixed with spike activity were often seen on the record while the patients were drowsing. On no occasion was an actual seizure captured on EEG.

    In all cases, early disappearance of the EEG spike was noted shortly after medication was started. In fact, it is suspected that in many patients whose case histories barred them from this survey, the nonappearance of a rolandic spike at the initial EEG was attributable to the fact that very early initiation of an anticonvulsant regimen, before neurologic referral, had suppressed the seizures and also the EEG spike activity.

It should be noted that several patients whose anticonvulsant medication was discontinued somewhat prematurely did not manifest EEG spikes upon removal of the drugs but nevertheless experienced occasional seizures. This tendency for seizures to recur was immediately suppressed by reinstituting the anticonvulsant regimen. However, 24-hour EEG monitoring was not done in these patients.

Anticonvulsant Medication

As indicated previously, suppression of seizures with an anticonvulsant regimen was effected with ease in all patients. Often this was effected on dosages that seemed far below the therapeutic levels, and although drug levels were measured initially, it rapidly became apparent that drug suppression of seizures could be effected on levels well below those usually accepted as the therapeutic range. Later patients in this series were not managed with periodic blood levels; for the most part patients had been controlled on 100 to 200 mg of sodium phenytoin at bedtime.

As mentioned above, complete success was achieved with this therapeutic regimen, and no patients in the survey needed anticonvulsants at follow-up.

Migraine Symptoms (Table 9.2).

The high frequency of headache symptoms was noted in a 1974 series (Bladin and Papworth, 1974), and this present series presents the same findings.

Presentation

Table 9.2 shows that, when specific questions were asked at initial presentation, 21 patients gave a history of recurrent headaches and also of recurrent abdominal pain, and 4 gave a history of recurrent abdominal pain alone. In addition, 16 patients at that time lateralized the headache to one or the other side of the cranium. Classical migraine with teichopsia was found in only two cases at first clinical presentation. However, final follow-up interview data showed that in four patients the symptom of recurrent headache had indeed already been noted by the parents when the patient presented with seizures, but since the appropriate question was not asked, such information was not tendered. As pointed out by one parent, "There was enough to worry about with the child's seizures, not to mention the headache!" This, no doubt, goes a long way toward explaining why such a reasonably well-defined juvenile seizure syndrome has not been commonly reported as being associated with recurrent headache.

Table 9.2 Benign Rolandic Epilepsy—Migraine. A Summary of 30 Cases Including 19 Males and 11 Females Between Ages Six and Ten

Presentation	
Recurrent abdominal pain only	4
Recurrent sick headaches	20
Unilateral ache	16
Ache nonlateralized	4
"Classical" migraine	2
Follow-up history, migraine	
Recurrent: "sick headache," pallor, prostration	24
"classical"	4
Occasional recurrent abdominal pain	3
No migraine admitted to	3
Family history of migraine	21
Headache lateralization	
Total patients	16
Ache and spike ipsilateral	10
No lateralization	6
Possible speech maturation problem	
Left-sided sylvian spike	14
Speech maturation problems	7

Review Findings

Follow-up neurologic examinations and interviews after the passage of years showed that of 30 patients, 24 now admitted to ongoing migraine and 4 of these suffered from the occasional classical migraine, with the attacks being ushered in by teichopsia. There were three patients who had suffered only from recurrent abdominal pain and nausea, pallor, and vomiting of unknown cause, and no migraine or migraine equivalent was admitted in three other patients. Review of the family history of migraine showed that in 20 cases there was a positive history of migraine in one or the other parent or in a sibling (most often in both). However, one patient was adopted, with the family history unknown, and in another case the patient's mother had had occasional attacks of headache labeled migraine but it was uncertain whether the patient himself had manifested the condition.

Lateralization of Headaches

In 16 patients the headache was lateralized to one side or the other. In 10 patients, the side of lateralization was ipsilateral to the appearance of the EEG spike, and in 6 cases there was no lateralization of the headache. It should be pointed out that in every case in which focalized clinical seizures had been reported, this was in complete accord with the lateralization of the spikes. In only one case, however, was simultaneous lateralized headache and contralateral focal ictal activity reported.

Medication

Anticonvulsant medication did not provide protection against the occurrence of headache in any of these patients. Despite complete suppression of seizures, recurrent headaches continued. In three patients, pizotifen was deemed necessary as a temporary prophylaxis against the appearance of recurrent and inconveniencing headache. In no case was antimigrainous therapy substituted for anticonvulsant therapy.

Speech Problems

In 14 patients, the rolandic spike was lateralized to the left side. It was noted that of these 14 patients, 7 manifested a speech maturation difficulty far out of proportion to any other cognitive functional impairment. All these children were in fact right-handed and became the subject of an ongoing neuropsychological review to determine the permanence of this phenomenon. This may well be one of the aspects of the condition of "acquired aphasia" or the syndrome of "epileptic speech arrest" (Sato and Dreifuss, 1973; Shoumaker et al., 1974; Landau and Kleffner, 1957; Worster-Drought, 1971).

DISCUSSION

The nature and behavior of the seizures in benign rolandic epilepsy have been well enough documented in many previous series that they need not be further elaborated on here. Suffice it to say that the seizures in this group of patients closely resembled the classic pattern described in the literature on this subject. In passing, it is worth commenting on the much larger number of patients excluded from this study whose seizures presented in exactly the same form and circumstances, but whose EEGs were devoid of rolandic spikes because of the premature initiation of anticonvulsant therapy. This is undesirable, since such action clouds the issue of diagnosis and especially prognosis. The association of a history of recurrent headache and benign rolandic epilepsy has not attracted much comment in the literature to date. Blom et al. (1972) noted that 2 patients out of 40 suffered from migraine, and Beaumanoir et al. (1974) commented that there was "a fairly frequent history of migraine" (4 patients out of 26). Without a doubt, this is due to the general paucity of migrainous symptoms in this age group and, consequently, the lack of historical inquiry at clinical examination. In this group of patients the bulk of cases was found to exhibit recurrent headache, and this was confirmed by parents and bolstered by a positive family history. "Classical migraine" was uncovered in a very much smaller number of patients in this series.

Whatever the true etiology of the headache, its recurrent nature, its familial occurrence, and the positive response to antimigrainous therapy reported by some patients and affected family members alike, argue strongly for a migrainous basis.

Finally, the congruity of lateralization of headache and lateralization of EEG spikes are worthy of comment. Despite the fact that at times both the EEG abnormality and the headache manifested bilaterally, in 64% of those patients in whom the headache was noticeably unilateral, this corresponded to the lateralization of the EEG spike.

It is also to be noted that 50% of the patients with left hemisphere sylvian spikes were found to have had problems with speech maturation. Whether this can be attributed to a process similar to that reported by previous authors (Landau and Kleffner, 1957; Worster-Drought, 1971; Gascon et al., 1973; Shoumaker et al. 1974; Sato and Dreifuss, 1973) will be investigated in the near future. Indeed, a genetic basis for benign rolandic epilepsy has been postulated (Heijbel et al., 1975) and thus its concomitance with migraine and other disorders is perhaps not so surprising. Mild behavior and learning problems are commented on by Lerman and Kivity (1975). Heijbel and Bohman (1975) did not find verbal problems in any patients in their series, although scholastic difficulties in some patients were noted by Beaussart (1972). Retarded speech development was found by Blom et al. (1972) in one patient in their series, and Blom and Brorson (1966) pointed out that developmental abnormalities can be found in association with rolandic spikes.

Therefore, it might be that the "benign" appellation be applied specifically to the outcome of the seizure condition and not to its accompaniments in other areas of cerebral function.

REFERENCES

Beaumanoir A, Ballis T, Varfis G, Ansari K. Benign epilepsy of childhood with rolandic spikes. A clinical, electroencephalographic and telencephalographic study. Epilepsia 1974;15:301–15.

Beaussart M. Benign epilepsy of children with rolandic (centro-temporal) paroxysmal foci: a clinical study of 221 cases. Epilepsia 1972;13:795–811.

Beaussart M, Faou R. Evolution of epilepsy with rolandic paroxysmal foci: a study of 324 cases. Epilepsia 1978;19:337–42.

Bladin PF, Papworth G. "Chuckling and glugging" seizures at night—sylvian spike epilepsy. Proc Australian Assoc Neurol 1974;11:171–5.

Blom S, Brorson LO. Central spikes or sharp waves (rolandic spikes) in children's EEG and their clinical significance. Acta Paediatr Scand 1966;55:385–93.

Blom S, Heijbel J, Bergfors PG. Benign epilepsy of childhood with centro-temporal

EEG foci. Prevalence and follow-up study of 40 patients. Epilepsia 1972;13: 609–19.

Blom S, Heijbel J. Benign epilepsy and children with centro-temporal EEG foci. A follow-up study in adulthood of patients initially studied as children. Epilepsia 1982;23:629–31.

Gascon G, Victor D, Lombroso CT, Goodglass H. Language disorder, convulsive disorder and electroencephalographic abnormalities. Arch Neurol 1973;28:156–62.

Heijbel J, Blom S, Rasmuson M. Benign epilepsy of children with centro-temporal EEG foci. A genetic study. Epilepsia 1975;16:285–93.

Heijbel J, Bohman M. Benign epilepsy of children. Intelligence, behaviour and school adjustment. Epilepsia 1975;16:679–87.

Landau WM, Kleffner FR. Syndrome of acquired convulsive disorder in children. Neurology 1957;7:520–3.

Lerman P, Kivity S. Benign focal epilepsy of childhood: a follow-up study of 100 recovered patients. Arch Neurol 1975;32:261–4.

Lombroso, CT. Silvian seizures and mid-temporal spike foci in children. Arch Neurol 1967;17:52–9.

Sato S, Dreifuss FE. Electroencephalographic findings in a patient with developmental expression aphasia. Neurology 1973;23:181–5.

Shoumaker RD, Bennett DR, Bray PF, Curless RG. Clinical and EEG manifestations of an unusual syndrome in children. Neurology 1974;10–16.

Worster-Drought C. An unusual form of acquired aphasia in children. Dev Med Child Neurol 1971;13:563–71.

10

Electrographic Observations on Migraine and Transient Global Amnesia, Confusional Migraine, and Migraine and Epilepsy

Tommaso Sacquegna
Pietro Cortelli
Anna Baldrati
Piero de Carolis
Paolo Tinuper
Elio Lugaresi

The association between migraine and clinical events such as transient global amnesia, confusional states, and epileptic seizures is known, but electroencephalographic (EEG) studies during such events are rarely described. We report three patients who presented these unusual clinical phenomena. The first developed transient global amnesia following an attack of classical migraine status. The second had a confusional state that occurred during a classical migraine attack. The third had an attack with combined features of migraine and epilepsy.

Clinical and EEG studies of these three cases provide some objective information that may help us understand the pathophysiology of these clinical events in relation to the migraine attack.

CASE REPORTS

CASE 1   The patient, a 31-year-old man, had an 11 year history of classical and common migraine attacks. One morning, he developed recurrent attacks of classical migraine consisting of right visual field photopsias, right hand and forearm paresthesias and left-sided headache. Migraine attacks followed one another for several hours. His wife then noted that he could not recall recent events and kept repeating the same questions over and over. This episode of memory loss lasted about 90 min.

Neurologic examination was normal. He recalled that his last aura was similar to those previously experienced, but was totally amnesic for the attack itself. Computerized tomography (CT) brain scans performed 3 hours after the attack and 2 days later were both normal. An EEG performed that day showed slow waves over temporal regions with prevalence of sharp delta waves on the left. Serial EEGs revealed decrease and subsequent disappearance of the abnormalities over the next few days (Fig. 10.1).

Comment

This man presented with recurrent serial attacks of classical migraine followed by acute onset of short-term memory impairment and retrograde amnesia. The clinical picture, characteristic of transient global amnesia, seemed to be precipitated by the classical migraine status.

CASE 2   This intelligent 17-year-old girl began to have recurrent headaches before the age of 10. From the age of 11, she developed 20 to 30 minute episodes of visual hallucinations in one half of the visual field and, at times, spreading paresthesias on the same side of the body. This was followed by headache and on some occasions the attacks progressed to slight confusion. The attacks usually ended in deep sleep. Neurologic examination, brain CT scans, a left carotid arteriogram, and EEG were all normal.

On the day of the ictus she developed a migraine attack with a visual scotoma followed by right homonymous hemianopia. Within 30 minutes the visual deficit subsided, followed by left-sided headache associated with migrating paresthesias in the right arm and the right side of the face. She appeared drowsy and was slow to speak and reply, 2 hours after the onset. She showed minor disorientation for time and space, but neurologic examination was otherwise normal.

The first EEG, recorded 30 minutes later, showed marked asymmetry with decreased occipital activity and slow waves at 1 to 2 Hz over the left hemisphere. The slow abnormalities had an anterior prevalence and were also present over the frontal regions of the right hemisphere (Fig. 10.2). Two hours later, she slept for 3 hours. On awakening she was completely free of symptoms but did not remember having been examined.

A brain CT scan was normal on the following day and also a few days later. The EEG abnormalities gradually resolved, but 72 hours later some slow activity persisted over the left posterior regions. An EEG on the 10th day was completely normal.

Comment

This girl had a classical migraine attack leading to a confusional state. The neurologic symptoms and EEG findings in the acute phase indicated dysfunction of the left cerebral hemisphere.

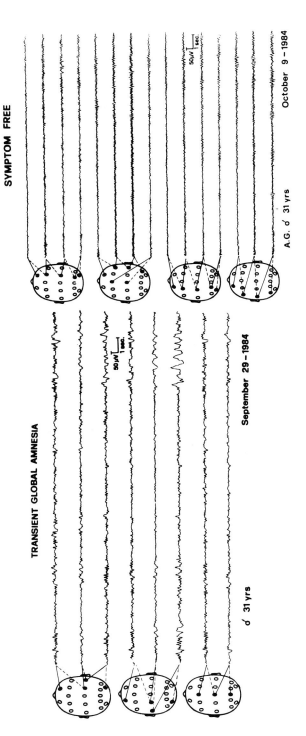

Figure 10.1 The EEG during an attack (left) showed irregular posterior activity on the left side and bursts of slow waves predominating over the left temporal region. After an attack (right) the EEG showed no abnormality.

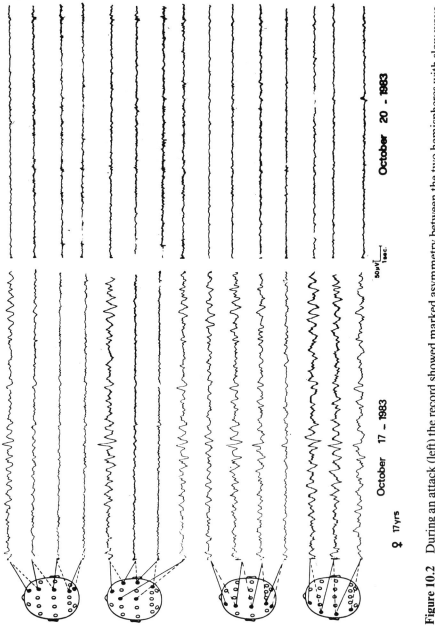

Figure 10.2   During an attack (left) the record showed marked asymmetry between the two hemispheres with slow wave activity predominating over the left and spreading to the frontal regions of the right. Note the poorly regulated, low amplitude left occipital activity. Four days later (right), while the patient was symptom-free the EEG was normal.

CASE 3   This 42-year-old woman had a history of perimenstrual migraine attacks since adolescence. Her father had common migraine and her cousin suffered from epileptic seizures. At age 29, she began to develop migraine attacks complicated by drowsiness and slight confusion that lasted for hours. During these attacks she sometimes complained of visual disturbance. The attacks recurred preferentially during the menstrual period or in association with highly emotional experiences. An interictal EEG performed after sleep deprivation showed bursts of sharp waves with left anterior predominance. Her brain CT scan and cerebral arteriography were normal.

One morning this woman developed a headache and underwent EEG recording. The tracing showed slowing of background activity with bursts of delta waves. The headache began to throb and the patient became drowsy. Suddenly she complained of blurred vision. The EEG showed a generalized decrease in amplitude and rhythmic paroxysmal theta activity at 4 Hz appeared over the left occipital region. At this point the patient spoke slowly and could only count by repeating; she also made mistakes. The discharge lasted 4 minutes and stopped abruptly; at that point the patient became fully alert and had no disturbance of vision or headache (Fig. 10.3). Slow activity persisted over both hemispheres. After a few minutes, photic stimulation induced pronounced bilateral driving intermingled with sharp waves over both hemispheres but with posterior predominance. This pattern was never observed during subsequent EEGs.

The patient never had episodes of blurred vision and/or disturbance of consciousness except in association with her headaches. These attacks did not respond to antiepileptic treatment, but improved with flunarizine therapy.

Comment

The recorded attack presents the clinical and electrographic aspects of confusional migraine with an overlapping occipital seizure.

DISCUSSION

The clinical features and course of the first case are consistent with a diagnosis of transient global amnesia (TGA) (Fisher and Adams, 1964). The exact nature of the mechanism underlying TGA remains uncertain. Most authors (Matthew and Meyer, 1974; Shuping et al, 1980) have attributed it to transient ischemia of cerebral memory structures, especially of the mesial temporal lobes and hippocampal regions, while others (Cantor, 1971; Fisher, 1982) have suggested an epileptic etiology. Our observation is similar to other reports (Olivarius and Jensen, 1979; Crowell et al, 1984) describing TGA in association with migraine. Caplan et al (1981) reviewed 12 personal cases of TGA related to migraine; they found that the headache was left-sided in 8 and bilateral in 4. They suggested that migrainous vascular dysfunction of the dominant temporal lobe, which is correlated with verbal memory, could explain TGA. The EEG findings are also similar to previous reports. Rowan and Protass (1979) and Gilbert (1978) have reported EEG abnormalities such as bitemporal delta activity or transient temporal spikes, especially when nasopharyngeal recording was performed.

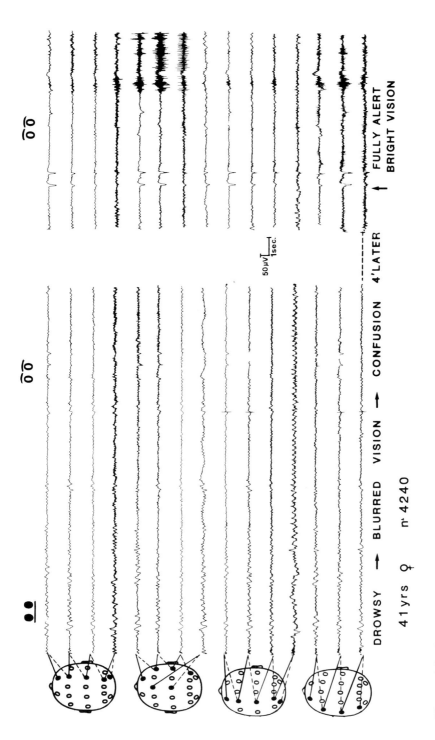

Figure 10.3   The EEG during the attack (left) showed a generalized slow background activity with bursts of delta waves followed by a sudden decrease in amplitude and a rhythmic paroxysmal theta activity at 4 Hz in the left occipital region. This discharge lasted four minutes and then stopped abruptly (right).

The cerebral blood flow studies of Olesen et al (1981) and their colleagues (Lauritzen and Olesen, 1984) showed that classical migraine attacks have a typical pattern of spreading hypoperfusion. The pathophysiologic substrate could be Leão's spreading depression, although this interpretation is still debated (Gloor, 1986). It seems reasonable to speculate that metabolic and/or vascular impairment typical of classical migraine may have spread to mesial temporal structures, thus triggering a TGA episode.

Our second case illustrates a long-lasting confusional state following a classical migraine attack. Since the first description by Bickerstaff (1961) of the clinical picture of "basilar artery migraine," impairment of consciousness has been described in association with transient cerebellar and brain-stem symptoms and has been attributed to transient dysfunction of the reticular formation. Some authors (Emery, 1977; Ehyai and Fenichel, 1978) have pointed out that the clinical and EEG findings during attacks of confusional migraine suggest hemispheric rather than brainstem dysfunction. In our case the focal neurologic symptoms originated in the left hemisphere, as did the electrographic abnormalities. Clinically, the patient's disturbance of consciousness appeared to be a state of "clouding" with reduced wakefulness and awareness, poor attention, and memory disturbance. Our observation, as well as others, indicate that impairment of consciousness during a migraine attack may be due to hemispheric cerebral dysfunction.

The third patient had complex attacks with combined features of migraine and epilepsy. The question of possible relationships between migraine and epilepsy has been a source of continuing controversy since the time of Gowers (1907). The hypothesis of such a relationship has been supported by reports on patients who developed an epileptic seizure during an attack of classical or basilar migraine. Many questions arise from the patients reported by Slatter (1968), Camfield et al (1978), Swanson and Vick (1978), and Panayiotopoulos (1980) to have basilar migraine and epilepsy. These cases share several features such as on-going spike and slow-wave activity from occipital regions, blocked or attenuated by eye opening; occurrence of visual symptoms, at times followed by convulsive seizures; and good response to anticonvulsants. These features are also characteristic of "benign partial epilepsy of childhood with occipital spike waves." An alternative explanation is that these patients have occipital lobe epilepsy followed by headache (Gastaut, 1982).

This patient presented several unusual features: the headache always preceded the episodes of blindness and impairment of consciousness; no disturbance of vision or consciousness occurred outside the migraine attack; there was no interictal occipital focus. The impairment of consciousness was very likely due to propagation of occipital discharges towards the temporal lobe. The disturbance underlying the confusional migraine attack may have caused a breakdown of inhibitory mechanisms in the occipital cortex. Thus, the migraine attack could have activated a potentially epileptic lesion too small in itself to induce an occipital seizure.

The electroclinical study of the first two patients indicates a causal relationship between classical migraine, transient global amnesia, and a confusional state. It is likely that the pathophysiological mechanism is a reversible dysfunction of the temporal lobes or other portions of the cerebral hemispheres. Confusional migraine would have been labeled or diagnosed as basilar migraine had we not recorded the attack. Our case shows that a confusional state may follow a classical migraine attack and may be caused by a cerebral hemispheric dysfunction; this may be the case in other patients as well.

Our last case illustrates that the metabolic impairment of confusional migraine may trigger an epileptic seizure.

REFERENCES

Bickerstaff ER. Impairment of consciousness in migraine. Lancet 1961;2:1057–59.

Camfield PR, Metrakos K, Andermann F. Basilar migraine, seizures, and severe epileptiform EEG abnormalities. Neurology 1978;28:584–88.

Cantor F. Transient global amnesia and temporal lobe seizures. Neurology 1971;21:430–1.

Caplan L, Chedru F, Lhermitte F, Mayman C. Transient global amnesia and migraine. Neurology 1981;31:1167–70.

Crowell GF, Stump DA, Biller J, McHenry LC, Toole JF. The transient global amnesia-migraine connection. Arch Neurol 1984;41:75–9.

Ehyai A, Fenichel GM. The natural history of acute confusional migraine. Arch Neurol 1978;35:368–69.

Emery ES. Acute confusional state in children with migraine. Pediatrics 1977;60:110–14.

Fisher CM. Transient global amnesia: precipitating activities and other observations. Arch Neurol 1982;39:605–8.

Fisher CM, Adams RD. Transient global amnesia. Acta Neurol Scand 1964 (suppl. 9);40:1–83.

Gastaut H. L'épilepsie bénigne de l'enfant à pointe-ondes occipitales. Rev EEG Neurophysiol 1982;12:179–201.

Gilbert GJ. Transient global amnesia: manifestation of medial temporal epilepsy. Clin Electroencephalogr 1978;9:147–52.

Gloor P. Comments on "Migraine and regional cerebral blood flow". Trends in Neuroscience 1986;9:21.

Gowers WR. The borderland of epilepsy. London: Churchill, 1907.

Lauritzen M, Olesen J. Regional cerebral blood flow during migraine attacks by xenon-133 inhalation and emission tomography. Brain 1984;107:447–61.

Matthew NT, Meyer JS. Pathogenesis and natural history of transient global amnesia. Stroke 1974;5:303–11.

Olesen J, Larsen B, Lauritzen M. Focal hyperemia followed by spreading oligemia and impaired activation of rCBF in classic migraine. Ann Neurol 1981;9:344–52.

Olivarius B, Jensen TS. Transient global migraine amnesia in migraine. Headache 1979;19:335–8.

Panayiotopoulos CP. Basilar migraine? seizures, and severe epileptic EEG abnormalities. Neurology 1980;30:1122–25.

Rowan AJ, Protass LM. Transient global amnesia: clinical and electroencephalographic findings in 10 cases. Neurology 1979;29:869–72.

Shuping JR, Rollinson RD, Toole JF. Transient global amnesia. Ann Neurol 1980;7:281–85.

Slatter KH. Some clinical and EEG findings in patients with migraine. Brain 1968;91:85–8.

Swanson JW, Vick NA. Basilar artery migraine. Neurology 1978;28:782–86.

11

Electrographic Observations during Attacks of Classical Migraine

Anne Beaumanoir
Mira Jekiel

Reports dealing with electroencephalographic (EEG) recordings during or immediately after migrainous attacks are rare compared with those describing EEG findings between attacks. As previously stated by Barolin (1966), the scarcity of such observations has added to the difficulty of understanding the pathophysiologic mechanisms underlying the migraine attack. We studied 66 EEGs recorded during the ictal or postictal phases of a migrainous attack in an attempt to define possible relations between epilepsy and migraine.

MATERIAL AND METHODS

A total of 66 EEG records from 30 subjects — 18 male and 12 female — obtained during, immediately after, within 48 hours, or during the week after a migrainous attack constitute the material of this study (Table 11.1).

All 30 patients had classical or basilar migraine according to the Friedman classification (1962). More than half had been followed for several years. They agreed to come to the EEG laboratory during the development of, or immediately after, an attack. This method of recruitment probably introduced a bias in favor of younger subjects, not yet regularly employed. In our study, the prevalence of males derives from our collaboration with the physician of a boys' boarding school.

Thirty-one cases (1 patient was studied twice during an attack) were divided into three groups.

Table 11.1   Temporal Relationship of EEG Recordings to Migraine Attacks*

Time of EEG Recording	Group 1	Group 2	Group 3	Total
Ictal	7	9	8	24
≤ 48 hr after	10	11	7	28
> 48 hr after < 1 week	4	6	4	14
Total	21	26	19	66

Note: *66 recordings in 30 patients

First Group.   Migraine attacks with visual symptoms, most often unilateral, followed by hemicrania, sometimes associated with other signs or vegetative disturbances. This group was comprised of 11 patients, 7 male and 4 female, aged 12 to 28 years (mean: 16 years) at the time of recruitment (Cases 1 to 11) (Table 11.2).

Second Group.   Migraine attacks with bilateral visual symptoms accompanied or followed by vegetative symptoms; vertigo; impairment of consciousness, or ataxia followed or accompanied by headache, usually occipital (basilar migraine). This group included 11 patients, 5 male and 6 female, aged 7 to 25 years (mean: 13 years). (Cases 12 to 22) (Table 11.3).

Third Group.   Migraine with vertebrobasilar symptoms associated with clinical signs suggesting involvement of other vascular territories. This group consisted of 8 patients but resulted in 9 cases (one patient (Cases 23 and 24) was studied during one attack at age 9 and during another attack when he was 13). Six patients were male and two were female. At the time of recording they were aged 9 to 25 years (mean: 17.5 years) (Cases 23 to 31).

In the course of the study 24 EEGs were performed during a migraine attack, 28 were performed less than 48 hours after the end of a paroxysm, and 14 were performed between the 3rd and 7th day following the acute event (Table 11.4).

Tables 11.2, 11.3, and 11.4 show results for each group, considered by type of migrainous symptoms and associated EEG data. The latter are represented in the table as follows:

A.   Polymorphous delta activity, continuous and nonreactive, alternating between the two parieto-temporo-occipital regions and superimposed on a diffusely abnormal EEG.

B.   Polymorphous delta activity associated with more abundant theta over one temporoparietal area.

A'B'.   Abnormal activity of the same type as in A and B, clearly less pronounced, and associated with reappearance of normal background activity.

Table 11.2   EEG Findings in 11 Patients Who Had Migraine Attacks with Visual Symptoms and Hemicrania (Group 1)

Characteristic	1	2	3	4	5	6	7	8	9	10	11
						Case Number					
Sex	F	M	M	M	M	M	M	F	F	F	M
Age (yrs)	12	13	13	13	14	14	15	16	19	20	28
Ictal EEG											
Number	2	1	0	0	1	0	0	1	1	1	0
Prodromal phase	AB	ABE'			B			A	AB	ACE'	
During headaches	B										
Postictal EEG											
Number	1	2	1	1	1	2	2	0	2	1	1
≥12 h				A'B'		B'	A'B'				
<24 h						B'					
<48 h	B'	A'B'	B'				N		B'	B'C'	B'
<1 wk		N			N		N		N		
Interictal EEG	N	N	N	N	N	N	N	N	N	N	N

For key to table, see pages 164 and 168.

Table 11.3 EEG Findings in 11 Patients Who Had Migraine Attacks with Bilateral Visual Symptoms and Other Sensory or Motor Signs and Residual Headache (Group 2)

Characteristic	Case Number										
	12	13	14	15	16	17	18	19	20	21	22
Sex	F	F	M	F	F	M	F	F	M	M	M
Age (yr)	7	8	9	10	12	13	13	13	16	17	25
Ictal EEG											
Number	1	1	1	1	0	1	0	1	2	0	1
Prodromal phase											ACE
During headaches	AC	CD	C	C		CD		C	CC'D		
Postictal EEG											
Number	1	1	1	3	1	2	1	2	2	2	1
≥12 h		C'D'				C'D'		BE'		C'	
<24 h	C'B'			C'							
<48 h				D'	D'E'	D'	D'		D		
<1 wk			N	D'						sleep	
Interictal EEG	N	OccSW	N	N	OccSW	N	N	N	D'	N	N
								N	N	N	N

For key to table, see pages 164 and 168.

Table 11.4 EEG Findings in 9 Patients* Who Had Migraine with Vertebrobasilar Symptoms and Signs of Involvement of Other Vascular Territories (Group 3)

Characteristic	Same patient 23	Same patient 24	Case Number 25	26	27	28	29	30	31
Sex	M	M	M	M	M	F	M	F	M
Age (yr)	9	13	13	13	15	23	24	25	25
Ictal EEG									
Number	1	2	0	1	1	2	0	0	1
Prodromal phase	A'BE'	B B'			ABE				
During headaches				BE'	A'C	A'BC			C
Postictal EEG									
Number	1	1	1	1	1	1	1	1	0
≥ 12 h									
< 24 h			A'B'						
< 48 h	B'			D'E'	C'	Sleep asym.	A'	B p.C'E'	
< 1 wk		B'							
Interictal EEG	N	N	N N	Rol. spike	N N	N	N	Occ. spike	N N

*One patient (Cases 23/24) had recordings at different ages and is counted twice. For key to table, see pages 164 and 168.

C.   Monomorphic delta replacing the background activity over both parieto-occipital, and to a lesser extent temporal, regions. This activity usually occurs as part of a diffusely abnormal EEG. Monomorphic delta waves could be inhibited over one or both hemispheres by external stimuli, particularly eye opening.
D.   The same anomalies as in C but reactive to eye opening.
C'D'. Similar delta activity as in C and D but of lower voltage and discontinuous.
E.   Discontinuous rhythmic or almost rhythmic spike and wave complexes or focal spikes over posterior head regions.
E'.   Isolated spikes over posterior head areas.
N.   Normal.

In two cases (Cases 22 and 28), the EEG was recorded during the migraine aura. Results will be presented by group for the three groups of patients. One or two cases from each group will illustrate the data. Interictal tracings are discussed only if they were abnormal.

RESULTS

First Group (Cases 1 to 11; Table 11.2)

Records obtained between attacks were normal in all patients. EEGs were performed during attacks with hemicrania in five cases and during diffuse headache in two others.

Although the EEG obtained during attacks was always taken during the vasodilatation phase, it differed according to the time elapsed from the beginning of the attack. EEG anomalies during the headache phase were at first bilateral, then tended to focalize in the parieto-occipital regions, contralateral to the symptoms of the attack, as they became more distant from the beginning of the episode. The EEG performed within the first hour (as in Cases 1, 2, and 8) was diffusely abnormal. Although visual symptomatology was unilateral and the headache was localized, slow polymorphous and monomorphous nonreactive anomalies occupied both parieto-occipital regions. These anomalies focalized progressively, whereas the background rhythm reappeared, superimposed on the slow waves. Hours or days following the attack, the focal anomalies persisted but were less marked.

In two cases (Cases 2 and 10), sporadic spikes were observed during the vasodilatation phase; these were parietal in one case and left temporo-occipital in the other. In Case 2 the attacks began with unilateral scotomata followed by a painful sensation of sparkling and hemianopia. In Case 10, visual and painful symptoms were accompanied by anarthria.

CASE 9   The patient was a female, born in 1961, and had no family history of migraine. Since the age of 9, she had both common and classical migraine. After 1975 the attacks became more frequent. Arteriography provoked a 48-hour-long migraine attack. Migraines were characterized by scotomata followed by hemianopia and hemicrania, usually on the left. One migrainous episode occurred on February 2, 1980. The first EEG was performed less than 2 hours after the beginning of left hemicrania (Figure 11.1a). The second EEG was performed about 36 hours after the headache was gone (Figure 11.1b).

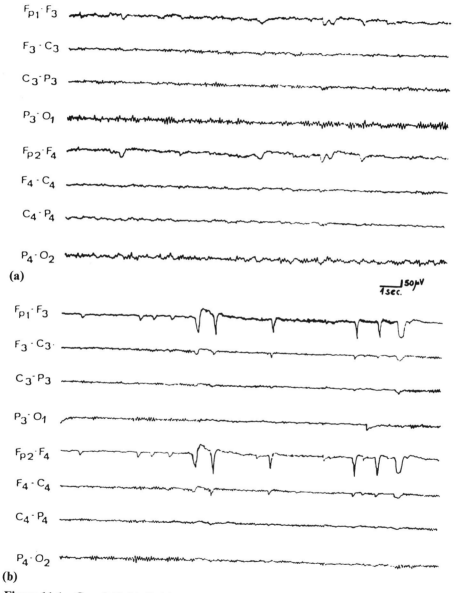

Figure 11.1 Case 9, Table 2. (a) The first EEG was performed less than two hours after the beginning of left hemicrania. Note asymmetry of amplitude and monomorphic slow waves on the right. $P_4O_2 - C_4P_4$. (b) The second EEG was performed about 36 hours after the headache was over. The EEG is normal.

Second Group (Cases 12 to 22; Table 11.3)

EEGs Obtained between Attacks

Two patients of this group (Cases 13 and 16) showed a focus of posterior spikes. Neither of them had ever had seizures. In Case 13 there was no family history of either migraine or epilepsy. The child had febrile convulsions at 18 months, and the first migraine attack occurred at age 6. She was amblyopic. Case 16 had suffered from migraine for 2 years; her brother and her mother had migraine, and she was amblyopic too. (Case 18, whose EEG between attacks was normal, was also amblyopic.)

EEG Pattern during Migraine

With the exception of Case 22, who will be reported in detail, all recordings were performed during the headache or during vegetative manifestations and, in three cases, during a confusional state. The nine ictal EEGs were different from those recorded in the first group. They were characterized by high-amplitude monomorphic slow posterior activity, showing a tendency to spread less and less anteriorly as the time interval from the beginning of the attack increased.

In Cases 13, 17, and 20, clear lateralization of the abnormalities was seen during the attack. In all the EEG recordings, with the exception of those obtained less than 1.5 hours after the beginning of the attack (Cases 20 and 22), the posterior slow waves were blocked by eye opening. Their morphology and their reactivity suggested that they were related to occipital intermittent rhythmic delta activity (OIRDA). No spikes were recorded during the vasodilatation phase.

CASE 17   The patient was a male, born in 1966, and had a family history of one sister with migraine. His first episode of common migraine occurred at age 7. A second episode occurred when he was 9. He complained of bright flashing lights followed by a gleaming, motionless, broken image before his eyes. He then seemed unable to see for a short time. During later, similar attacks he also complained of dysesthesias in both hands and that his head felt cold. The aura lasted about ½ hour and was followed by occipital headache, vertigo, nausea, and marked confusion alternating with episodes of somnolence lasting 3 to 24 hours.

The first EEG (Figure 11.2a) was performed about 2 hours after the beginning of an episode. The patient was confused and nauseated, and complained of diplopia. The second EEG (Figure 11.2b) was performed 12 hours after the beginning of the attack. The patient was still sleepy and had a headache. The third EEG was obtained between attacks (Figure 11.2c).

CASE 19   The patient was a female, born in 1968 to a mother with migraine. The patient's first migraine occurred at age 13. She complained of altitudinal hemianopia following a period of micropsia. The child was nauseated and vomited. She also had ataxia and diarrhea. On the way to the hospital she said she saw a red ball before her eyes and then complained of occipital headache.

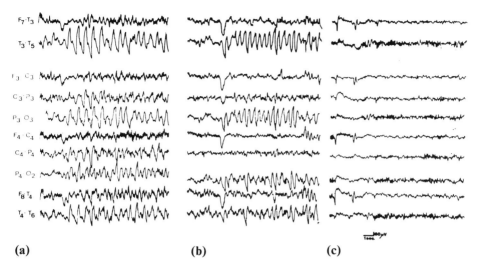

F₇ T₃

T₃ T₅

F₃ C₃

C₃ P₃

P₃ O₃

F₄ C₄

C₄ P₄

P₄ O₂

F₈ T₄

T₄ T₆

(a) (b) (c)

Figure 11.2 Case 17, Table 3. (a) The first EEG was performed about two hours after the beginning of the migraine. Note bilateral monomorphic slow waves on the temporo-parieto-occipital scalp derivation. (b) The second EEG was performed 12 hours later. The patient was still sleepy and had a headache. Note bilateral OIRDA. (c) The third EEG, a normal interictal record, was obtained between attacks.

The first EEG was performed 1½ hours after the beginning of the attack, during the headache phase and while she still had vertigo (Figure 11.3a). The second recording was done about 3½ hours later when she was still nauseated and the headache had just disappeared (Figure 11.3b).

Third Group (Cases 23 to 31; Table 11.4)

Records obtained between attacks were normal except for Cases 26 and 30. Case 26 had rolandic spikes and a history of nocturnal seizures. This patient began to have migraine at age 11, whereas the last seizure had occurred at age 9. Case 30 had occipital spikes and was amblyopic.

Seven EEGs were obtained during migraine attacks in five patients. In Case 28 it was recorded during the aura. In cases with basilar migraine the EEG was identical to that described for the second group. When visual symptoms were not associated with dysfunction of the rostral part of the midbrain, the slow anomalies were similar to those described for the first group but were usually more diffuse (for example, EEGs 23 and 24, obtained from the same patient examined at the ages of 9 and 13).

CASES 23 & 24   The patient was a male born in 1967. His father had migraine with an identical pattern. The patient's first migrainous attack occurred at age 8.

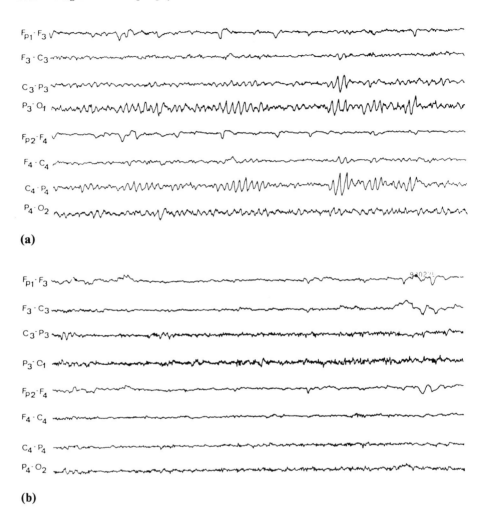

(a)

(b)

Figure 11.3 Case 19, Table 3. (a) The first EEG was performed one-and-a-half hours after the beginning of the attack. Note bilateral parieto-occipital monomorphic slow waves. (b) The second recording was done about three-and-a-half hours later. Note some posterior slow waves.

The second one, two years later, was recorded. The attack began with "holes" in the left visual field followed by "blurred" vision, as if he were in a bright white cloud; this lasted a few minutes. Initially he could speak but had word-finding difficulty; after 1 to 2 minutes he could no longer speak. Vision gradually returned to normal and he had nausea and vomiting. The visual aura and aphasic state lasted about 60 minutes. The EEG was performed about 60 minutes after the visual symptoms began (Figure 11.4a). The second EEG was performed the next day (Figure 11.4b). It was normal.

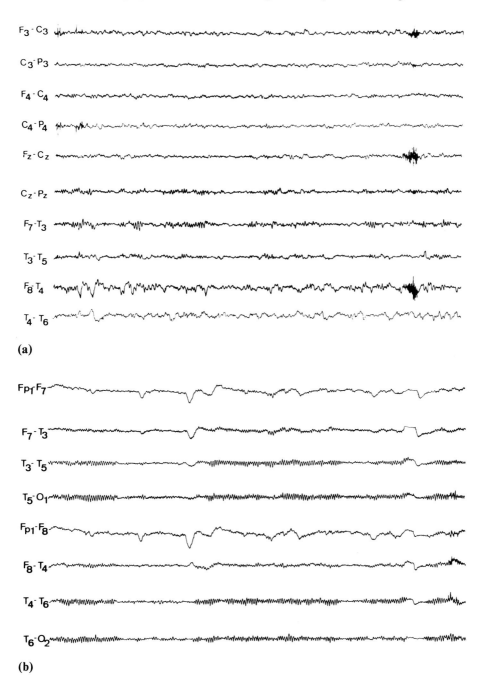

(a)

(b)

Figure 11.4 Case 23/24, Table 4, age 11. (a) The first EEG was performed during the attack, about one hour after its beginning. Note diffuse slow waves and focal temporal abnormalities. (b) The second EEG was performed the next day.

DISCUSSION

These observations show that basilar migraine, in spite of a sometimes identical visual aura, may have different EEG correlates. If we distinguish the patterns of abnormality described as A and B from those termed C and D, we observe that for 12 patients with the clinical syndrome described by Bickerstaff (1961), the EEG contained OIRDA in 10 of 11 recordings. These data confirmed our earlier results (Matthis et al., 1980) which were obtained in 17 young patients with migraine, including 4 with classical migraine and 4 with basilar migraine. These eight cases were included in the present study.

During vasodilatation, two types of EEG were recorded. The first (Figure 11.1) was characterized by monomorphic and polymorphic slow waves. Low-amplitude background activity sometimes persisted. The slow anomalies appeared over a progressively smaller area in the parieto-temporo-occipital territory. At first they were seen bilaterally, even in cases with lateralized head pain; then they became more unilateral as the interval from the beginning of the attack increased. Such EEG changes have been described for classical migraine by many authors: Engel et al. (1945), Dow and Whitty (1947), Barolin and Karbowski (1973). Apart from their topographic distribution, these anomalies are comparable to the ones described by Navarranne et al. (1967) and Gastaut et al. (1974).

The second EEG pattern characteristic of the vasodilatation stage (Figure 11.2) consisted of high-amplitude monomorphic slow delta waves replacing the normal patterns seen over posterior quadrants. These slow waves were blocked promptly in response to eye opening and were elicited by rapid intermittent photic stimulation. They were never triggered by low-frequency stimuli. This EEG pattern, which we described in 1976, was reported earlier by Ziegler and Wong (1967) in one case, and later by Lapkin et al. (1977) in two cases of basilar migraine. The morphology of this slow activity, its reactivity to external stimuli, and its resemblance to occipital intermittent rhythmic delta activity (OIRDA) suggest that it originates in cortical rather than deep midline structures, as suggested by some authors.

These electrographic abnormalities were recorded during the phase following the aura of migrainous attacks or during a period of vasodilatation, whereas it had been assumed, and later was shown, that the classical migraine aura is associated with vasoconstriction. The majority of EEGs performed during migraine can be compared only with EEGs performed in the postictal phase of epileptic attacks. That phase, like the focal epileptic seizure itself, is usually of short duration, whereas the vasodilatation phase, corresponding to the state following the migraine aura, is prolonged.

In considering any possible relationship between epilepsy and migraine, one has to study the EEG data gathered during the migraine aura. Ictal EEGs are common, but EEGs recorded during the aura of classical migraine are rare and are most often obtained by chance. In our material, 24 EEGs were obtained during the headache phase of migraine because of the cooperation of patients who came to the EEG laboratory on our request; only twice, because of the patient's proximity to the EEG laboratory when the migraine began, were we able to record a patient during a migraine aura. Once, the recording began before the first signs of migraine were present. These two patients are reported in detail.

CASE 28   The patient was a female, born in 1948. Her mother had migraine. Her own migraine started at age 13 or 14. At first the migraine attacks were often catamenial; then they gradually became less frequent. Only a few have occurred over the last 4 years.

Arteriography and other investigations during attacks were normal. Her first pregnancy was in 1971. During her second month of this pregnancy she had one attack; no more attacks occurred for the next year. An attack began in the hospital where she was working as a nurse. An EEG was performed less than ½ hour after the beginning of the episode, which was characterized by "sparkles" with left retro-orbital pain followed by "bright balls dancing" before her eyes while the orbital pain was fading away. Left periorbicular twitching started, and she had vertigo and ataxia. She was led to the EEG laboratory by a colleague, to whom she suddenly said, "This time I'm completely blind!" about 5 minutes after the beginning of the attack, which lasted more than an hour. After ½ hour of complete blindness, there were brief periods when blurred vision returned.

The EEG (Figure 11.5a) was recorded about ½ hour after the beginning of the attack, during the period of blindness. Bilateral spike and slow wave epileptic discharges were seen over both posterior regions with left-sided prepoderance. She had vertigo and vomited when she was moved. At the end of the recording, after the spikes had disappeared from the tracing, she began to experience headache, somnolence, nausea, and vertigo. These symptoms lasted about 48 hours (Figures 11.5b and 11.5c).

CASE 22   A male, born in 1954, had the first of his long-lasting migraine attacks when he was 14 or 15 years old. Investigations in 1972, including an EEG, were normal. During his attacks he saw flashing bright lights that were followed by scintillating scotomata and blindness lasting 10 to 30 minutes. An aura was recorded by chance during a follow-up EEG (Figure 11.6) that was taken while he was in the hospital after a ski accident without head injury. The resting EEG was normal. The migraine began 1 minute after the end of, not during, intermittent photic stimulation, as in the cases described by Swanson and Vick (1978).

The patient first noted gleaming spots before his eyes that were associated in the EEG with monomorphic slow waves confined to posterior head regions. While experiencing these scintillating scotomata, he refused to close his eyes. After 6 minutes he began to repeat continuously, "I see everything white," and sometimes, "I'm going to see everything white." Pseudorhythmic spike and wave activity was seen over the left parieto-occipital region and, occasionally, on the right.

After 9 minutes the patient felt violent occipital pain, which later diminished, and he said, "That's it, I'm blind!" While the blindness persisted, spikes were seen to decrease on the left. The patient spoke with difficulty. It was impossible to determine whether he was confused or dysphasic. After 17 minutes the

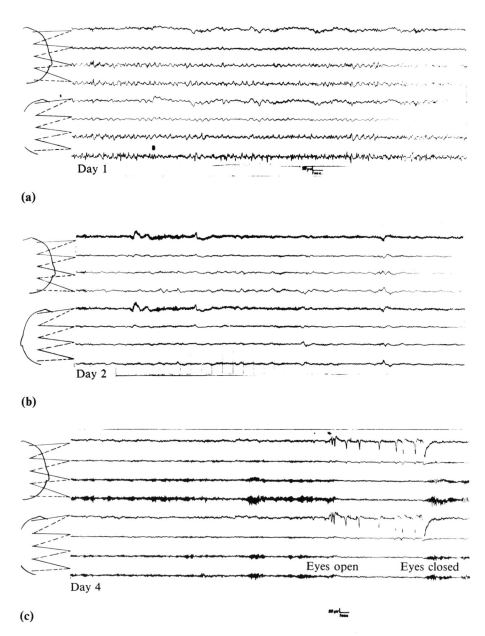

(a)

Day 1

(b)

Day 2

(c)

Day 4

Eyes open   Eyes closed

Figure 11.5   Case 28. (a) The first EEG was recorded about half an hour after the beginning of the attack, during the period of blindness. (b) A sleep EEG was performed 24 hours later. (c) A normal EEG was recorded two days later.

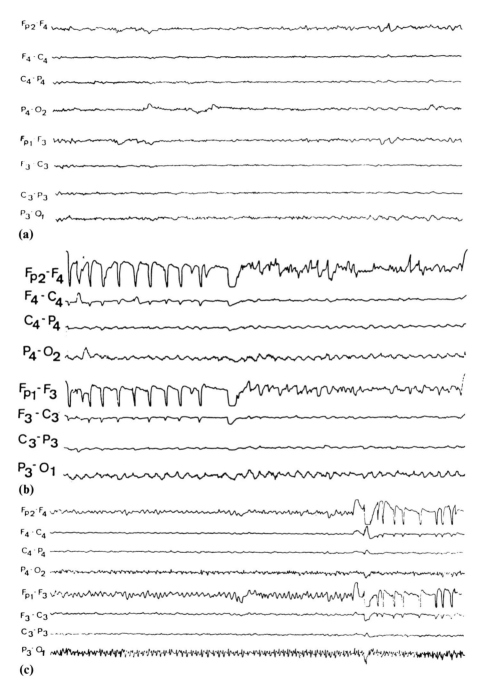

Figure 11.6 Case 22. (a) Record before the attack, (b) 2 minutes after the beginning, (c) 17 minutes after the beginning, (d) 20 minutes after the beginning, (e) 32 minutes after the beginning, (f) 1 hour after the beginning.

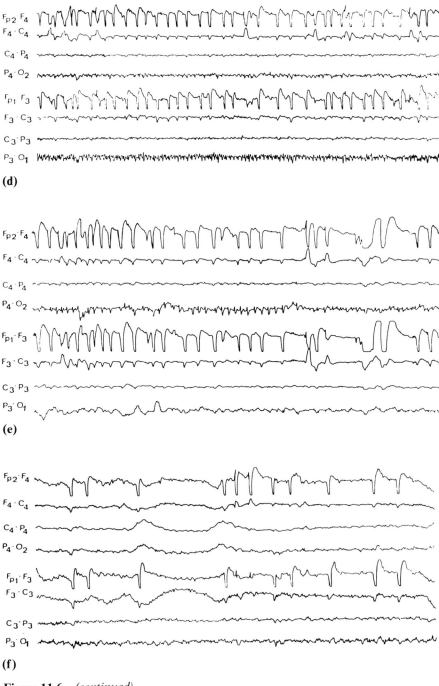

(d)

(e)

(f)

Figure 11.6   *(continued)*

repetitive spike and wave activity was noted only over the right parieto-occipital region. The patient said, "I'm still blind, but it's soon going to cease." Then he said, "I'm starting to see red!" At that moment, in the 20th minute of the aura, the EEG again showed spikes in the right parieto-occipital region, and these were quite rhythmic for about 1½ minutes. As the EEG activity became slower, the spikes disappeared completely. He began to recognize objects presented in his right visual field. After 30 minutes the headache began, and slow waves were seen over both occipital regions. The recording lasted 1½ hours (Figure 11.6f).

The EEG records during the migraine aura in two of our patients, as in one of the cases of Huott et al. (1974) and in the patients of Swanson and Vick (1978), suggest a similarity between epileptic discharge and the electrophysiological changes accompanying the vasoconstriction phase of migraine. The repetitive spikes were not seen at the onset; indeed, the first EEG sign of the migraine aura were the monomorphic slow waves, which in our Case 28 appeared before the repetitive spikes. This preexistence of monomorphic slow waves has never been described in epileptic attacks, in which the first electroencephalographic signs are the spikes, usually at about 10 per second. On the other hand, the repetitive nature of and morphology of the spike and wave discharges accompanying the migraine aura liken them to those described as pseudoperiodic lateralized epileptiform discharges (PLEDs) by Naquet et al. (1965) and by Gastaut et al. (1971), during ischemia. The slow pseudorhythmic spikes recorded between the 6th and 17th minutes of the attack could reflect local hypoperfusion in the cortical territories supplied by the vertebral arteries with resulting blindness (Figure 11.6). Kogure and Schwartzmann (1980) concluded that PLEDs occur during the phase of greatest metabolic abnormality related to the ischemic hypoxia. In Case 22, the spike recruitment began 10 minutes after the migraine had started. This EEG pattern (Figure 11.6) suggests an epileptic process, lasting 90 seconds, correlated with positive visual phenomena that preceded the return of vision. Such an irritative phenomenon at the junction of the hypoperfusion and hyperperfusion phases resembles the seizures occurring between the aura and the headache phase of classical migraine attacks as reported by Manzoni et al. (1979).

The findings obtained by EEGs recorded during the aura of classical migraine provide some objective evidence for the sequence of events in this process, which Basser (1969) compared to the "spreading depression" of Leão. The ionic intracellular and extracellular neuronal and glial modifications involved in the genesis of cortical seizure propagation, as shown by Dietzel et al. (1982) and previously by Sypert and Ward (1974), could explain the occurrences of epileptic seizures in some cases at the time of transition from the vasoconstriction to the vasodilatation phase of the migraine attack. In headache with vegetative or brain stem symptoms, the monomorphic slow waves recorded during the aura and the postictal phase of migraine attack may reflect dysfunction of midbrain structures implicated in basilar migraine.

REFERENCES

Barolin GS. Migraines and epilepsies, a relationship? Epilepsia 1966;7:53–66.

Barolin GS, Karbowski K. Okzipitale Krisen im "Grenzland der Epilepsie." Z EEG EMG 1973;4:1–8.

Basser LS. The relation of migraine and epilepsy. Brain 1969;92:285–300.

Bickerstaff E. Basilar artery migraine. Lancet 1961,1:115–7.

Dietzel UH, Hormeier G, Lux HD. Stimulus-induced changes in extra-cellular Na⁺ and Cl⁻ concentration in relation to changes in the size of extracellular space. Exp Brain Res 1982;181:1–12.

Dow DH, Whitty CWM. Electroencephalographic changes in migraine. Lancet 1947;2:52–4.

Engel L, Ferris B, Romano J. Focal electroencephalographic changes during the scotomas of migraine. Am J Med Sci 1945;209:650–7.

Friedman AP et al. Classification of headache. JAMA 1962;179–717.

Gastaut H, Naquet R, Vigouroux RA. The vascular syndrome of the parieto-temporo-occipital "triangle." In: Zulch E, ed. Cerebral circulation and stroke. Heidelberg: Springer, 1971:82–92.

Gastaut JL, Giraud J, Saint-Jean M. Expression électroencéphalographique des migraines hémiplégiques. Revue EEG Neurophysiol Clin 1974;4:2.

Huott AD, Madison DS, Niedermeyer E. Occipital lobe epilepsy: a clinical and electroencephalographic study. Eur Neurol 1974;11:325–39.

Kogure K, Schwartzmann RJ. Seizure propagation and ATP depletion in the rat stroke model. Epilepsia 1980;21:63–72.

Lapkin M, French J, Golden G, Rowan J. The electroencephalogram in childhood basilar artery migraine. Neurology 1977;27:580–3.

Matthis H, Perriaud P, Jekiel M, Beaumanoir A. Serial EEG records during migrainous attacks. Proceedings of the 2nd European Congress of EEG and Clinical Neurophysiology, Salzburg, Austria, Lechner H, Aranibar A, eds. Amsterdam; Excerpta Medica, 1980;267–71.

Manzoni GC, Terzano MG, Mancia D. Possible interference between migrainous and epileptic mechanism in intercalated attacks. Case report. Eur Neurol 1979;18:124–8.

Naquet R, Franck G, Vigouroux R. Données nouvelles sur certaines décharges paroxystiques du carrefour pariéto-temporo-occipital rencontrées chez l'homme. Zbl Neurochir 1965;25:153–80.

Navarranne P, Simon Y Canton L, Gastaut H. Données électroencéphalographiques sur les crises cérébrales migraineuses. Rev Neurol 1967;116:319–28.

Swanson JW, Vick NA. Basilar artery migraine. 12 patients with an attack recorded electroencephalographically. Neurology 1978;28:782–6.

Sypert GW, Ward AA Jr. Changes in extracellular potassium activity during neocortical propagated seizures. Exp Neurol 1974;45:19–41.

Ziegler DK, Wong G. Migraine in children: clinical and electroencephalographic study of families. The possible relation to epilepsy. Epilepsia 1967;8:171–87.

12

Juvenile Migraine and Epilepsy: EEG and Neuropathological Findings in a Fatal Case

Peter F. Bladin
Sam F. Berkovic

The association between migraine and epilepsy has been discussed a great deal in the literature (Basser, 1969; Jay, 1982; Slatter, 1968) and, indeed, throughout this volume. The prognosis for certain migraine-epilepsy syndromes has been reported as benign, with infrequent seizures and acceptable responses to anticonvulsants (Camfield et al., 1978; Panayiotopoulos, 1980).

On the whole, migraine attacks and seizures are reported as occurring independently of one another, but occasionally patients are seen with seizures that are ushered in by an attack of migraine (Camfield et al., 1978; Slatter, 1968; Terzano et al., 1981). The case we will relate in this chapter involves a child with recurrent intractable seizures ushered in by attacks of migraine with resultant bouts of status epilepticus, one of which proved fatal. This case is reported in order to illustrate the possible fatal outcome of a migraine-epilepsy syndrome. In addition, this patient afforded a unique opportunity for ictal electroencephalographic (EEG) studies and neuropathological examination.

CASE REPORT   The propositus presented for evaluation and treatment of recurrent bouts of unconsciousness starting at age 5 and culminating in death at age 10 years, 8 months. The patient had a past history of mild maternal preeclampsia, mild neonatal jaundice, and some feeding difficulties. Developmental milestones were normal apart from delayed speech; at age 4, he was assessed as having the communication skills of a 2-year-old. Repeated examinations showed some impairment of language development, but there was an absence of definitive neurologic signs or evidence of mental retardation.

At age 5, the patient was found stuporous and covered in vomit. He had been off-color, sweaty, and feverish that day. A presumptive diagnosis of a febrile convulsion was made by the attendant medical practitioner, but at that stage no eyewitness proof of the convulsive elements was obtainable.

After 9 months had passed, an episode of abdominal pain, nausea, and pallor culminated in a major tonic-clonic convulsion for which parenteral diazepam was given by the emergency physician. He was subsequently transferred to the Austin Hospital. Shortly after admission, jerking of the right limbs was noted and after some time this proceeded to a secondary generalized tonic-clonic seizure. Postictally, right-sided weakness was noted. An EEG performed 2 days after admission showed infrequent spiking over centrotemporal regions with right-sided predominance (Figure 12.1). A presumptive diagnosis of benign rolandic epilepsy of childhood was made, and phenytoin was prescribed. Over the next 2½ years, nine similar attacks occurred. All of these began with a prolonged episode of

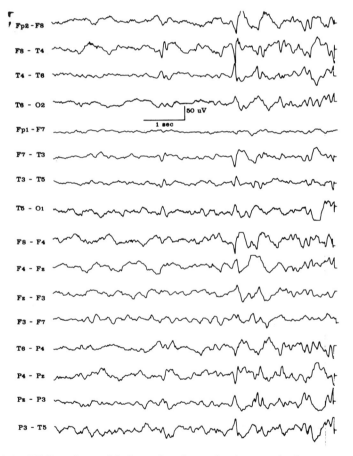

Figure 12.1   EEG performed 2 days after the patient's second seizure at age 6. There was an increased amount of slow activity in the record, and a high-voltage spike was present in the centrotemporal regions, favoring the right side.

abdominal pain accompanied by pallor and retching and culminated in severe vomiting, oncoming stupor, and tonic stiffening. This would usually be followed by clonic jerking, especially of the right-hand side, but often spreading to involve all four limbs, with a secondary generalized major tonic-clonic seizure.

At age 8, the patient reported that severe left-sided headache would usher in the whole symptom complex. At that time a diagnosis of basilar migraine and convulsive syncope was made, but owing to uncertainty and faulty reporting there was still some doubt if true epileptic phenomena were present.

At age 8 years, 8 months, one attack culminated in status epilepticus, and this was documented clinically and electrically (Figure 12.2). Intravenous diazepam (10 mg) was not sufficient to stop the seizure, but an additional 4 mg of intravenous clonazepam was effective. A transient but very noticeable postictal right hemiparesis occurred. Investigations including blood sugar levels, serum electrolytes, urinary amino acids, and a computerized tomography (CT) scan were all normal. It was obvious that both migraine and epileptic seizures were occurring, and therapy with combinations of anticonvulsants and antimigrainous medication was tried: phenytoin, carbamazepine, sodium valproate, propranolol, pizotifen, and finally, a year later, methysergide. It was noted that some attacks consisted simply of headache, pallor, anorexia, and vomiting but that others involved stupor and right-sided convulsions often spreading to secondary generalized seizures.

The course of methysergide given for 6 months in the patient's 10th year seemed to limit his attacks to only one migraine and no seizures at all during this period. However, when methysergide was withdrawn for a month during the mandatory "drug holiday" period, seizures ushered in by headache and nausea occurred again. Methysergide was restarted at the end of the month, but three

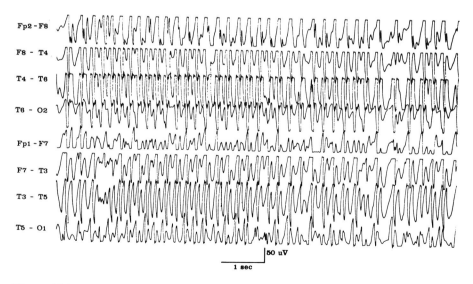

Figure 12.2 EEG performed at age 8 years, 8 months. Tonic-clonic status epilepticus was present clinically and electroencephalographically.

full-blown migraine-epileptic episodes occurred over the next 6 months. An EEG record obtained immediately after one such attack showed marked postictal slowing over the left hemisphere, in accordance with clinical observation of postictal right hemiparesis, dysphasia, and right-sided neglect (Figure 12.3).

At the age of 10 years, 5 months, carbamazepine monotherapy was started, and the patient experienced only one headache in the following 4-month period and had no seizures. This period ended with a severe attack of headache followed by abdominal pain and vomiting and culminating in status epilepticus and cardiorespiratory arrest. Despite persistent resuscitative attempts by paramedical ambulance personnel, the patient was dead on arrival at the hospital.

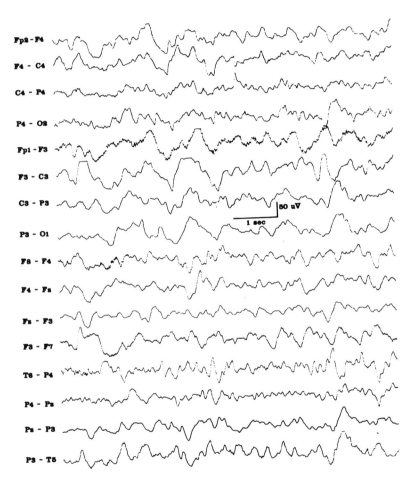

Figure 12.3   EEG performed at age 10 years, 4 months, 60 minutes after a convulsion ushered in by migraine. There was marked slowing over the left hemisphere; mild hemiparesis, dysphasia, and right-sided neglect were seen clinically.

NEUROPATHOLOGY

The formalin-fixed brain weighed 1400 g. The external surface of the brain and the cerebral vessels appeared normal. Multiple coronal sections of the cerebrum did not reveal any pathologic changes, and sections of the brain stem and cerebellum were normal.

Histologic examination of brain sections showed no significant abnormality other than in the left hippocampus (Figure 12.4). This showed extensive neuronal loss and reactive gliosis in Sommer's sector and adjacent prosubiculum, with lesser degrees of neuronal dropout, in Rose's sectors H3-5. There was preservation of neurons in H2. The right hippocampal formation showed no significant neuronal loss (Figure 12.5).

DISCUSSION

The relationship of migraine and epilepsy has been a subject of debate for 75 years, ever since Gowers (1907) gave migraine a place in the borderland of epilepsy. Both are common conditions, and some authors have attributed any association to chance (Lance and Anthony, 1966; Lees and Watkins, 1963). In these studies, epilepsy was regarded as an homogenous disorder, thus diluting the effect of associations between migraine and specific epileptic syndromes. It is now apparent that migraine is associated with a number of epileptic syndromes occurring in childhood and adolescence, as documented elsewhere in this volume. In the majority of these cases, migraine and epilepsy do not occur at the same time and statistical methods are required to confirm the association. Of special interest are the uncommon cases where migraine ushers in seizures. Such cases should be particularly useful in understanding the relationship between migraine and certain forms of epilepsy.

The clinical history of the patient reported here showed that he suffered from both migraine and epilepsy, and that migraine appeared to precipitate every seizure. Although migrainous symptoms sometimes occurred without an epileptic attack, the converse never occurred. This form of migraine-epilepsy syndrome is relatively uncommon.

Three other clinical features were of interest. First, the postictal hemiplegia was always on the right side. Second, from the age of 8, when headache became a prominent part of his migraine attacks, it was referred to the left side of his head. Third, the patient's original presentation was of delayed speech maturation in a right-handed boy with no other evidence of cognitive impairment. It is therefore tempting to invoke a unitary pathology to account for all the patient's clinical manifestations.

The EEG findings lend support to the clinical lateralization and focalization of symptoms. Although there was some suspicion of benign rolandic epilepsy when we considered the electroclinical findings after the first record (Figure 12.1), the subsequent history made it obvious that this was not the

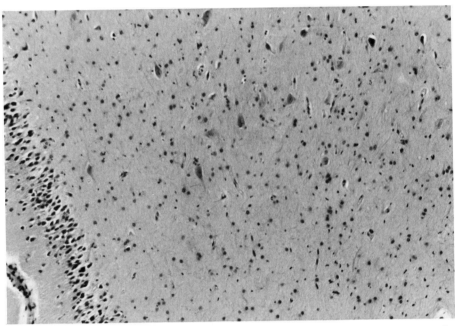

Figure 12.4   Left hippocampus. Rose's sectors H4 and H5 are shown, in which there is considerable neuronal loss and gliosis. The molecular and neuronal layers of the dentate gyrus are seen on the left, and are normal (Luxol fast blue × 300).

correct diagnosis. Indeed, spiking in the central and pararolandic areas has been reported in 9% of children with a clinical history of migraine who have never had seizures (Kinast et al., 1982). The profound postictal disturbance in the left hemisphere (Figure 12.3) was an obvious indication of the lateralizing emphasis given to the cerebral disturbance. Observers of the episodes of status, especially at its onset, reported clinical right-sided jerking initially, so that although the electrical activity recorded consisted of bilaterally synchronous recruited paroxysmal components (Figure 12.2), the clinical facts suggested that the status epilepticus was secondary generalized. We are aware of only one previous case of documented status epilepticus in a patient suffering migraine and epilepsy (Slatter, 1968).

Computed tomography indicated no organic pathology in the left hemisphere that could account for these symptoms as a basis for either the seizures or the headaches. Although the neuropathologic finding of left-sided mesial temporal sclerosis is obviously of great interest, the nature of the seizures indicated that the form of the patient's epilepsy was not temporal lobe epilepsy. Although nausea and vomiting can occasionally form part of a temporal lobe seizure, both the duration of these symptoms and the form of the seizures negated this diagnosis. It is far more likely that mesial temporal sclerosis was a result of the repeated bouts of status epilepticus rather than the cause of the seizures.

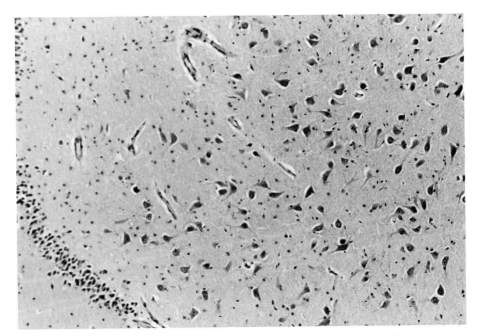

Figure 12.5   Right hippocampus. A comparable section of the right hippocampus shows no abnormality (Luxol fast blue × 300).

The lack of response to treatment was remarkable in this patient. Previous studies, and our own experience, have shown that migraine-epilepsy syndromes are effectively treated by simple drug regimens (Camfield et al., 1978). Despite good compliance, this patient continued to have repeated bouts of migraine, seizures, and status epilepticus. Anticonvulsants and antimigrainous drugs were used singly and in combination. For periods of a few months, both methysergide alone and carbamazepine alone appeared to be effective, but the patient ultimately relapsed on all forms of therapy. Attacks of migraine in this patient held the potential for inducing status epilepticus. This potential emphasizes the necessity for complete suppression of migraine in such patients and cautions us not to regard this migraine-epilepsy syndrome as totally benign.

REFERENCES

Basser LS. The relation of migraine and epilepsy. Brain 1969;92:285–300.

Camfield PR, Metrakos K, Andermann F. Basilar migraine, seizures and severe epileptiform EEG abnormalities: a relatively benign syndrome in adolescents. Neurology 1978;28:584–8.

Gowers W. The borderland of epilepsy. London: Churchill, 1907.

Jay GW. Epilepsy, migraine and EEG abnormalities in children: a review and hypothesis. Headache 1982;22:110–4.

Kinast M, Lueders H, Rothner AD, Erenberg G. Benign focal epileptiform discharges in childhood migraine (BFEDC). Neurology 1982;32:1309–12.

Lance JW, Anthony M. Some clinical aspects of migraine. A prospective survey of 500 patients. Arch Neurol 1966;15:356–67.

Lees F, Watkins SM. Loss of consciousness in migraine. Lancet 1963;2:647–50.

Panayiotopoulos CP. Basilar migraine? seizures and severe epileptic EEG abnormalities. Neurology 1980;30:1122–5.

Slatter KH. Some clinical and EEG findings in patients with migraine. Brain 1968;91:85–98.

Terzano MG, Manzoni GC, Maione R, Moretti G, Mancia D. Association patterns between epileptic and migraine attacks. Acta Neurol (Napoli) 1981;36:587–98.

13

Alternating Hemiplegia in Childhood

B. Dalla Bernardina
G. Capovilla
E. Trevisan
V. Colamaria
G. Andrighetto
E. Fontana
C. A. Tassinari

The syndrome of alternating hemiplegia in children is rarely reported in the literature (Table 13.1) and is little known in clinical practice. The etiology and nature of this syndrome are much debated, particularly its relationship to basilar migraine. Our clinical and polygraphic studies of three cases allow us to delineate further the features of this syndrome and to add some data to the discussion of its pathophysiology.

CASE REPORTS

CASE 1 A girl aged 8 years whose gestation and delivery had been normal had no family history of migraine or epilepsy. At age 3 months, when she had her first attack, her psychomotor development was normal. During this attack she turned up one of her eyes and turned her head to the same side; this episode lasted 2 to 3 minutes. There was no residual deficit, and an electroencephalogram (EEG) was normal.

    After two months, another attack occurred; psychomotor development remained within normal limits. At 7 months she started to have episodes of monocular horizontal nystagmus accompanied by stiffening of the ipsilateral arm and plaintive crying. Within a few minutes flaccid hemiplegia was noted, and it lasted from a few hours to a maximum of 3 days. During these episodes, consciousness remained intact. The affected side could alternate from one attack to

189

Table 13.1   Summary of Published Reports of Alternating Hemiplegia in Infants

Report	Case Number	Number of Cases
Verret and Steele (1971)	Cases 1–3	3
"Alternating hemiplegia in childhood"		
Golden and French (1975)	Case 2	1
"Basilar artery migraine in young children"		
Hosking et al. (1978)	Cases 1–6	6
"Alternating hemiplegia"		
Hockaday (1979)	Case 2	1
"Basilar artery migraine in childhood"		
Dittrich et al. (1979)	Cases 1–3	3
"Paroxysmal hemiparesis in childhood"		
Krägeloh and Aicardi (1980)	Cases 1–5	5
"Alternating hemiplegia in infants"		
Total cases		19

another or even during the same episode; sometimes she had bilateral involvement with flaccid quadriplegia and severe autonomic disturbances. Initially the attacks occurred every 15 days. At 8 months phenobarbital (PB) and then valproate (VPA) and phenytoin (PHT) were prescribed without effect. Until age 3, when she was admitted to the Pediatric Clinic of Verona, the episodes of alternating hemiplegia, and more rarely quadriplegia, continued to occur about once a week. A computerized tomography (CT) scan at 11 months was normal. Psychomotor development deteriorated progressively.

When first admitted to the hospital at age 3 she had generalized hypotonia. This was predominantly axial, with marked dystonic and athetoid movements of the limbs; she was unable to walk without assistance. She was intellectually retarded; speech was poor and restricted to two or three bisyllabic words. Head circumference was 47 cm (−1 standard deviation [SD]). The fundi were normal. Repeated investigations showed no evidence for a degenerative or metabolic disease. Blood electrolytes, lactate, pyruvate, and blood and urinary amino acids were normal, even when measured during an attack. Between episodes glucose, calcium, blood urea nitrogen, hemoglobin, hematocrit, platelets, lipids, protein electrophoresis, hepatic enzymes, tri-iodothyronine, thyroxine, thyroid stimulating hormone, creatine phosphokinase, lactic acid dehydrogenase, ammonia, copper, and iron levels were all normal. Blood levels of PB and PHT were within the therapeutic range. Visual and auditory evoked potentials, EMG, and motor and sensory conduction velocities were all normal. EEGs recorded between attacks were within normal limits both during wakefulness and in all stages of nocturnal sleep. Concomitant EMG records showed continuous polymorphous intentional abnormal movements. EEGs recorded during the hemiplegic attacks showed asymmetrical background activity with decreased alpha activity over the hemisphere contralateral to the hemiplegia. This asymmetry gradually resolved with recovery from the neurologic deficit. During recovery from an attack, a cold stimulus applied to the slightly weak arm induced a reactive effort. A few minutes later marked flaccid weakness reappeared. Deep tendon reflexes were always easily elicited during hemiplegic attacks.

During hospitalization, probably as a consequence of repeated stressful investigations, a unilateral attack became bilateral. Respiratory distress as well as swallowing difficulties developed during this attack disappearing only after several hours of complete rest and sleep.

Antiepileptic drugs were gradually withdrawn and a rehabilitation program started. Different anti-migraine drugs failed to modify the course of the hemiplegic attacks. At age 5 the child was able to walk without assistance but was ataxic and had choreoathetoid movements at rest. She could speak only a few simple words. She continued to have hemiplegic episodes about once a month. These were usually shorter than they were before, but sometimes lasted 4 to 5 hours. From the age of 6, the attacks were preceded by severe and sudden migraine that was clearly described by the child.

At the same age, treatment with 7.5 mg/day of Flunarizine was started; afterwards the attacks became less frequent (1–2/month), shorter (1–3 minutes) and less severe (the child was able to walk during attacks). The neurological disturbances progressively improved. The child is now 8 years old and her neurologic status and scholastic proficiency are normal for her age.

CASE 2   The monozygotic female twin of Case 3 had no family history of migraine or of epilepsy. Birth weight was 2500 g.

Feeding difficulties were noted during the first week of life. Early psychomotor development was not well documented. The infant smiled and had good contact with the environment but was clearly hypotonic: by 4 months she had not acquired head control.

At this age the first paroxysmal episode developed. It was described as a sudden appearance of horizontal nystagmus accompanied by brief tonic generalized stiffening with crying, followed within a few minutes by generalized hypotonia that improved in about 15 minutes. After 15 days another better-described attack occurred. She had right horizontal monocular nystagmus, hypertonia of the right arm, and crying, followed by flaccid right hemiplegia lasting 2 hours, without impairment of consciousness. An EEG recorded some days later during wakefulness was normal. At the age of 6 months, because of increasing frequency of attacks, which by then occurred weekly, she was admitted to another hospital.

She was hypotonic, with dystonic movements of her limbs, and had still not acquired head control. Her head circumference was 1 SD below the mean. The fundi were normal. Blood count, glucose, blood urea nitrogen (BUN), electrolytes, hepatic enzymes, protein and cerebrospinal fluid (CSF) electrophoresis, amino acids, thyroid hormones, urinary screening for neurometabolic disease, skin biopsy, and CT scan were normal. An interictal EEG showed abnormal slow activity in the left occipital region.

A diagnosis of partial epilepsy was made, and the baby was given PB, 5 mg/kg/day. Despite this, the frequency and intensity of the episodes did not change. VPA, 20 mg/kg, was added without effect. The attacks occurred every 4 to 5 days and lasted from a few hours to 3 days. Hemiplegia could involve either side of her body, even during the same attack. At times, flaccid quadriplegia appeared with dysphagia and dyspnea. As the baby grew, developmental delay became apparent, with marked language deficit and hypotonia.

At age 2, when first seen in our institution, she was having weekly attacks. There was severe axial hypotonia with dystonic and choreiform movements of the legs and arms. She was not able to sit without help. Pyramidal signs were absent. The baby was intellectually dull, but there was no evidence of progressive deterioration. Her speech was poor and limited to two or three bisyllabic words. Head circumference was still 1 SD below the mean. Hemoglobin, hematocrit, platelets, lipids, hepatic enzymes, protein electrophoresis, creatine-phosphokinase (CPK), ammonia, copper and iron levels, blood electrolytes, lactate, pyruvate, and amino acids, measured during an attack, did not show any abnormality. Auditory and visual evoked potentials, EMG, and motor and sensory conduction velocities were normal. Blood levels of PB and VPA were within the therapeutic range.

The EEG recorded between attacks showed bilateral well-organized normally reactive background activity without paroxysmal abnormalities during both wakefulness and sleep. The simultaneous EMG showed, during wakefulness, frequent asynchronous bursts of muscular activity without an EEG correlate (Figure 13.1). A polygraphic recording from the onset of an attack of right hemiplegia showed a decrease of alpha activity and slowing over the left hemisphere (Figure 13.2a). Consciousness was not impaired, and the child continued to play with a puppet using her left arm. She fell asleep 40 minutes after the onset of the attack. The EEG asymmetry diminished (Figure 13.2a, right) and completely disappeared during slow-wave sleep (Figure 13.2b, left). After 4 hours of sleep the

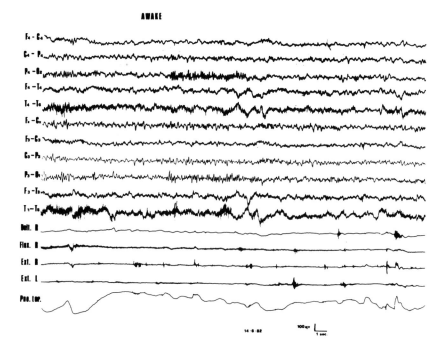

Figure 13.1 Case 2. Between attacks the EEG is normal. The EMG shows frequent asynchronous bursts corresponding to repeated dystonic movements.

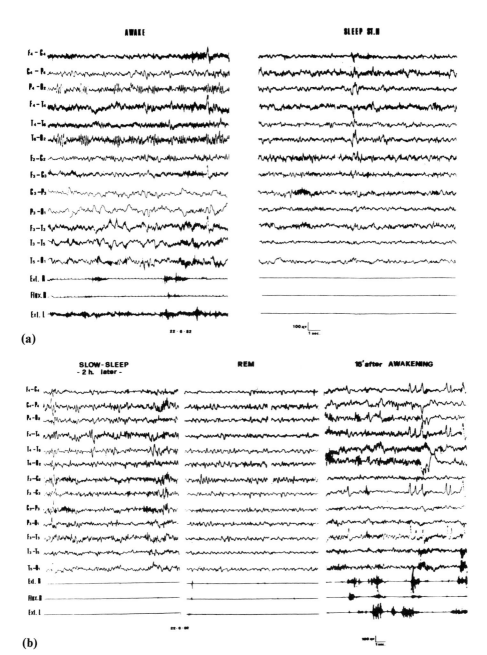

AWAKE

SLEEP ST.II

(a)

22 · 6 · 82

100 μV

1 sec

SLOW-SLEEP
- 2 h. later -

REM

15' after AWAKENING

(b)

22 · 6 · 82

100 μV

1 sec

Figure 13.2 Case 2. (a) (*left*) During an attack with right hemiplegia, the EEG during wakefulness shows depression of alpha activity with theta and delta activity over the left hemisphere. On attempted volitional bilateral arm movement, the EMG shows little muscle activity in the right extensor and flexor muscles compared with normal muscle activity in the left extensors during the right hemiplegia. During sleep (*right*) the EEG asymmetry becomes progressively less evident. (b) Two hours later, no asymmetry is seen during slow and rapid eye movement (REM) sleep. After awakening, 4 hours after onset of sleep, the right hemiplegia is absent for a few minutes but then reappears. The EEG shows persisting voltage depression and slowing over the left hemisphere.

right-sided deficit seemed to have recovered, but a few minutes later it reappeared and the EEG asymmetry was still present (Figure 13.2b, right). The deficit disappeared completely only on awakening the following day. Because her affected twin sister had epileptic seizures during this time, PB was continued.

At age 3 the child was able to walk alone but was ataxic and had significant psychomotor retardation. She was severely hypotonic, had choreoathetoid movements, and was without speech. In spite of multiple trials of anti-migraine drugs, hemiplegic attacks recurred several times monthly but were shorter and much less severe than before. Despite PB treatment, at the age of 3.5 years rare but long lasting partial epileptic seizures with occipital symptomatology appeared. When she was 4.5 years old, the baby was given Flunarizine (5 mg/day). This treatment decreased the frequency and severity of hemiplegic attacks.

Nevertheless, epileptic fits and particularly neuropsychological deficits have not improved. Now, at age 6, she is unable to walk alone and her speech is restricted to some bisyllabic words.

CASE 3   The monozygotic twin of Case 2 had a birth weight of 2400 g. In the first days of life she was tremulous and had feeding difficulties. The clinical history was quite similar to that of her sister, but the first attack occurred at 5 months of age. An EEG performed shortly after an attack showed left occipital slow activity. As with her sister, a diagnosis of partial epilepsy was made, and PB was started without any improvement in the frequency or duration of her hemiplegic episodes. Initially the frequency was one per week, lasting from a few hours to 2 days.

When first seen by us at age 2, she had marked hypotonia, predominantly axial, and dystonic-athetoid movements of the limbs and mouth. Pyramidal signs were not present. She was unable to sit by herself, had no speech, and head circumference was 1 SD below the mean. All investigations performed with her sister were also normal in her case.

An EEG recorded between attacks was normal during wakefulness and sleep. A record obtained during a right hemiplegic episode showed left hemisphere slowing, predominantly over the occipitotemporal regions. As with her sister, the asymmetry was clearly present in wakefulness and in stage 1 of sleep. It became much less evident during slow-wave sleep, but the clinical picture and the EEG improved only after a prolonged period of sleep.

At 2 years, 7 months, alternating hemiplegic episodes continued to occur about once weekly. She was not able to walk alone, and her vocabulary was limited to two to three bisyllabic words. Two attacks were observed when she was in the hospital. Suddenly she became irritable, cried, and had left monocular horizontal nystagmus. Within a few minutes left hemiplegia developed; it lasted 24 hours. On examination, tendon reflexes were present. Respiratory distress, pallor, and swallowing difficulty were noted, but she remained conscious and responsive, although very irritable and plaintive.

A polygraphic sleep record showed that after 4 to 5 hours of sleep the asymmetry and hemiplegia disappeared for a few minutes, only to reappear 10 minutes after awakening, as her parents had previously observed. The EEG showed slowing contralateral to the hemiplegia, affecting mainly posterior head regions.

During hospitalization the child had her first febrile status epilepticus, characterized by brief but repeated partial seizures, alternately involving both sides of the body. The seizures consisted of conjugate lateral deviation of the eyes and unilateral rhythmic clonic jerks with loss of contact. After intravenous diazepam the seizures remained subclinical. The ictal EEG (Figure 13.3) showed paroxysmal discharge of high-amplitude, 2 to 2½ per second spike and wave activity, lasting 1 to 2 minutes and involving alternately the temporo-occipital regions of both hemispheres.

In spite of intravenous diazepam the seizures persisted, stopping only after intramuscular PB was given. Ictal or postictal hemiplegia was not observed, and there was no electrographic postictal depression — confirming that these epileptic attacks differed from her habitual hemiplegic episodes.

Because of the partial seizures, PB was continued with a blood level of 22 micromol/ml. At age 3 her hemiplegic episodes continued at the same frequency but were much shorter. She was able to stand and walk with support but was ataxic and hypotonic with dystonic and choreoathetoid movements. Speech was still limited to a few bisyllabic words. Like her sister, this child was given Flunarizine (5 mg/day). The hemiplegic attacks decreased in frequency and severity but partial epileptic fits and neurological disturbances have not been modified.

Now the child at age 6 years, is able to walk but is still ataxic with dystonic and choreoathetoid movements and her speech is very poor.

DISCUSSION

The clinical features and course of the three patients reported here are consistent with the diagnosis of alternating hemiplegia. Similar observations have been reported under different labels (Table 13.1).

Comparison of the 19 previously described cases with the 3 presented here confirms, as outlined by Krägeloh and Aicardi (1980), that alternating hemiplegia in infants is a clinically well-defined and easily recognizable syndrome with characteristic features. Both sexes are equally represented (12 girls and 10 boys). There is no family history of epilepsy, but a family history of migraine has been elicited in more than a third of the cases (Table 13.2).

Neuropsychologic development before the onset of attacks may be either normal or delayed; however, in half the cases it has not been described adequately (Table 13.2), possibly because the early onset makes precise assessment difficult.

The mean age of onset of hemiplegic attacks is 7 months, with a range from 1 to 18 months. At onset the attacks were generally characterized by abnormal ocular movements, most often monocular nystagmus; plaintive crying; and a sudden but variable tonic or dystonic stiffening of one side of the body which later becomes weak, sometimes with ipsilateral head turning or tilting. Impairment of consciousness is described in only a few cases. These brief spells are followed by flaccid hemiplegia lasting from minutes to days, usually hours. One side alone or both simultaneously are involved in most patients; only rarely is involvement exclusively unilateral or bilateral (double hemiplegia) (Table 13.3). Frequently the attacks, particularly if bilateral and/or of long

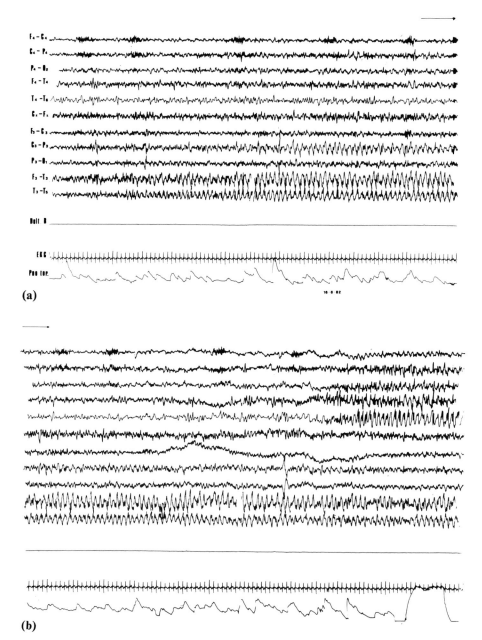

Figure 13.3   Case 3. (a) After diazepam, seizures persist without clinical manifestations. The paroxysmal activity consists of 2 to 2½ per second spike and wave activity with onset over the left hemisphere. (b) Continuation of the seizures as described in 3a. While the discharge over the left hemisphere progressively decreases, independent discharge appears on the right side.

Table 13.2   Pertinent Family History and Psychological Development of Infants with Alternating Hemiplegia

Patient Data	Published Cases (N = 19)	Personal Cases (N = 3)	Total Cases (N = 22)
Family history			
Epilepsy	—	—	—
Migraine	8	—	8
Neuropsychological development at onset			
Normal	5	1	6
Delayed	3	2	5
Not described	11	—	11

duration, are accompanied by striking autonomic disturbances such as tachycardia, sweating, mydriasis, paroxysmal severe respiratory distress, and sometimes difficulty in swallowing. In some cases the symptoms seem to be relieved by sleep. Attacks are usually frequent at the outset, in spite of different medications (Table 13.3), but frequency and severity progressively decrease with age. In no cases were the hemiplegic attacks followed by permanent gross deficit attributable to a specific attack. Although the frequency of attacks decreases, soon after onset neuropsychologic deficits become apparent even in those children who were normal at the onset. Progressive deficits consist of axial hypotonia with dystonia and dyskinesias of variable severity, with mild spasticity in some cases, intellectual impairment of variable degree, and delayed speech.

The etiology of this peculiar syndrome remains unknown. Laboratory and neuroradiologic investigations were normal even when performed during

Table 13.3   Distribution of Hemiplegia during Its Evolution and Frequency of Attacks

Patient Data	Published Cases (N = 19)	Personal Cases (N = 3)	Total Cases (N = 22)
Distribution of attacks			
Only unilateral	4	—	4
Unilateral and bilateral	8	3	11
Only bilateral	3	—	3
Not described	7	—	7
Frequency of attacks			
Several per day	4	—	4
Several per week	5	3	8
Several per month	4	—	4
Not described	6	—	6

the attacks. No evidence for dysmetabolic or structural pathology was found. We think that the repeated diurnal and nocturnal polygraphic records, performed in our patients during and between hemiplegic attacks, yielded some useful information on the possible nature of these peculiar paroxysmal events.

1.   *Alternating hemiplegia is certainly not a form of epilepsy, and the attacks are not epileptic.* Verret and Steele (1971) and Hosking et al. (1978) referred to the frequent recurrence of epileptic seizures in their patients, but in no case did they find paroxysmal EEG abnormalities. Dittrich et al. (1979) referred to the presence of "epileptic foci" in two of their patients, but the EEG excerpts reproduced in their paper are not suggestive of epilepsy. Krägeloh and Aicardi (1980) thought that the hypothesis that alternating hemiplegia is epileptic could not easily be discounted. Nevertheless, they described no paroxysmal EEG abnormalities in the tracings obtained between and during attacks.

In our three patients many attacks of hemiplegia were polygraphically recorded from their onset; paroxysmal discharges were never observed throughout the attacks, and in no case were paroxysmal EEG abnormalities observed between attacks during either wakefulness or sleep.

The repeated partial epileptic seizures recorded in our Case 3 were clinically different from hemiplegic attacks. In particular, hypotonia was never observed during or after these seizures. Moreover, the EEG confirmed the epileptic nature of these seizures, constituting definite proof that alternating hemiplegia is not epileptic, and that it cannot be considered to represent a "unilateral atonic seizure" such as described by Gastaut and Broughton (1972), or a hemiparetic seizure (Hanson and Chodos, 1978). The absence of paroxysmal abnormalities just before the hemiplegia, and of postictal deficits after repeated epileptic events (Case 3), make it unlikely that alternating hemiplegia could be analogous to Todd's paralysis.

Thus, Case 3 shows that alternating hemiplegia is not epileptic, even in the presence of the epileptic seizures that can appear in some cases.

2.   At the onset, in some cases, one might consider the diagnosis of *vertiginous attacks* similar to those of paroxysmal torticollis (Snider, 1969) or benign paroxysmal vertigo (Dalla Bernardina et al., 1982) of infancy. These diagnostic possibilities are easily excluded after the appearance of the typical flaccid alternating hemiplegia, which is never observed in these two syndromes.

3.   *Alternating hemiplegia may be related to migraine,* especially to basilar migraine (Bickerstaff, 1961). Such a relationship has been suggested by Verret and Steele (1971), Golden and French (1975), and Hosking et al. (1978). This theory is supported by:

a.   The high incidence of a family history of migraine
b.   The appearance of headache in some patients with alternating hemiplegia
c.   Symptoms of acute and transient involvement of the brain stem with-

out clinical or radiologic signs of fixed lesions, suggesting a vascular mechanism

d. EEG slowing during attacks, similar to that described in migrainous patients (Lerique-Koechlin and Mises, 1964; Smyth and Winter, 1964; Bruyn, 1968), especially in cases with hemiplegic migraine (Rosenbaum, 1960; Slatter, 1968; Gastaut et al., 1974) or with basilar migraine (Slatter, 1968; Lapkin et al., 1977; Lapkin and Golden, 1978).

In our cases, EEG slowing during the attacks was contralateral to the hemiplegia. However, the slowing was not as marked as that observed in patients during attacks of hemiplegic migraine or basilar migraine. Nevertheless, it is difficult to suggest that vascular involvement of the brain stem would produce the unilateral symptoms that are so frequently observed. We do not include the cases of basilar migraine and epilepsy reported by Camfield et al. (1978), Panayiotopoulos (1980), and Terzano et al. (1981), who probably have observed partial epilepsy similar to that more recently described by Gastaut (1982), Beaumanoir (1983), and Dalla Bernardina et al. (1984).

Autonomic phenomena and neurologic sequelae and death have been reported in migraine, especially basilar migraine (Connor, 1962; Guest and Woolf, 1964; Buckle et al., 1964; Neligan et al., 1977; Petersen et al., 1977), but there are no descriptions in migrainous patients of the characteristic neurologic syndrome that appears in the infants with alternating hemiplegia.

The literature contains some accounts of extrapyramidal paroxysmal movements during attacks of complicated migraine or at their end (Infeld, 1901; Pakozdy, 1929; Schob, 1917, quoted by Bruyn, 1968), but these descriptions are not sufficiently clear to permit comparison with cases of alternating hemiplegia.

4. *Alternating hemiplegia could be related to paroxysmal dyskinesias.* Dittrich et al. (1979) proposed a possible relationship between the miscellaneous group of paroxysmal dystonic conditions and alternating hemiplegia. Others have not taken this possibility into consideration. Krägeloh and Aicardi (1980) thought that these conditions were definitely distinct. Moreover, even if sporadic cases (Gordon, 1980) of early-onset paroxysmal choreoathetosis exist, neurologic and intellectual deterioration have not been reported. Alternating hemiplegia cannot be considered an atypical manifestation of paroxysmal kinesigenic choreoathetosis (Kertesz, 1967) or of familial paroxysmal dystonic choreoathetosis (Lance, 1977).

Even though the significance of the syndrome of alternating hemiplegia remains unknown, it must be considered (Krägeloh and Aicardi, 1980) as a clinically well-defined and easily recognizable disorder; it should be recognized early because of its characteristic neurologic and developmental prognosis. Treatment with calcium channel blockers may be effective in preventing recurrence of attacks (Casaer and Azou, 1984). This further supports a relationship of this syndrome to migraine.

ADDENDUM

After the first writing of this paper, Casaer and Azou (1984) and Curatolo and Cusmai (1984), outlined the possible effectiveness of calcium channel blockers in preventing recurrence of alternating hemiplegia attacks.

Following these reports, we started treating our patients with Flunarizine. In all cases (including three other patients) this appeared effective in decreasing the frequency and severity of the attacks. Improvement of neurological deficits following Flunarizine treatment occurred only in cases with normal initial development and who were treated within a few months of the onset of hemiplegic attacks. In a few cases suffering from epileptic seizures (2/6 personal cases), Flunarizine appeared ineffective in treatment of the seizures.

REFERENCES

Beaumanoir A. Infantile epilepsy with occipital focus and good prognosis. Eur Neurol 1983;22:43–52.

Bickerstaff GR. Basilar artery migraine. Lancet 1961;1:15–7.

Bruyn GW. Complicated migraine. In: Vinken PJ and Bruyn GW, eds. Handbook of clinical neurology. Amsterdam: North Holland, 1968;5:59–95.

Buckle RM, Du Boulay GH, Smith B. Death due to cerebral vasospasm. J Neurol Neurosurg Psychiatry 1964;27:440–4.

Camfield PR, Metrakos K, Andermann F. Basilar migraine, seizures and severe epileptiform EEG abnormalities. Neurology 1978;28:584–8.

Casaer P, Azou H. Flunarizine in the treatment of alternating hemiplegia in childhood. Lancet 1984;9:579.

Connor RC. Complicated migraine: a study of permanent neurologic and visual defect caused by migraine. Lancet 1962;2:1072–5.

Curatolo P, Cusmai R. Drugs for alternating hemiplegia migraine. Lancet 1984;10:980.

Dalla Bernardina B, Colamaria V, Santoni PI, Bondavalli S, Capovilla G, Gattoni MB. Vertigine parossistica benigna dell'infanzia. Boll Lega It Epil 1982;37/38:67–70.

Dalla Bernardina B, Colamaria V, Capovilla G, Bondavalli S. Sleep and benign partial epilepsies of childhood. In: Degen R, Niedermeyer E., eds. Epilepsy, sleep and sleep deprivation. Amsterdam: Elsevier 1984;119–33.

Dittrich J, Havlova M, Nevsimalova S. Paroxysmal hemiparesis in childhood. Dev Med Child Neurol 1979;21:800–7.

Gastaut H, Broughton R. Epileptic seizures, clinical and electroencephalographic features, diagnosis and treatment. Springfield, Ill.: Thomas, 1972:85–109.

Gastaut JL, Giraud J, Saint Jean M. Expression électroencéphalographique des migraines hémiplégique. Rev EEG Neurophysiol 1974;1:23–8.

Gastaut H. A new type of epilepsy: benign partial epilepsy of childhood with occipital spike-waves. Clin Electroencephalogr 1982;13:13–22.

Golden GS, French JH. Basilar artery migraine in young children. Pediatrics 1975;56:722–6.

Gordon N. Choreoathetosis of genetic origin. Dev Med Child Neurol 1980;22:521–3.

Guest IA, Woolf AL. Fatal infarction of the brain in migraine. Br Med J 1964;1:225–6.

Hanson PA, Chodos R. Hemiparetic seizures. Neurology 1978;28:920–3.

Hockaday JM. Basilar artery migraine in childhood. Dev Med Child Neurol 1979;21:455–63.

Hosking GP, Cavanagh NPC, Wilson J. Alternating hemiplegia: complicated migraine of infancy. Arch Dis Child 1978;53:656–9.

Kertesz A. Paroxysmal kinesigenic choreoathetosis. Neurology 1967;17:680–90.

Krägeloh I, Aicardi J. Alternating hemiplegia in infants: report of five cases. Dev Med Child Neurol 1980;22:784–91.

Lance JW. Familial paroxysmal dystonic choreoathetosis and its differentiation from related syndromes. Ann Neurol 1977;2:285–93.

Lapkin ML, French JH, Golden GS, Rowan AJ. The electroencephalogram in childhood basilar artery migraine. Neurology 1977;27:580–3.

Lapkin ML, Golden GS. Basilar artery migraine. A review of 30 cases. Am J Dis Child 1978;132:278–81.

Lerique-Koechlin A, Mises J. L'EEG dans une manifestation paroxystique non-épileptique de l'enfant: la migraine. Electroencephalogr Clin Neurophysiol 1964;16:203–4.

Neligan P, Harriman DGF, Pearce J. Respiratory arrest in familial-hemiplegic migraine. Br Med J 1977;2:732–4.

Panayiotopoulos CP. Basilar migraine? Seizures and severe epileptic EEG abnormalities. Neurology 1980;30:1122–5.

Petersen J, Scrutton D, Downie AW. Basilar artery migraine with transient atrial fibrillation. Br Med J 1977;2:1125–6.

Rosenbaum HE. Familial hemiplegic migraine. Neurology 1960;10:164–70.

Slatter KH. Some clinical and EEG findings in patients with migraine. Brain 1968;91:85–9.

Smyth VOG, Winter AL. The EEG in migraine. Electroencephalogr Clin Neurophysiol 1964;16:194–202.

Snider CH. Paroxysmal torticollis in infancy. Am J Dis Child 1969;14:117.

Terzano MG, Manzoni GC, Maione R, Moretti G, Mancia D. Association patterns between epileptic and migraine attacks. Acta Neurol Scan, New Series 1981;4:587–98.

Verret S, Steele JC. Alternating hemiplegia in childhood: a report of 8 patients with complicated migraine beginning in infancy. Pediatrics 1971;47:675–80.

14

Classical Migraine, Intractable Epilepsy and Multiple Strokes: A Syndrome Related to Mitochondrial Encephalomyopathy

G. S. Dvorkin
Frederick Andermann
Stirling Carpenter
Denis Melanson
Simon Verret
J. C. Jacob

Allan Sherwin
Sabah Bekhor
Elio Lugaresi
Chris Sackellares
John Willoughby
Daune MacGregor

One of the patients (Case 8) described in this chapter was presented by the late Dr. Wilder Penfield at a seizure conference at the Montreal Neurological Institute 26 years ago. This boy had both severe migraine and severe seizures, and this unusual association impressed one of us (F.A.), who attended the conference as a junior resident. The diagnosis of diffuse gray matter disease eventually made in this patient and the diagnosis of Alpers disease (poliodystrophia cerebri progressiva) entertained in the patient's brother, who died after a similar illness, did not seem to explain well the patient's intense migrainous manifestations followed by a malignant epileptic disorder. Over the years we have become aware of seven additional patients with a very similar syndrome of malignant migraine, severe epilepsy, and bilateral cerebral lesions. These nine patients from seven neurologic centers on three continents are the subject of this chapter. In two of the patients a diagnosis of mitochondrial encephalomyopathy with lactic acidosis was made.

CASE REPORTS

CASE 1   This was a 19-year-old right-handed male whose mother had common migraine. At age 13 he developed generalized tonic-clonic seizures associated with myoclonic jerks. An occipital spike focus was found on his electroencephalogram (EEG). He was treated with phenytoin, valproic acid, and clonazepam but still had occasional seizures. At age 18, he experienced an episode of throbbing headache associated with nausea and vomiting. Six months later he developed biocciptal headache associated with scotomata in both visual fields followed by profuse vomiting. For 3 days his family noticed that he was somnolent and confused. Generalized convulsions followed and he was taken to the hospital. Physical examination documented a confused and inattentive young man with a dense right homonymous hemianopia. He had almost continuous spike wave discharges from the left posterior quadrant on EEG. Computerized tomography (CT) revealed a hypodense lesion suggesting an infarct in the left occipital lobe (Figure 14.1a). Angiography demonstrated a complete block of the left calcarine artery (Figure 14.2). The headache resolved on the 4th hospital day, and he was discharged 3 weeks later with a persistent right homonymous hemianopia.

Two months later that he again developed pounding occipital headache, which interrupted sleep. He found himself to be completely blind. On admission to the hospital he complained of nausea, vomited, and had severe occipital headache. He was found to have cortical blindness. He was treated with intravenous (IV) decadron but remained lethargic and nauseated; he complained of severe pounding headache for 3 days. Investigations revealed acellular CSF with protein of 59 mg/dl. A CT scan showed a right occipital hypodense lesion suggesting infarction (Figure 14.1b), and an angiogram demonstrated attenuation of the right calcarine artery. His vision gradually improved, although he remained unable to read.

Four months later, he was noted to have visual acuity of 20/200 bilaterally with inferior arcuate field defects. There was mild flattening of the left nasolabial fold, and fine movements on the left were clumsily performed. His reflexes were slightly diminished on the left and plantar responses were flexor.

Laboratory examination revealed normal sedimentation rate, CBC, PT, PTT, fibrinogen, clotting-time, bleeding-time, platelet retention, platelet aggregation, antithrombin III, factor VIII, hemoglobin electrophoresis, cholesterol, C3, C4, rheumatoid factor, ANA, and cryoglobulins. Triglycerides were 245 mg/dl, and protein electrophoresis indicated a type IV hyperlipidemic pattern. The electrocardiogram showed a Wolff-Parkinson-White pattern, and the EEG revealed an intermittent generalized paroxysmal disturbance without epileptic activity.

Visual evoked responses indicated bilateral latency delay: P 100 OD–

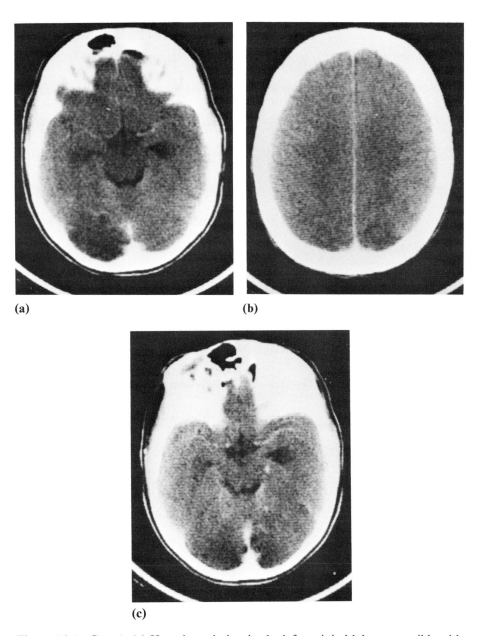

(a)

(b)

(c)

Figure 14.1 Case 1. (a) Hypodense lesion in the left occipital lobe compatible with infarction. (b) Right occipital hypodense lesion suggesting infarction. (c) Bioccipital hypodense lesions later in the course of the illness.

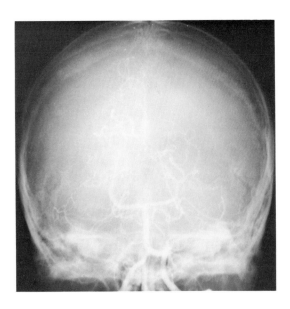

Figure 14.2   Case 1. Vertebral arteriogram showing complete block of the left calcarine artery.

180msec, P 100 OS–184msec. A CT scan suggested the presence of bioccipital infarcts (Figure 14.1c). Repeat angiogram confirmed the persistent occlusion of the left calcarine artery.

His vision improved somewhat, but he continued to have episodes of migrainous headache followed by generalized seizures. A year and a half later he had an episode of status epilepticus. He was intubated and treated with intravenous diazepam, phenytoin, and phenobarbital, leading to cessation of the clinical manifestations, but he continued to have electrical seizure activity. He could not be weaned from the respirator and developed repeated pulmonary infections and septicemia. He did not respond to treatment and died at age 20.

Autopsy showed lesions consistent with infarcts in all the lobes of the brain (Figure 14.3). They appeared to be of various ages, the oldest ones being in the occipital lobes. There the lesions resembled old cavitated cortical infarcts (Figure 14.4), but they had one somewhat atypical feature in that the molecular layer tended to be destroyed over the lesion. Some of the lesions appeared as laminar rarefaction in the cortex, particularly in the fifth layer. More recent lesions were sharply defined foci of necrosis with macrophages and hyperplastic endothelium. Some of these necrotic foci extended up to the pial surface, whereas others spared the outer two cortical layers. One small, more recent focus was recognizable only by eosinophilia of neurons and vacuolation of the neuropil. No vascular occlusion was identifiable, although many arteries were filled with red cells. The thalamus and brain stem were normal.

Summary.   Easily controlled occipital seizures started at age 13 in a boy with a family history of common migraine. At age 18 he developed severe

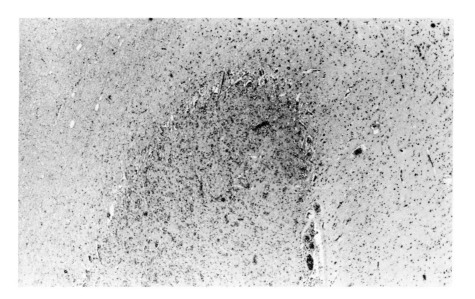

Figure 14.3   Case 1. This photomicrograph shows one end of a sharply demarcated area of recent massive necrosis that occupies the full thickness of the cortical ribbon at one side of the bottom of a sulcus (H&E × 35).

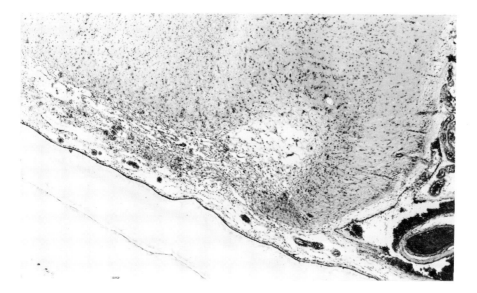

Figure 14.4   Case 1. Old cavited lesions were also found in the same case. They resemble old cortical infarcts (H&E × 35).

migraine leading to left occipital and later to right occipital infarcts. He died at age 20 following status epilepticus. Multiple cortical infarcts were found at autopsy.

CASE 2   This was an 18-year-old right-handed girl with a family history of common migraine. At age 9 she had developed seizures that started with visual changes and went on to secondary generalization. An occipital EEG spike focus was found. She was treated with phenytoin and phenobarbital with good control. At age 17 she developed daily episodes of flashing lights in the right visual field. One of these episodes was followed 1 month later by a generalized seizure. Her seizures became refractory, and she began to have both generalized seizures and partial simple status epilepticus with involvement of the right arm and leg. During her neurologic exam she had episodes of occasional staring and right facial twitching. She had profound nonfluent dysphasia with good comprehension, right homonymous hemianopia, right central facial weakness, and mild hemiparesis, as well as hemisensory loss to all primary modalities. During hospitalization she developed epilepsia partialis continua arising from the left posterior temporal and parietal areas. These seizures were temporarily controlled with large doses of carbamazepine (2200 mg per day), phenytoin, and phenobarbitone.

Investigations revealed leukocytosis, elevated sedimentation rate (52), and raised liver enzymes, all of which returned to normal spontaneously. CSF protein was 83 mg/dl, 135 mg/dl, and 104 mg/dl on three different occasions. CSF IgG was 7.6 mg/dl. Platelet count was elevated at 561,000 (N140/440,000). PT, PTT, fibrinogen, factor VIII, serum protein electrophoresis, and immunoelectrophoresis were normal. Rheumatoid factor and ANF were negative, C3 was 245 (slightly increased); CT scans revealed a hypodense nonenhancing lesion in the left occipital lobe. Four-vessel angiography showed delayed circulation in the distal branches of the left posterior cerebral artery. The middle inferior temporal branch of the posterior cerebral acted as collateral circulation supplying the posterior, inferior, and medial aspect of the occipital lobe. This suggested the presence of an infarct, although no definite occlusion was seen.

She continued to have episodes of left-sided partial status epilepticus with secondary generalization. A left temporal brain biopsy was carried out. There was lymphocytic cuffing of several vessels in the subcortical white matter and deep layers of the cerebral cortex. Many of the neurons in the fifth and sixth cortical layers had shrunken eosinophilic cytoplasm as if they were undergoing acute ischemic change. There was some diffuse gliosis in the cortex. She gradually improved, but her right hemiparesis and hemianopia persisted. She continued to have occasional episodes of flashing lights followed by generalized seizures.

Six months after discharge she began having seizures from the opposite, right, occipital region, documented by EEG studies. These became uncontrollable and culminated in status epilepticus from which she died. No autopsy was performed.

Summary.   Easily controlled occipital seizures started at age 9 in a girl with a family history of common migraine. Eight years later she developed frequent headaches, exacerbation of epilepsy, and recurrent focal status. First a left, then a right occipital lesion developed. She died at age 19 in status epilepticus.

CASE 3 A 41-year-old, right-handed, Indian male engineer with the β-thalassemia trait had a long history of classical migraine with visual aura. One brother had a similar history. The patient began having generalized seizures at age 27. His initial EEG and brain scan were normal. He was treated with phenytoin and phenobarbital.

At age 30, he suffered an episode in which he saw "stars and colors" throughout his visual field and his head turned to the right. This was followed by a generalized tonic-clonic seizure. During the following 3 years he had one seizure per year similar to the one just described. He was completely seizure-free for 3 years, then again began to have one attack yearly.

At age 38 he experienced three of his typical seizures in one day. On examination he was in a postictal state without focal signs. A month later, the patient experienced an episode of migraine status lasting 10 days. This consisted of visual phenomena — stars and colors — associated with severe, generalized, pounding headache. There was no overt convulsive activity during this 10-day period. The family felt that his hearing was impaired, and physical examination revealed receptive aphasia. An EEG showed delta activity throughout the left cerebral hemisphere. A recording taken 5 days later showed depression of cerebral activity over the left occipital lobe and the left temporal region. A CT scan revealed asymmetry of the lateral ventricles, the left being smaller than the right.

Over the next few weeks, he gradually improved and his speech became normal. EEGs showed improved background activity but continued to show paroxysmal irregularities over the left temporal region with depression of cerebral activity over the left temporo-occipital areas.

One month later, he again developed a confusional state, nausea, and vomiting. This time a left hemiparesis and homonymous hemianopia also developed. His EEG now showed sharp-and-slow-waves over the right temporal and parieto-occipital regions. A CT scan with and without contrast showed luxury perfusion in the territory of the right posterior cerebral artery and the posterior insular region. He was treated with steroids in high doses. A CT scan one month later showed a hypodense lesion in the right temporal and right capsular lenticular areas. He again improved gradually, with resolution of the left hemiparesis, although the hemianopia remained as a static deficit. Repeated EEGs during this time paralleled the clinical improvement. A Ga[68] PET scan revealed no focal abnormalities.

Four months later, he suffered a relapse with sudden loss of vision and hearing, as well as aphasia. An EEG revealed severe left frontal slow wave activity with epileptogenic bursts. A CT scan suggested the breakdown of the blood-brain barrier in the left temporal, posterior parietal, and occipital regions.

The patient underwent a left parietal brain biopsy. Sections showed abnormalities that varied in intensity from area to area but had no sharp boundaries. The most widespread change, involving both cortex and white matter, was an increase in astrocytes, many of which had enlarged cytoplasm (Figures 14.5 and 14.6). Elongated microglial nuclei were numerous in some cortical areas. There was patchy neuronal loss, mainly in the second and third cortical layers. Vessels were not increased in number and showed no endothelial hyperplasia, although venules in the white matter were dilated. Lymphocytic cuffing was found around one subarachnoid vein. There were a few mineral deposits in cortex and white matter and some in the walls of vessels.

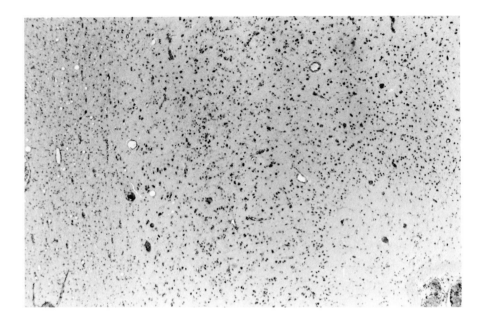

Figure 14.5   Case 3. Both cortex and white matter are abnormal and slightly hypercellular. The abnormality is diffusely present in the biopsy specimen (H&E × 35).

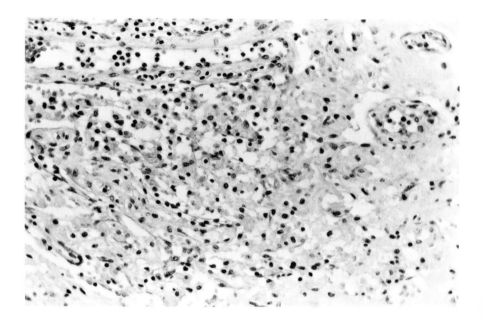

Figure 14.6   Case 3. Several reactive astrocytes are present in this field of cortex where there has been moderate neuronal loss (H&E × 220).

Hemoglobin, platelets, PTT, cholesterol, triglycerides, C3, C4, IgG, IgA, rheumatoid factor, ANA, B12, echocardiogram, and VDRL were normal. Serum IgG was elevated at 490 (N50–200). CSF was acellular, with a protein of 86 mg/dl. CSF IgG was 13 mg/dl and oligoclonal banding was positive.

When seen at age 41, the patient was dysphasic, cortically blind, and had cortical deafness. He was psychotic with violent rage reactions. The psychosis was considered to be secondary to his deafferented state and chronic steroid therapy. The steroids were gradually decreased, and he improved over the ensuing 3 weeks. Six months later resting lactic and pyruvic acid were 11 mg/dl (N 9–16) and 0.7 mg/dl (N 0.5–0.9), respectively. Post-exercise arterial lactic acid was 110 and 90 and 1 hour later 2 mg/dl. Pyruvic acid was 5.2, 5.5, and 0.83, respectively. CSF lactate was 18 mg/dl (N 9–16). A muscle biopsy specimen showed mild denervation and no ragged red fibers. Visual, auditory, and somatosensory evoked responses were abnormal but were difficult to evaluate in the presence of visual and auditory cortical deficit.

Summary.   Seizures developed at age 27 in a man with classical migraine and a family history of classical migraine. Exacerbations of migraine led 11 years later to a left temporo-occipital, then to a right-sided, and later to a second left-sided lesion. A cerebral biopsy specimen revealed lesions of uncertain origin. At age 41 he had cortical deafness, blindness, dysphasia, and profound mental changes.

CASE 4   A 17-year-old boy had developed headaches associated with prominent gastrointestinal symptoms at age 5. His father and paternal uncle had severe classical migraine. The patient's mother, between ages 20 and 40, had generalized seizures with atypical spike and wave discharges. She also suffered from recurrent headaches. At age 11, he had a series of right-sided migraine attacks with throbbing pain radiating from the orbit to the ear. These lasted 2 to 3 hours and occurred several times a day for 10 days. At age 12, he experienced his first seizure, which was generalized and nocturnal. A month later he had a number of right-sided sensory-motor partial simple seizures followed by transient hemiparesis. Then, 2 months later, he experienced left partial simple sensory-motor seizures that resulted in transient left hemiparesis. A CT scan showed a right occipital lucent area (Figure 14.7a). Right partial simple seizures, again followed by transient hemiparesis, recurred 3 weeks later. He was treated with phenobarbitone and phenytoin.

Seven months after the onset of seizures, he had a second series of migraine attacks. After 10 days of almost continuous migrainous phenomena, he had a residual left homonymous hemianopia. ASA therapy was added.

At age 13, he had a third series of migraine headaches that lasted 12 days. These were followed by right homonymous hemianopia and dyslexia as a static neurologic deficit. A week later, right partial simple seizures followed by transient hemiparesis recurred. A CT scan revealed a hypodense lesion in the left occipital region (Figure 14.7b), which diminished in size over the next month. A vertebral angiogram was normal and a left carotid angiogram showed poor distal vascularization, with slow perfusion and irregular caliber of the collaterals of the plica curva and parietal arteries. Prednisolone, 12 mg/day, was administered for 6 months. During that time the patient had two further episodes of left partial simple seizures with transient postictal hemiparesis.

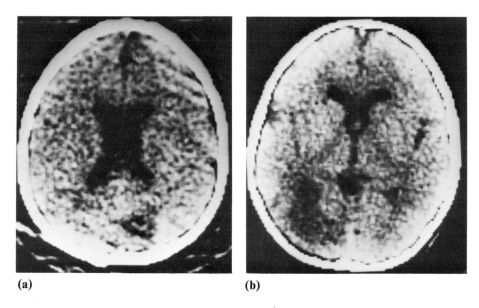

(a)   (b)

Figure 14.7   Case 4. (a) Lucent area right occipital region following a series of seizures. (b) Hypodense lesion, left occipital region, following status and transient hemiparesis.

At age 15, he again experienced left partial simple seizures. Clobazam, 20 mg/day, was added to his treatment. Three months later, he experienced a series of attacks characterized by vertigo, ataxia, and confusion, followed by left-sided headache. These lasted 3 to 4 hours and occurred several times per day for 3 days. Following these he was found to have cortical blindness. CT scans revealed extensive bioccipital hypodensities that were larger on the left.

Attempts to change anticonvulsant therapy resulted in partial simple motor status involving the right bucco-facial region. He was treated with clonazepam, 2.5 mg/day, ASA, 300 mg/day, and propranolol, 80 mg/day. He remained free of migraine and vertiginous attacks for 1 year. He did, however, continue to have multiple right partial simple seizures and developed persistent myoclonic seizures in the right orofacial region. Carbamazepine, 600 mg/day, was added to his treatment.

At age 17 he had cortical blindness and persistent myoclonic jerks involving the peribuccal region and the right side of his neck. He had a distal tremor resembling asterixis. An EEG revealed slow background activity, with degraded spike and wave discharges sometimes following a periodic pattern. Polygraphic analysis with simultaneous EEG and EMG recordings revealed no relationship between the EEG events and the facial myoclonus or the distal tremor.

The patient's condition continued to deteriorate, with random episodes of headache and serial seizures. A later attack ushered in by prolonged and recurrent headaches left him cortically deaf. A muscle biopsy specimen showed ragged red fibers. Cytochrome c oxydase, succinate cytochrome reductase, NADH cytochrome c reductase, citrate synthase, NADH dehydrogenase and succinate dehydrogenase were measured by Dr. DiMauro and were found to be within normal limits.

Summary.   Migraine developed at age 5 and seizures at age 12 in a boy with a family history of classical migraine and of epilepsy. Prolonged migraine at age 13 led to a left occipital lesion and, following a similar episode 2 years later, he had bilateral lesions. At age 17 he had cortical blindness and deafness, mental deterioration, and seizures, which remained difficult to control. Ragged red fibers, evidence of mitochondrial disease, were present in his muscle fibers.

CASE 5   This 28-year-old man developed episodes of pounding headache with nausea and vomiting associated with alternating hemianopia at age 17. A year later, the frequency and severity of his headaches worsened, and they became associated with expressive dysphasia. Later that year he was found to have expressive aphasia, right homonymous hemianopia, right central facial weakness, and bilateral papilledema. Serial EEGs revealed delta activity over the left temporal lobe, and an angiogram was reported to show an avascular lesion in that area. He had a left temporal cerebral biopsy, which revealed nonspecific changes. He continued to have series of prolonged headaches. His language function deteriorated; he suffered a decline in intellectual function and did not return to work. He was noted to be ataxic and clumsy on the right, and his handwriting deteriorated. He had his first seizure 6 months later, which was a right partial motor seizure with secondary generalization. Attacks were treated with phenytoin, carbamazepine, and valproic acid, resulting in poor control. His multiple seizure patterns included a Jacksonian march, staring spells, choking, and apneic spells.

At age 25 he had a ventriculoatrial shunt for "obstructive hydrocephalus." He continued to have prolonged attacks of headache, and his speech became incomprehensible. At age 28 he was incapable of understanding language and began to have difficulty swallowing. He was alert, of small stature, and oriented to person only. His speech was dysarthric and limited to a few words. He understood simple commands. He had a bilateral tremor and a pseudobulbar palsy. There was bilateral hemiparesis that was more marked on the left.

CSF was acellular with protein of 320 mg/dl. CSF IgG was 5.3 mg/dl and oligoclonal banding was positive. The sedimentation rate was normal. EEGs showed multifocal epileptiform activity maximal from the left temporal and central areas. A CT scan showed multiple focal areas of atrophy, mainly in the left temporal, occipital, and right parieto-occipital regions; there was also moderate diffuse atrophy. Carotid angiography revealed rapid transit time, especially over the left cerebral hemisphere. A GA[68] EDTA PET scan revealed increased transit time in both hemispheres, with moderate focal decrease in cerebral perfusion in the left temporal and both occipital areas. An EMG showed diminished amplitude, increased dispersion, moderately slowed nerve conduction velocity, and decreased recruitment, with linked potentials suggesting a polyneuropathy of axonal type. EKG revealed right axis deviation, and an echocardiogram showed asymmetric septal hypertrophy. Muscle, skin, and nerve biopsy specimens showed denervation atrophy and axonal degeneration. In an attempt to reduce his uncontrollable seizures, a left temporal lobectomy was carried out. Sections showed five sharply circumscribed cortical lesions characterized by destruction of neurons and neuropil, presence of macrophages, and hyperplasia of vessels (Figure 14.8). No vascular occlusion could be found. There was only slight improvement in seizure tendency. His condition continued to deteriorate.

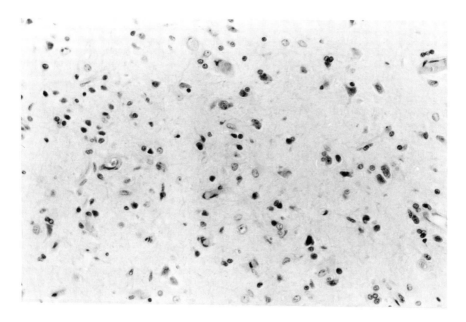

Figure 14.8   Case 5. This small circumscribed cortical lesion filled with macrophages appears consistent with a cortical infarct (H&E × 220).

Summary.   The patient's severe migraine with alternating hemianopia developed at age 17. A left temporal lesion was diagnosed at age 18 and was followed by increasingly frequent seizures. At age 28 he had evidence of multiple lesions in both posterior cerebral artery territories. A biopsy specimen showed focal cortical necrosis consistent with infarction. He remained severely disabled.

CASE 6   The patient was a 27-year-old man of low intelligence (IQ 70–80). At age 19 he developed severe headache and vomiting followed by two generalized seizures. Investigations were unrevealing and phenytoin was prescribed.

For 3 years he was free of headaches and seizures. He was referred at this time because of his clumsiness and lethargy. Mild nystagmus, slight ataxia of the arms and legs, and loud orbital, carotid, cardiac, and abdominal systolic murmurs were apparent. His blood pressure was 180/60. Investigations, including carotid, vertebral, aortic, and renal angiograms, were normal and an EEG was nonspecifically abnormal. A CT scan revealed enlargement of the fourth ventricle. Thyroid function tests, electrolytes, urea, creatinine, serum calcium, phosphorus, magnesium, complete blood count, and ESR were normal. Cardiac output was 9 liters/min, and there were no shunts. Echocardiogram revealed myocardial hypertrophy. Red cell transketolase, arterial blood gases, plasma, and urinary noradrenaline and metanephrines were normal. Phenytoin was discontinued, and propanolol was initiated. Several weeks later he became confused and aggressive after developing a visual disturbance (seeing colors) and complaining of headache. He slept for a brief period and then awoke blind and agitated. On examination, blindness was confirmed, and he vomited several times. Status epilepticus developed and continued for 24 hours. He recovered consciousness 2 days later but exhibited bizarre behavior for 2 to 3 weeks, thought to be due to postanoxic encephalopathy. A CT scan was normal. Carbamazepine was prescribed, and he has taken this drug ever since. His vision gradually recovered. He remained asymptomatic for 4 to 5 years, when a period of impaired consciousness accompanied by confusion, aggression, and auditory hallucinations occurred, lasting 3 to 4 weeks. On occasion he appeared mute, and he had one brief generalized seizure. No firm diagnosis of the nature of this episode was made.

Three months later, the patient was brought to the hospital because of acute onset of blindness. He was cortically blind. Speech was abnormal, containing nonsense words, and he had a tendency to repeat phrases. Over the next 2 days, he developed headache and became uncommunicative. There were no motor signs, and cortical sensory testing was not possible. A CT scan revealed extensive hypodensity of the posterior halves of both cerebral hemispheres (Figure 14.9). Extensive investigation proved unhelpful; carotid and vertebral angiography were normal 20 days later.

He remained uncommunicative, unable to respond to language, and apparently blind. He explored his room by touch continually and therefore probably without memory. He required institutional care.

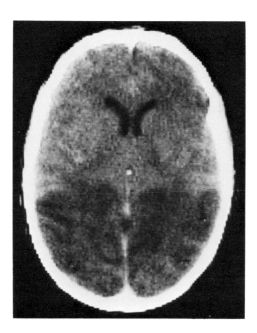

Figure 14.9 Case 6. CT scan showing extensive hypodensity of the posterior halves of both hemispheres.

Summary. A 27-year-old man with subnormal IQ presented at age 19 with migrainous symptoms followed by generalized seizures. During phenytoin therapy he remained asymptomatic for 3 years. A hyperdynamic circulation was found and investigated extensively without a cause being found. He suffered an episode of total visual loss followed by status epilepticus three weeks after cessation of phenytoin. Five years later, he presented with acute cortical blindness, which had developed in association with severe headache. A CT scan revealed extensive hypodensity bilaterally in the territory of the posterior cerebral arteries. He remained totally disabled and required institutional care.

CASE 7   A 13-year-old boy whose mother suffers from migraine hit his head while playing with friends and 3 hours later felt nauseated and complained of flashing lights in front of his eyes. The next morning his parents were awakened by gagging noises. He had a left-sided partial seizure, secondarily generalized, requiring intravenous diazepam. Postictally, he had right-sided pounding headache, left sided weakness involving the face, arm, and leg, and left homonymous hemianopia. His deep tendon reflexes were equal and his toes down going. He was treated with phenobarbitone and phenytoin and continued to vomit intermittently for 2 days. His neurologic examination became normal.

An EEG showed slow activity over the right hemisphere but no epileptogenic activity. Lumbar puncture, CBC, sedimentation, rate, skull and chest x-ray, viral studies, and CT scan were normal.

For 2 months he had occasional headaches. Then he complained of flashing lights appearing at approximately 10-minute intervals and lasting for a total period of 3 hours. Following this he developed severe bitemporal pounding headache accompanied by nausea and vomiting. The next day he had a left-sided seizure that was preceded by blurred vision and lasted 2 to 3 minutes. Following this he had a left homonymous hemianopia but no other abnormal physical findings.

EEGs showed slow waves and some paroxysmal seizure activity, mainly on the right. A CT scan showed a hypodense lesion in the right occipital lobe extending to the posterior parietal region. Right carotid and right vertebral angiography showed narrowing of vessels compatible with infarction of the medial right occipital lobe. Echocardiography, ECG, chest x-ray, clotting factors, protein eletrophoresis, cholesterol, and triglycerides were all normal.

A month later he complained of numbness in the right side of the chest, followed by twitching of the left hand and leg, rolling back of the eyes, and three left-sided seizures with subsequent left-sided weakness. Renal and liver function tests, LE prep, ANF, VDRL, Coombs test, immunoglobulins, and serum lead were all normal. CSF was acellular and protein was 59 mg/dl. A CT scan showed edema of white matter and enhancement of the gray matter involving the entire right hemisphere, with a slight shift of the frontal horn to the left and compression of the right frontal horn. Edema was most severe in the inferior occipital region. Angiography of both carotids showed delayed and decreased perfusion of the right parietal, occipital, and posterior temporal regions and evidence of mild cerebral edema. Another CT scan 15 days later showed diminished but persistent edema in the right cerebral hemisphere, most marked in the right occipital and posterior parietal areas.

Four months later, he complained of flashing lights. He became sleepy and had a generalized convulsion lasting less than 1 minute. Postictally he complained of right-sided headache. He then had a seizure involving the right face, arm, and leg, that became generalized and required intravenous diazepam. The next day he still complained of flashing lights and had a right homonymous hemianopia. He continued to have intermittent twitching of the left hand and complained of seeing flashing lights for several days. A CT scan showed a residual small infarction in the right occipital area and an area of decreased density in the contralateral, left, occipital lobe, suggesting infarction. The right homonymous hemianopia was permanent.

He was treated with high-dose steroids tapered over a four-month period. Pyzotiline and methysergide were initiated and phenytoin continued. Headaches became infrequent. He had another severe attack 2 years later. A muscle biopsy specimen showed ragged red fibers. Blood lactate levels of 4.2 mg/dl (N < 2.0) were found. Cytochrome c oxydase, succinate cytochrome reductase, NADH cytochrome c reductase, citrate synthase, NADH dehydrogenase and succinate dehydrogenase were measured by Dr. DiMauro and found to be within normal limits.

Summary.   Migrainous attacks, quickly followed by partial seizures with generalization, started at age 13 in a boy with a family history of migraine. These involved the right occipitoparietal region and led to a destructive lesion with severe edema of this area. Later, migrainous symptoms were followed by left parieto-occipital damage. While receiving vigorous antimigraine therapy he had no further attacks. He had a stable clinical picture for 2 years but then had another catastrophic attack. A muscle biopsy specimen showed ragged red fibers, evidence of mitochondrial disease.

CASE 8   This patient, the son of a Cuban pathologist, was investigated by Dr. Wilder Penfield in 1958, and we quote verbatim from his notes:

"The outstanding features as I understand them, are as follows: Normal young man aged 18. He has had migraine, which is regularly left-sided, from childhood. Age 9: Operation for obstruction of the intestinal tract by Dr. Gross in Boston. In 1954, age 15: Fell from a motorcycle. He was riding on the back, and when he was picked up he was found to be having a seizure, and an old lady says that the movement was in the right hand. Attacks at intervals following this usually associated with left-sided migraine headaches, and with stars of a scintillating variety. The side of the stars is not certain. This is followed by nausea and at times convulsive movements of the right hand.

"October 20, 1957: While watching a moving picture, his friend noticed that he was covering his eyes. He asked him what was the matter and he said he was seeing stars. A little later, he was having a severe left-sided headache and the friend noticed that the right hand was jerking. The friend became alarmed and insisted on his leaving the moving picture. They walked out together. On October 23, he went into frequent attacks which were followed by hemiparesis or a hemiplegia, lasting about 3 weeks. On November 13, there was vomiting due to intestinal obstruction. On December 1, the attacks became severe. On December 9, he had an abdominal operation following which he was free of attacks for 5 days. At the end of the 5th day, the attacks returned and have been continuous up to the present in spite of medication which he was given in very large amounts; phenobarbital and dilantin and intravenous paraldehyde.

"As seen this morning, he is having clonic movements of the right shoulder, right abdominal musculature and sometimes in the right leg at the hip. This may spread so that there is twitching of the eyelids and of the hands at times. On inquiry, he says that there is a tingling numbness of the right arm. He seems to have a right homonymous hemianopsia as judged by a very rough test. He showed no evidence of aphasia although he is right-handed.

"X-rays showed slight comparative smallness of the left cranial chamber. In the pneumogram carried out last October in Havana, there was very slight comparative enlargement of the anterior part of the left lateral ventricle. The inferior horns appear quite symmetrical. There was a superficial collection of air in the central region of Rolando near the midline; side not quite certain. There is an unusual bony vascular channel in the left occipital region. The electrogram shows spike activity in the left occipital and left central areas, sometimes appearing independently.

"Family history: All members of the family including mother and father who are first cousins and the other three children have migraine. In the father's case, it is either right-sided or left-sided, interchangeably.

"Investigations of J.R.: CSF protein 76 mg% with 2WBC, Lange curve 0012332100. Left carotid angiogram was normal. Left vertebral angiogram revealed, despite adequate injection of contrast, non-filling of the basilar system with the dye remaining in the vertebral artery, compatible with either partial or complete occlusion of the upper left vertebral artery. EEG demonstrated focal electrographic status from the posterior half of the left hemisphere involving the left occipital and left central region."

The patient underwent a left craniotomy with removal of the left occipital lobe. Again we quote from Dr. Penfield's operative note: "There was true abnormality of the occipital lobe particularly in the vicinity of the calcarine fissure. There was very marked electrographic abnormality of the epileptogenic type. There was a second area in the region of the precentral gyrus, where shoulder movement could be produced. The occipital lobe has been removed. . . . Progress very guarded." The operative specimen showed microscopic changes similar to those seen at autopsy.

He continued to deteriorate and died 3 weeks later. Aside from operative defects, gross abnormality of cortex was seen in the left parietal and both occipital lobes. Microscopic abnormalities were present as far forward as the right rolandic cortex. The lesions here were poorly demarcated and alternated with normal areas. There were varying degrees of neuronal loss, astrocytic hypertrophy, and microglial infiltration (Figures 14.10, 14.11, 14.12). His cortical vessels were mildly increased in size in affected areas. His hippocampi, basal ganglia, and cerebellum were all normal.

Summary.   Migraine started in childhood in a boy with strong family history of classical migraine. Seizures developed at age 15 leading to left occipital and central status epilepticus. A left occipital lobectomy was carried out in an attempt to reduce the epileptogenic abnormality. He died 3 weeks later. Extensive cortical lesions were found during the autopsy.

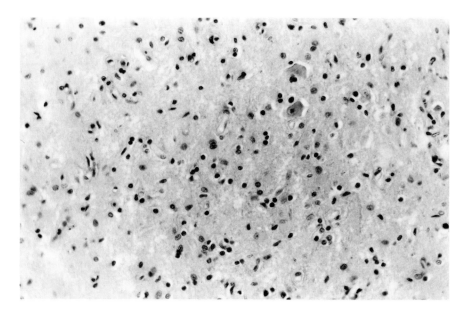

Figure 14.10   Case 8. This section of cortex shows severe neuronal loss with increase in astrocytes and microglia (H&E × 220).

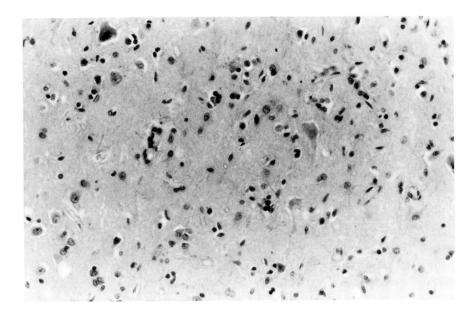

Figure 14.11   Case 8. This area of cortex is abnormal because of the astrocytic and microglial reaction but it is adjacent to an almost normal area (H&E × 220).

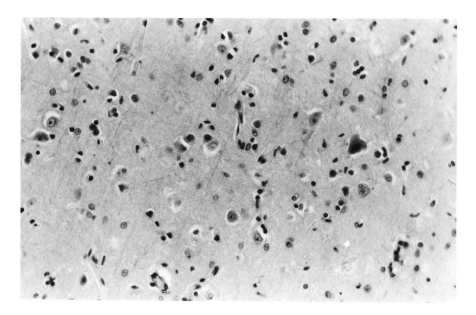

Figure 14.12   Case 8. The cortex here is almost normal, although it is adjacent to the abnormal area in the previous figure (H&E × 220).

CASE 9   The patient was a 9-year-old boy, the brother of the previous patient. Again we quote from Dr. Penfield's history obtained from the parents in 1958:

"The brother of J.R. was normal until, as a boy of 8 or 9, he had a seizure beginning in the right hand at the time of a very severe febrile illness. The illness was due to an intestinal parasite which produced dysentery. He spent from July 1945 to March 1946 in the Boston Children's Hospital. When he left the hospital, he was normal physically and mentally. On leaving, however, the father pointed out to Dr. Lennox and to Dr. Bronson Crothers, that if they held the boy's right hand quietly they would feel a periodic contraction of the grip which came at regular intervals of some seconds. The patient was changed from Phenobarbital to Dilantin and that same day or the next day, he called to his mother and when she went to him he was having a seizure. Following this, he continued to have attacks which consisted in bilateral symmetrical simultaneous jerking of the arms and perhaps the legs but without loss of consciousness. When he was anaesthetized to try to stop them the attacks returned, first on the right."

The attacks continued until he died. An autopsy of the brain was carried out at Boston Children's Hospital in 1947. There was severe loss of nerve cells from the cerebral cortex, especially in the deeper layers, associated with swollen bodied astrocytes and microglia. The white matter was normal. There was also loss of Purkinje cells and of some neurons in the pons and medulla.

Summary.   The brother of the previous patient developed seizures at age 8 or 9 progressing to status epilepticus and death at age 10. Neuronal degeneration and gliosis were found at autopsy. A diagnosis of Alpers' disease was entertained by the pathologist, Dr. Betty Banker.

DISCUSSION

These nine patients all have a history of migraine, usually classical in its features and often associated with occipital symptoms. They all had seizures. In some, the seizure disorder initially appeared benign, but all progressed to malignant partial epilepsy, and all developed cerebral lesions, particularly, but not exclusively, in the posterior cerebral territory. The course was unrelentingly progressive, leading to severe bilateral cerebral dysfunction and neurologic deficits. The striking clinical similarity of these nine patients, with their tendency to develop bilateral occipital lesions, suggests a common pathogenesis.

Among the patients there was a strong predominance of males, eight, and only one female. Onset was early in life. Four developed symptoms in the first decade, four in the second decade, and only one in the third.

Three patients initially presented with seizures. These were occipital with localized foci in two and a history of visual phenomena at the onset of the attacks in the third. Migrainous symptoms preceding the seizures were not reported in these three patients but the retrospective information available about this part of the history might not be reliable. Initially, the seizures were easily controlled, recurred at long intervals, and had no particular precipitation. They had little resemblance to the episodes of partial status or repetitive attacks that became prominent later in the course of the illness.

In the other patients, the illness started with migraine which was usually classical and severe. These early attacks were often followed by prolonged but not permanent neurologic deficits, and this was noted in four cases (Cases 1, 4, 5, and 8). Visual manifestations were prominent in seven, and a clear history of sensory symptoms or dysphasia was lacking. Case 9 had no clear history of migraine; his brother, Case 8, had severe and prominent migraine and their consanguinous parents both had classical migraine. The history of Case 9 is old and posthumous; when it was recorded, attention was mainly focused on the seizures and the pathologic findings.

The response of migraine to medication in the early stages could not be well assessed in this group of patients as they were usually seen at a time when they already had neurologic deficits; no reliable retrospective information was available. Vigorous antimigraine treatment in the later stages of the illness did not prevent recurrence of attacks (Cases 3, 4, and 7).

The patients then proceeded to develop increasingly severe seizures, often ushered in or triggered by prolonged migrainous symptomatology such as headache, prostration, and vomiting. At times, the migrainous symptoms amounted to migrainous status and lasted for many days. They were associated with recurrent visual phenomena in seven cases. These visual changes were at times difficult to distinguish from focal occipital epileptic manifestations and were usually superimposed on severe ongoing headaches, nausea, and vomiting.

When the epileptic attacks were especially prolonged and lasted for more than 1 day, they led to permanent neurologic deficits. Seizure patterns in this

Table 14.1   Nine Patients with Classical Migraine, Intractable Epilepsy, and Multiple Strokes

Case Number	Onset of Seizures (yr)	Onset of Intractable Seizures (yr)	Onset of Migraine (yr)	Onset of CNS Deficit (yr)
1	13	18	18	18
2	9	17	17	18
3	27	38	Early	38
4	12	12	5	13
5	18	18	17	18
6	19	19	19	?
7	13	13	13	13
8	15	18	Childhood	18
9	8	8	8	8

phase of the illness were varied and included generalized attacks, partial simple seizures with or without secondary generalization, myoclonic seizures, and epilepsia partialis continua.

Once permanent neurologic deficits were present, severe and prolonged partial status epilepticus with secondary generalization developed in six pa-

Pathology	Lactic H⁺	Muscle	Present Status
Autopsy: multiple cortical infarcts	—	—	Died at 20 yrs
Biopsy: inconclusive	—	—	Died at 19 yrs
Biopsy: diffuse lesions	Serum N CSF ↑	N × 2, denervation	41 yrs, demented
—	Serum ↑	Ragged red fibers	17 yrs, blind, deaf, demented
Biopsy: consistent with microstrokes	—	Denervation atrophy; Nerve: axonal degeneration	28 yrs, severe epilepsy, demented
—	—		27 yrs, blind, demented
—	Serum ↑	Ragged red fibers	15 yrs, deteriorating
Autopsy: diffuse lesions	—	—	Died at 19 yrs
Autopsy: diffuse lesions	—	—	Died at 9 yrs

(Continued on page 224)

tients, despite treatment with high doses of antiepileptic medication. The status proved difficult to control and death was attributable to complications arising from it in four patients. Antiepileptic medication also did not seem to prevent the recurrence of episodes of status epilepticus. Despite intensive questioning, no obvious trigger leading to the bouts of migraine or epileptic status that

Table 14.1   *(continued)*

Case Number	Computerized Tomography (CT)	Angiography	Other
1	Bioccipital hypodensities	Nonfilling right calcarine artery; attenuation left calcarine artery	Hyperlipidemia type IV
2	Left occipital hypodensity	4-vessel study: delayed circulation in distal branches of left posterior cerebral artery	
3	Right temporal lobe hypodensity; left parieto-occipital edema	—	Thalassemia trait
4	Bioccipital hypodensities	Left carotid: poor distal vascularization with slow perfusion and irregular caliber of collaterals of plica curva and parietal arteries; normal vertebral	
5	Focal atrophy, bioccipital	Carotid: rapid transit time	
6	Hypodensity posterior half of both hemispheres	Normal carotid and vertebral	
7	Bioccipital hypodensities	Right carotid, right vertebral; narrowing of vessels suggesting infarction, medial occipital lobe; carotids: delayed and decreased perfusion right parietal, occipital, posterior temporal regions, mild edema	
8	Pre-CT era	Left carotid: normal; left vertebral: nonfilling basilar system	
9	Pre CT era		

preceded the cerebral infarctions could be determined.

Clinical events clearly referable to migrainous symptomatology were headache, nausea, vomiting, abdominal pain, confusion, aphasia, and scintillations with fortification spectra. The patients' migraine in this series had no outstanding clinical features that would lead one to suspect that they were going to develop this syndrome. In the literature there are rare case reports of migraine associated with severe neurologic deficit or death (Ferguson and Robinson, 1982; Guest and Woolf, 1964). These differ from the cases reported here by virtue of their sudden apoplectic presentation, as opposed to the stepwise deterioration seen in our patients, by the absence of seizures, and by involvement of more anterior vascular territories.

A family history of migraine was present in seven patients from six families. Classical migraine occurred in four families. In the two cases where there was no family history of migraine this was not specifically asked for, since the significance of such a history was not appreciated at the time. Two of the patients were brothers and in this family the parents were consanguinous. Both parents had inherited severe classical migraine from their common ancestor and the siblings who did not develop this syndrome also suffered from migraine. A family history of epilepsy was found in only one patient and the histories may be incomplete in this regard.

Hemiplegic migraine was often considered in the differential diagnosis. It is inherited as an autosomal dominant, and the tendency to recurrent hemiplegia is found in affected family members. Epilepsy, particularly severe epilepsy, is not a feature of hemiplegic migraine (Bradshaw and Parsons, 1965) and we do not feel that these patients have this disorder.

The bilaterality with a tendency to symmetry and the localization of the lesions led to unusually severe neurologic deficits. Cortical blindness and deafness were prominent and were seen in four cases. Other disorders of mentation such as dementia and psychotic behavior were striking. Long tract signs were not a predominant feature.

Blood laboratory data in these patients were negative. There was no evidence for thrombogenesis. Case 1 had type IV hyperlipidemia and this was probably not significant. There was no evidence of vasculitis. Case 2 had a raised ESR and Case 3 had consistently raised serum IgM.

Cerebrospinal fluid analysis showed consistently raised protein in the six patients in whom this was measured. Two patients also had positive oligoclonal banding. Case reports of cerebral infarction in complicated migraine as a single event with subsequent good recovery usually mention normal CSF (Dorfman et al., 1979). Likewise, hemiplegic migraine, a dominantly inherited disorder with repeated, stereotyped attacks, also shows normal CSF (Bradshaw and Parsons, 1965). When complicated migraine has been unusually severe, (Ferguson and Robinson 1982) with frequent attacks (Cohen and Taylor, 1979), or associated with infarction (Murphy, 1955), the raised CSF protein reflects breakdown of the blood-brain barrier. Lumbar punctures in our patients were done late in the course of the disease when the process accelerated, and permanent neurologic deficits remained following attacks of migraine and seizures. Thus, the CSF profile in the setting of migraine and cerebral infarction may simply reflect both the severity of the attacks and the chronicity of the problem.

The EEG abnormalities were severe but not specific for the syndrome. Two patients who had early seizures had occipital spike foci. With severe migrainous episodes, there was much lateralized or generalized delta activity, and with late fixed lesions and frequent seizures there was active focal epileptic discharge. Electrographic discharge during status epilepticus was also not specific, and there was at such times much delta activity with more or less prominent spike discharge.

The radiologic changes do not suggest interference with brain growth dating from birth or early life or other preexistent structural abnormalities. At the time of severe neurologic deficits, the CT scans showed a remarkable consistency, with hypodense areas or lucencies in occipitotemporal or parieto-occipital regions in all seven patients in whom they were done. In four patients this correlated with nonfilling of arteries or impaired circulation, suggesting that the area of hypodensity represented cerebral infarction. The vascular territory involved the posterior cerebral artery or calcarine distribution. The lesions tended to occur first on one side and following another attack were often found on the other side.

As an isolated event, complicated migraine can lead to cerebral infarction, and corresponding CT changes have been previously reported (Dorfman et al., 1979; Castaldo et al., 1982; Hungerford et al., 1976). The vascular occlusions seen in two of our patients would be hard to ascribe to the status itself since they involved large arteries; the vertebral in one patient and the main trunk of the posterior cerebral in the other. There was a striking absence of morphologic changes in blood vessels and there was no radiographic abnormality to suggest the presence of angiitis. The vascular changes demonstrated radiologically were suggestive of a vasospastic etiology such as the type that might be expected in migraine and are similar to what has been described in other patients with vascular occlusion associated with this condition (Dukes and Vieth, 1964; Dorfman et al., 1979; Castaldo et al., 1982).

Awareness of the syndrome of mitochondrial encephalomyopathy lactic acidosis and stroke-like episodes or MELAS syndrome (Rowland, 1983) by one of us (D.McG.) led to a muscle biopsy in Case 7. The finding of ragged red fibers in this case and subsequently in Case 4 suggested the presence of a disorder of energy metabolism in this series of patients.

Mitochondrial dysfunction has been associated with a number of rare and incompletely defined disorders of both cerebral and muscle function. These include Alpers' disease (Sandbank and Lerman, 1972), Leigh's syndrome (Crosby and Chou, 1974), Kearns-Sayre syndrome (Karpati et al., 1973), Canavan's disease (Gambetti et al., 1969), the cerebrohepatorenal syndrome of Zellweger (Goldfischer, 1973), and myoclonus epilepsy syndrome with ragged red fibers (MERRF) (Shapira et al., 1975; Shapira et al., 1977).

The pathologic hallmark of mitochondrial cytopathies, ragged red fibers, is by itself a nonspecific finding and does not indicate an exact etiology. Abnormalities of mitochondria with concomitant lactic acidemia may be roughly translated into two phenotypic clinical groups; patients with purely myopathic features and those with both muscular and cerebral abnormalities. The biochemical lesions that underlie this clinical diversity appear to involve the respiratory chain.

Beginning in the early 1970s, individual case reports described varying biochemical abnormalities associated with an inconsistent array of phenotypic syndromes. More recently, DiMauro et al. (1985) have attempted to classify the mitochondrial myopathies by dividing them into disorders of substrate utilization, oxidation and phosphorylation coupling, and respiratory chain defects. The first two generally give rise to disorders in which the myopathic features are predominant. Respiratory chain abnormalities appear to be the underlying cause of the mitochondrial encephalomyopathies. The respiratory chain is divided into four complexes and defects among these four again are phenotypically inconsistent. For instance, defects in Complex 1 (NADH–coenzyme Q reductase), which carries hydrogens from NADH to coenzyme Q, have been reported in patients with pure myopathies as well as one with an encephalomyopathy (Morgan-Hughes et al., 1982; Morgan-Hughes and Landon, 1983). Defects in Complex 3 (reduced coenzyme Q–cytochrome c-reductase, responsible for carrying electrons from coenzyme Q to cytochrome-c) share the same heterogeneity (Morgan-Hughes et al., 1977, 1982; Hayes et al., 1984). The clinical spectrum associated with deficiencies in Complex 4 (cytochrome C oxidase) is even greater and ranges from fatal infantile mitochondrial myopathy with renal involvement (DiMauro et al., 1980, 1983) to patients with Leigh's Disease (Willems, 1977) and Alpers' Disease (Prick et al., 1983).

The literature on mitochondrial encephalomyopathy discloses a syndrome comprising patients of both sexes with normal early development who present in the first or second decade of life with growth failure, short stature, and intellectual deterioration. The children develop seizures, nerve deafness, alternating hemiparesis or hemianopia, cortical blindness, and cerebral infarcts (Pavlakis et al., 1984; Riggs et al., 1984; Kuriyama et al., 1984; Holliday et al., 1983). Increased lactate and pyruvate in blood, CSF, and urine, as well as abnormal mitochondria (ragged red fibers) complete the laboratory picture. Pavlakis et al. (1984) reviewed nine published cases and added two of their own to this syndrome of mitochondrial myopathy, encephalopathy, lactic acidosis, and stroke-like episodes (MELAS).

It is no accident that investigators whose expertise lies in the area of muscle metabolism described patients in whom various myopathies dominated the clinical presentation (Bland et al., 1981; DiMauro et al., 1980; Morgan-Hughes et al, 1979; Hudgson et al., 1972; Hart et al., 1977; Hackett et al., 1973, Tarlow et al., 1973). Most of our patients were referred to the Epilepsy Service of the Montreal Neurological Institute because of intractable partial seizures or status epilepticus. This mode of presentation heightened our awareness of the epileptic and migrainous components of the syndrome.

Since migraine was prominent in our patients, it is relevant to consider to what extent it has been present in patients with MELAS. One of the patients of Pavlakis et al. had intermittent headaches. Two of the reviewed nine cases had episodic vomiting, headache, and left homonymous hemianopia following right-sided headaches. Four of the others had episodic vomiting but no headache, and one was said to have had periodic losses of consciousness. The two patients with nausea, vomiting, and unilateral headaches were in their second decade; the patients with only intermittent vomiting were in their first decade. This is consistent with the natural history of migraine; autonomic symptoms often overshadow the headache early in life. Thus, a review of the literature of mitochondrial encephalomyopathy reveals that a number of the patients had either "pounding headaches" (Hart et al., 1977) or intermittent nausea and vomiting from an early age (Askanas et al., 1978). One case report describing patients with NADH – Co Q dehydrogenase deficiency mentions nausea, vomiting, and abdominal pain followed by unilateral pounding headaches (Holliday et al., 1983). Flashing lights then preceded generalized seizures. This case history is prototypical for the syndrome we are describing.

Pavlakis et al. (1984) conclude from their review that "all" patients had ragged red fibers and "most" had elevated blood lactate concentrations; the biological markers of MELAS syndrome. They studied mitochondrial enzymes in tissue obtained from four patients and found no consistent abnormality. In our patients we found that ragged red fibers and/or raised blood and CSF lactate and pyruvate levels appear to be mutually independent. One of our patients (Case 3) had raised CSF lactate without ragged red fibers, another, (Case 7), had both ragged red fibers and increased lactate. A third patient, (Case 4), had ragged red fibers and in a fourth, Case 5, a muscle biopsy specimen was normal (lactate and pyruvate were not measured). All the mitochondrial enzymes in our patients with ragged red fibers studied by Dr. DiMauro (cytochrome c oxidase, succinate cytochrome reductase, NADH cytochrome c reductase, citrate synthase, NADH dehydrogenase and, succinate dehydrogenase) were within normal limits.

Pavlakis et al. briefly discuss the so-called Hackett-Tarlow syndrome (Hackett et al., 1973) or juvenile mitochondrial myopathy. This group of patients also overlapped with MELAS in having short stature, epilepsy, episodic vomiting, and neurosensory hearing loss. They consider it to be heterogeneous and indistinct, mainly because the syndrome evolves gradually, accruing symptoms that culminate in an encephalopathic state. In our cases we have also been impressed by the progressive evolution of the disease toward a deteriorated state with severe fixed neurologic deficits.

Despite their striking clinical resemblance, the pathology of our cases is not homogeneous. In our series, the lesions of Case 1 are strongly suggestive of cortical infarcts of varying age. Those of Case 5 are consistent with infarcts. Changes in the biopsy specimen of Case 2 are too equivocal to be classified. The lesions of Case 3 are of uncertain origin, do not resemble those of Case 1, and are not suggestive of infarction. Those of Cases 8 and 9 are relatively similar to those of Case 3, except that they show more evident neuronal loss and lack involvement of the white matter. Adequate tissue for study was present from five patients. The lesions of two suggest ischemia; the lesions of the three others do not. Nevertheless, no clinical features were found to support a division among these five patients.

Pathologic information in the series of Pavlakis et al. was available for three patients. One showed a shrunken brain with cortical atrophy. There was severe loss of neurons in the cerebral cortex with microcystic and "spongy" alteration as well as gliosis. "Profound neuronal alterations" were present in the basal ganglia and the granular layer of the cerebellum. Mineral deposits in and around blood vessels were seen in the basal ganglia. Two siblings showed focal neuronal loss in the cerebral cortex with microcystic change, gliosis, and vascular proliferation. Mineralization was seen in and around vessels of the globus pallidus and putamen. In at least one of the three patients the hippocampus was examined and appeared normal.

A patient with features of both MELAS and MERFF syndromes reported by Kuriyama et al. (1984) had pathologic findings similar to those of our Cases 1 and 5. This patient, who died at age 18, had intermittent vomiting, seizures, cerebellar ataxia, myoclonus, dementia, deafness, macular degeneration, optic atrophy, ragged red fibers, increased lactate and pyruvate in blood and CSF. Autopsy showed solitary and continuous foci of infarction, involving all lobes of the brain but most extensive in the occipital region. Both old and fresh lesions were found. There was also massive calcification in the caudate, putamen, internal capsule, lateral thalamus, and dentate nucleus. Isolated mitochondria from brain and muscle revealed decreased oxygen consumption.

Few reports have laid emphasis on the migrainous phenomena with which we have been so impressed. However, many of the patients described in the literature were deteriorated at presentation and this may have obscured a diagnosis of migraine which by definition requires a competent witness and detailed family and clinical history. Also, some of the patients with mitochondrial encephalomyopathy presented at an early age when migraine phenomena are known to be varied and protean. Unfortunately, many of the reports in the literature do not document the family history of migraine. Our group of patients emphasize both the migrainous phenomena and the strong family history of this condition.

In the study of Pavlakis et al., four of the nine patients represented two pairs of siblings; two of our patients were brothers as well. In the other cases, the family history is either negative or not commented upon. In our series, eight of nine patients were male as were eight of the eleven reviewed by Pavlakis et al. In light of the accepted increased female to male ratio in migraine, and the known maternal inheritance of mitochondrial DNA, we agree with Pavlakis' suggestion that MELAS may be transmitted by non-Mendelian maternal inheritance. Parents of our fourth patient had muscle biopsies which were studied by Dr. Gambetti. The father's biopsy specimen was normal by light and electron microscopy. The mother's biopsy specimen showed minimal nonspecific myopathic changes and some increase of lipid vacuoles associated with clusters of mitochondria that were of normal appearance. These findings suggest that the patient's mother is also affected, though to a mild degree. Maternal inheritance has recently, also, been demonstrated in MERFF by Rosing et al. (1985).

The case histories that we have presented span 25 years and are derived from referral centers in three continents, attesting to the rarity of the condition. The syndrome described has been diagnosed as a mitochondrial disorder in two of our patients. Some of our patients presented and died too long ago to confirm the diagnosis. Many of the case histories documented in the literature have, for the reasons outlined, underplayed the striking clinical presentation that so impressed us: migraine, epilepsy, and multiple strokes.

Adequate classification of these cases will only be possible when pathogenetic mechanisms are known, but they and the patients with MELAS and MERRF syndromes as well as intermediate cases can be provisionally subsumed in the category of mitochondrial encephalopathies. It is not clear whether the variation in semeiology is related merely to variation in the distribution of abnormal mitochondria or whether there is variation in the mitochondrial component affected.

The similarities in the clinical presentation of our patients are such that the presence of this syndrome may now be strongly suspected on clinical grounds. The absence of ragged red ribers on biopsy evidently does not exclude the diagnosis: muscle symptoms were either not noted or absent in our patients. It is possible that in some, the process involved the central nervous system without being reflected in skeletal muscle. Involvement of the smooth muscle of cerebral arteries could explain both the stroke-like clinical features, the radiologic findings, and some of the pathologic lesions suggesting infarction; this, however, remains speculative. Migraine is genetically determined and common in the general population. Severe migraine may lead to this devastating syndrome in patients with borderline or abnormal energy metabolism who may otherwise remain asymptomatic. This view may reconcile the findings of a positive migraine family history with the exceptional development of this syndrome in one or two family members; however, this too must remain speculative until the basic mechanisms of this disorder are understood.

REFERENCES

Askanas V, Engel WK, Britton DE, Adornato BT, Eiben RM. Reincarnation in cultured muscle of mitochondrial abnormalities. Arch Neurol 1978;35:801–9.

Bland JM, Morgan-Hughes JA, Clark JB. Mitochondrial myopathy: biochemical studies revealing a deficiency of NADH-Cytochrome b reductase activity. J Neurol Sci 1981;50:1–13.

Bradshaw P, Parsons M. Hemiplegic migraine, a clinical study. Q J Med 1965;34:65–85.

Castaldo JE, Anderson M, Reeves SG: Middle cerebral artery occlusion with migraine. Stroke 1982;13(3):308–11.

Cohen RJ, Taylor JR. Persistent neurologic sequelae of migraine: a case report. Neurology 1979;29:1175–7.

Crosby TW, Chou SM. "Ragged-red" fibers in Leigh's disease. Neurology 1974;24: 49–54.

DiMauro S, Bonilla E, Zeviani M, Nakagawa M, DeVivo DC. Mitochondrial myopathies. Ann Neurol 1985;17:521–38.

DiMauro S, Mendell JR, Sahent Z et al. Fatal infantile mitochondrial myopathy and renal dysfunction due to cytochrome-c-oxidase deficiency. Neurology 1980;30:795–804.

DiMauro S, Nicholson JF, Hays AP et al. Benign infantile mitochondrial myopathy due to reversible cytochrome-c-oxidase deficiency. Ann Neurol 1983;14(2):226–34.

Dorfman LJ, Marshall WH, Enzmann DR. Cerebral infarction and migraine: clinical and radiologic correlations. Neurology 1979;29:317–22.

Dukes HT, Vieth RG. Cerebral arteriography during migraine prodrome and headache. Neurology 1964;14:630–40.

Ferguson KS, Robinson SS. Life threatening migraine. Arch Neurol 1982;39:374–5.

Gambetti P, Mellman WJ, Gonatas NK. Familial spongy degeneration of the central nervous system (Von Bogaert-Bertrand disease). An ultrastructural study. Acta Neuropathol 1969;12:103–15.

Goldfischer S. Peroxisomal and mitochondrial defects in the cerebro-hepatorenal syndrome. Science 1973;182:62–4.

Guest IA, Woolf AL. Fatal infarction of brain in migraine. Br Med J 1964;1:225–6.

Hackett TN, Bray PF, Ziter FA, Nyhan WL, Creer KM. A metabolic myopathy associated with chronic lactic acidemia, growth failure, and nerve deafness. J Pediatr 1973;83:426–31.

Hart ZH, Chang CH, Pervin E, Neerunjun JS, Aygar R. Familial poliodystrophy, mitochondrial myopathy, and lactate acidemia. Arch Neurol 1977;34:180–5.

Hayes DJ, Lecky BR, Landon DN, Morgan-Hughes JA, Clark JB. A new mitochondrial myopathy: biochemical studies revealing a deficiency in the cytochrome b-c_1 complex (Complex III) of the respiratory chain. Brain 1984;107:1165–77.

Holliday PL, Climie A, Gilroy J, Mahmud MZ. Mitochondrial myopathy and encephalopathy: Three cases—a deficiency of NADH-CoQ dehydrogenase? Neurology 1983;33:1619–22.

Hudgson P, Bradley WG, Jenkison M. Familial "mitochondrial" myopathy—a myopathy associated with disordered oxidative metabolism in muscle fibers. Part 1. Clinical, electrophysiological and pathological findings. J Neurol Sci 1972;16:343–70.

Hungerford GD, du Boulay GH, Zilkha KJ. Computerized axial tomography in patients with severe migraine: a preliminary report. J Neurol Neurosurg Psychiatry 1976;39:990–4.

Karpati G, Carpenter S, Larbrisseau A, Lafontaine R. The Kearns-Shy syndrome. J Neurol Sci 1973;19:133–51.

Kuriyama M, Umezaki H, Fukuda Y et al. Mitochondrial encephalomyopathy with lactate pyruvate elevation and brain infarction. Neurology 1984;34:72–7.

Morgan-Hughes JA, Darveniza P, Kahn SN et al. A mitochondrial myopathy characterized by a deficiency in reducible cytochrome *b*. Brain 1977;100:617–40.

Morgan-Hughes JA, Darveniza P, Landon DN, Land JM, Clark JB. A mitochondrial myopathy with a deficiency of respiratory chain NADH-CoQ reductase activity. J Neurol Sci 1979;43:27–46.

Morgan-Hughes JA, Hayes DJ, Clark JB et al. Mitochondrial encephalomyopathies—biochemical studies in two cases revealing defects in the respiratory chain. Brain 1982;105:553–82.

Morgan-Hughes JA, Landon DN. Mitochondrial respiratory chain deficiencies in man. Some histochemical and fine structural observations. In: Scarlato G, Gerri C, eds. Mitochondrial pathology in muscle disease. Padua; Piccin Medical Books, 1983;20–37.

Murphy JF. Cerebral infarction in migraine. Neurology 1955;5:359–61.

Pavlakis SG, Phillips PC, DiMauro S, De Vivo DC, Rowland LP. Mitochondrial myopathy, encephalopathy, lactic acidosis and strokelike episodes. A distinctive clinical syndrome. Ann Neurol 1984;16:481–8.

Prick MJJ, Gabreels FJM, Trijbels JMF et al. Progressive poliodystrophy (Alpers' Disease) with a defect in cytochrome aa_3 in muscle: a report of two unrelated patients. Clin Neurol Neurosurg 1983;85:57–70.

Riggs JE, Schochet SS, Fakadej AV et al. Mitochondrial encephalomyopathy with decreased succinate-cytochrome reductase activity. Neurology 1984;34:48–53.

Rosing HS, Hopkins LC, Wallace DC, Epstein CM, Weidenheim K. Maternally inherited mitochondrial myopathy and myoclonic epilepsy. Ann Neurol 1985;17:228–37.

Rowland LP. Molecular genetics, pseudogenetics and clinical neurology. The Robert Wartenberg lecture. Neurology 1983;33:1189–1195.

Sandbank U, Lerman P. Progressive cerebral poliodystrophy—Alpers' disease: disorganized giant neuronal mitochondria on electron microscopy. J Neurol Neurosurg Psychiatry 1972;35:749–55.

Shapira Y, Cederbaum, SD, Cancilla PA, Nielsen D, Lippe BM. Familial poliodystrophy, mitochondrial myopathy and lactate acidemia. Neurology 1975;25:614–21.

Shapira Y, Harel S, Russell A. Mitochondrial encephalomyopathies: a group of neuromuscular disorders with defects in oxidative metabolism. Isr J Med Sci 1977;13(2):161–4.

Tarlow MJ, Lake BD, Lloyd JK. Chronic lactic acidosis in association with myopathy. Arch Dis Child 1973;48:485–92.

Willems JL, Monnens LAM, Trijbels JMF et al. Leighs' encephalomyelopathy in a patient with cytochrome c oxidase deficiency in muscle tissue. Pediatrics 1977;60:850–7.

II

Ictal Headache

15

Ictal Pain: Unilateral, Cephalic, and Abdominal

Warren T. Blume
G. Bryan Young

In 1831, Bright described a patient whose epileptic attacks were preceded by a "peculiar cramp-like sensation" ascending from the leg. Autopsy revealed a tumor "indenting itself into the upper part of the posterior lobe of the left hemisphere of the brain." This may be the first description of ictal pain.

Gowers (1901) gave the first systematic description and study of pain as a symptom of epileptic seizures and discerned three groups of patients by type of pain: hemicorporeal (unilateral), cephalic, and abdominal.

Of the 858 patients seen at our epilepsy unit from 1973 to 1977, 24 (2.8%) described pain in their ictal symptomatology. Young and Blume (1983) found that these patients each fell into one of Gowers' groups, which were defined as follows: (1) unilateral pain in the face, arm, leg, or trunk (unilateral group); (2) pain restricted to the scalp or calvarial region (cephalic group); and (3) central abdominal pain (abdominal group). Patients with only postictal pain, e.g., headache, or preictal pain that did not appear to be part of the seizure, were not included in this series.

UNILATERAL GROUP

Clinical Features

Of the 24 patients in our epileptic population who experienced ictal pain, 10 (1.17% of our total population) had unilateral ictal pain. Patients described it as burning, cramping, stinging, achy, electric, throbbing, or like a vibrating knife. Each of these patients was able to localize its origin and occasional march. The pain appeared anywhere on the face, trunk, or limbs, but usually on the arm. It was the first ictal symptom in three cases and followed focal sensory and/or motor symptoms on the same side in all others except for one patient in whom right arm pain followed vocalization.

The following case illustrates unilateral ictal pain particularly well:

A 14-year-old girl with a congenital left hemiparesis developed seizures at age 10. The seizures began with a "burning, tingling pain" in the left forearm that progressed to a "shooting pain" in the left shoulder. This sometimes proceeded to macropsia and then a generalized tonic-clonic seizure. On examination, her paresis was most marked in her left arm and hand. Her small left hand was analgesic and anesthetic distal to the wrist, with pinprick sensation reduced but still perceived in the remainder of the left upper limb, left upper thorax, left side of the neck, and left lower face. Position sense was impaired in the left wrist. A seizure recorded on the EEG showed reduction in voltage in the right central region just prior to the onset of left arm pain (Figure 15.1). Quasi-periodic right central sharp waves followed this flattening.

During neurosurgery the right postcentral gyrus, precentral gyrus, and inferior parietal region (Figure 15.2) were discovered to be atrophic. It is likely that this shrunken area included the "hand area," as stimulation just above this area produced a sensation of tingling in the left forearm. Cortical epileptiform activity was present superior and posterior to the gliotic area on the postcentral gyrus. Resection of the atrophic area and immediately adjacent cortex relieved her of seizures. Her sensory deficit was only slightly increased. Histologically, neuroglial nodules were present in the meninges. The cortex showed a disorganized neuronal arrangement with dense gliosis and foci of calcification.

Other illustrative cases appear at the end of the chapter. In all 10 cases,

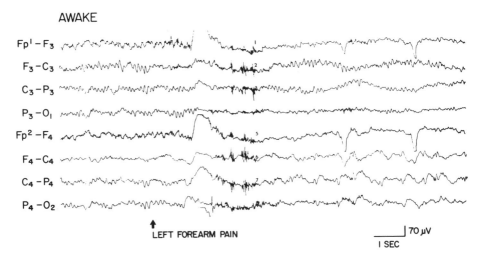

Figure 15.1   EEG recorded during a painful seizure in a 14-year-old girl. Right hemisphere EEG activity attenuates about 1 second before left forearm pain begins. Movement artifact partially obscures this attenuation. Sequential right central (C_4) spike waves constitute the remainder of the seizure.

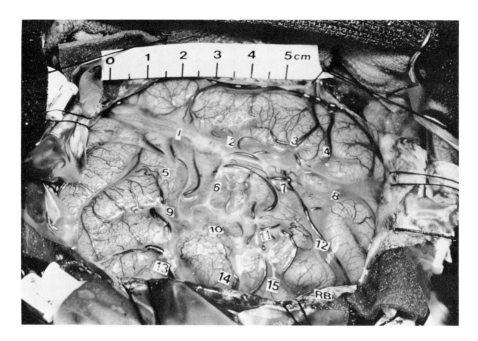

Figure 15.2   Right fronto-parieto-temporal region at surgery. Position 1 at antero-inferior corner of electrode "grid." Marked atrophy of: inferior portion of precentral gyrus, which, by stimulation, included 1, 6, 10, 14; postcentral gyrus (2, 11, 15) and anterior inferior parietal region (7, 8, 12). Epileptiform activity appeared principally at positions 11, 14, 15, and 7.

associated clinical and/or laboratory data indicated that the seizures originated in the hemisphere contralateral to the pain. Motor and sensory ictal events (6 patients) or motor phenomena alone (2 patients) appeared ipsilateral to the pain in 8 of these 10 patients. Such phenomena specifically implicated the contralateral rolandic and/or parietal regions in 7 of these 8 patients and simply lateralized the origin in the eighth patient.

Of the 5 patients with EEG-recorded painful seizures, 4 clearly involved or originated in the contralateral rolandic and/or parietal regions, including the 2 of these 10 patients whose ictal symptoms alone would not have definitely lateralized the origin. The fifth EEG-recorded seizure appeared to arise diffusely in the contralateral hemisphere.

Supporting evidence for involvement of the contralateral rolandic region came from neurologic examinations of 4 patients, all of whom had an associated hemiplegia or monoplegia. Two of these patients had sensory impairment in the same region as the motor impairment. Radiological and/or operative findings disclosed rolandic lesions in 5 patients. The above-described case provided the most convincing evidence of rolandic origin: epileptiform activity was localized to the postcentral gyrus at electrocorticography; excision of this gyrus abolished the painful seizures.

Similarly, the contralateral centroparietal region was the most common site for unilateral painful seizures in earlier series (Gowers, 1901; Head and Holmes, 1911; Michelsen, 1943; Lewin and Phillips, 1952; Russell and Whitty, 1953; Whitty, 1953; Fine, 1967; Wilkinson, 1973).

The seizures of only 2 of our 10 patients with unilateral pain were due to progressive lesions: metastatic melanoma in one and regional encephalitis (Rasmussen et al., 1958) in the other.

Mechanism

Duality of Ascending Pain Projections

Mountcastle (1974) proposed that two forebrain mechanisms exist that preserve the duality of pain carried by peripheral afferent $A\delta$ and C fibers. [$A\delta$ fibers carry sharp, pricking pain; C fibers mediate long-lasting, burning pain (Kelly, 1981)]. It is likely that the neospinothalamic system mediates short-latency, sharp, accurately localized pain via the posterior nuclear group of the thalamus to the somatosensory areas of the cerebral cortex (SI and SII). This posterior group of thalamic nuclei is a cytoarchitecturally heterogenous group of neurones lying medial to the medial geniculate body and extending rostrally to the nucleus ventralis posterior (ventrobasal complex). Neurones of the posterior nuclear group respond to noxious stimuli (see below).

In contrast, a phylogenetically older paleospinothalamic system is thought to mediate slow-onset burning pain that is difficult to localize precisely. Spinothalamic fibers of this system terminate in the medial and intralaminar thalamic nuclei either directly or indirectly via the bulbar and mesencephalic reticular formation. Noxious somatic stimuli elicit discharges of the nucleus gigantocellularis of the medullary reticular formation (Casey, 1969; Collins and Randt, 1958; Goldman et al., 1972) and the mesencephalic reticular formation (Collins and Randt, 1960; Young and Gottschaldt, 1976). Because these nuclei project to the diffuse thalamocortical system, the hypothalamus, and the limbic system, including the cingulate gyrus, the paleospinothalamic system may mediate the arousal and affective reactions to painful stimuli.

Descriptions of pain by our unilateral group of patients (sharp, stinging, shock-like; burning, cramp-like, achy) suggest that either or both systems may be involved in different patients.

Parietal Lesions and Pain

Considerable clinical and experimental data suggest that both the cortical and thalamic components of the neospinothalamic system are involved in appreciation of pain and therefore in producing painful seizures.

Parietal lobe lesions in humans have given rise to spontaneous pain (Biemond, 1956; Fields and Adams, 1974; Hamby, 1961; Marshall, 1951; Michelsen, 1943). Conversely, Kleist (1922, cited by Biedenbach, 1979) found impaired pain and temperature sensation in lesions involving areas 3a and 3b of Brodmann. Others, such as Marshall (1951) and Russell (1945), also have found that parietal lesions may be associated with an elevation of the pain threshold on the contralateral side.

Several authors (Erickson, Bleckwenn, and Woolsey, 1952; Lewin and Phillips, 1952; Hamby, 1961; Lende et al., 1971; Young and Blume, 1983) have reported abolition of painful seizures by surgical removal of the postcentral gyrus.

The hyperpathia that may develop after some parietal lesions (Marshall, 1951) may indicate a dual cortical role in pain appreciation, with some parietal corticofugal fibers inhibiting the response to nociceptive afferent impulses (Mountcastle, 1974). An experimental correlate is provided by Peele (1944), who found that lesions in area 3 of the parietal lobe of monkeys permanently elevated the pain threshold on the contralateral side. In contradistinction, lesions in areas 1, 2, 5, and 7 gave a transient hypalgesia but contralateral hyperpathia later developed.

Parietal Stimulation

Stimulation of the postcentral gyrus occasionally elicits contralateral pain (Erickson, Bleckwenn, and Woolsey, 1952; Lewin and Phillips, 1952; Hamby, 1961), especially when its sulcal portion is stimulated. Stimulation is apparently more likely to elicit pain in subjects with somatosensory cortical lesions that cause spontaneous pain, but only in the pain-producing lesion area (Hamby, 1961).

Pain-evoked Potentials

Biedenbach et al. (1979) stimulated the tooth pulp (a pain-specific stimulus) of nonhuman primates, and obtained evoked potentials within the somatosensory "face" area of the postcentral gyrus with a mean latency of 13.6 msec for single shocks and 24.9 msec for multiple shocks. These latencies suggest that the impulses traveled primarily by the neospinothalamic pathway. The main focus of both pulp-driven neurones was found at the base of the central sulcus corresponding to cytoarchitectonic area 3a. Andersson et al. (1973), stimulating the tooth pulp, elicited unitary activity at the lateral part of the coronal gyrus in the cat with a latency of 5 to 12 msec.

Human evoked potential data also suggest that the cortex participates in pain appreciation. However, the relatively long latencies raise questions about the pathway(s) involved. Chatrian et al. (1975) evoked two types of cerebral responses in humans to painful tooth pulp stimulation: low postcentral and vertex. The authors wondered if the apparently longer latency of postcentral potentials from these scalp recordings than in direct recordings from monkeys resulted from lack of scalp penetration by earlier potentials. Therefore, these potentials could have been transmitted by the neospinothalamic system via the posterior nuclear group of the thalamus. The vertex potentials may have been produced by the cingulate gyrus, having ascended via the paleospinothalamic system.

Carmon et al. (1976), Carmon et al. (1978), Chen et al. (1979), and Carmon et al. (1980) all correlated the amplitude of long-latency pain-evoked vertex potentials in humans with subjective estimation of pain intensity suggesting mediation via the polysynaptic paleospinothalamic system. This system is thought to be responsible for the estimation of pain intensity and for the affective reactions to pain (Mountcastle, 1974).

Role of the Thalamus

Cortically originating epileptic seizures might also elicit pain because of spread to thalamic nuclei. Wilder et al. (1969), Kusske and Rush (1978), Morillo et al. (1982), and others have demonstrated early and prominent spread of cortical epileptic discharges to thalamic and other subcortical nuclei. Gutnick and Prince (1972, 1974) recorded spike bursts in thalamocortical relay cells whose axons projected to a penicillin-induced cortical epileptogenic focus. Such spike bursts coincided with bursts of cortical spikes that were shown to travel antidromically to the thalamic nuclei. In an anatomical study, Jones and Powell (1968) showed that somatosensory cortical areas SI and SII each project in a topographically organized manner upon the nucleus ventralis posterior and upon the posterior group of thalamic nuclei.

Hassler (1970) found that repetitive stimulation of the posterior nuclear group of the thalamus gave localized pain in conscious humans. In this area, Poggio and Mountcastle (1960) found that 60% of cells responded only to noxious stimulation of large peripheral receptive fields. Curry (1972) found that only 3% of posterior nuclear group cells responded to noxious stimuli, but the difference may be due to his use of deeper anesthesia than that employed by Poggio and Mountcastle. Casey (1966) found cells in the posterior nuclear group that responded more actively to the noxious than to innocuous stimuli.

The paleothalamic system may also become involved in some cortically originating seizures as there are considerable corticofugal projections upon intralaminar thalamic nuclei (Brodal, 1981). McLachlan et al. (1984) recorded burst firing in centralis lateralis (an intralaminar thalamic nucleus) following burst firing of cortical neurones during generalized seizures in the cat. Casey (1966) obtained abundant cell discharges in intralaminar and medial thalamic nuclei from noxious peripheral stimuli, supporting their role in pain appreciation. Moreover, stimulation of the medial thalamus may give diffuse, burning pain in humans (Sano, 1977).

SUMMARY

The above data suggest that cortically originating seizures may cause pain by either or both of the following mechanisms: (1) epileptic discharge involving cortical areas shown experimentally and clinically to be involved in pain appreciation, and (2) spread of a cortically originating epileptic discharge ortho- or antidromically to thalamic areas involved in ascending nociceptive pathways.

CEPHALIC GROUP

Clinical Features

The 11 patients with cephalic ictal pain comprised 1.3% of our epilepsy patients, an incidence strikingly similar to that of Gowers (1.4%).

Only 2 patients described the pain as throbbing. Others described it as sharp or steady, but many were unable to ascribe quality to it. Cephalic pain initiated the seizure in 8 patients and accompanied other ictal symptoms in 3.

Although the pain was unilateral in 7 of these 11 patients, the site of pain bore no relationship to that of the known or presumed seizure origin.

All patients had partial seizures. The nature and location of EEG abnormalities varied considerably from patient to patient, but 4 patients had occipital EEG foci interictally. In 2 of these, the right occipital and right posterior temporal regions were the origins of recorded seizures with cephalic pain.

Similarly, Camfield, et al. (1978) described 4 adolescents with a triad of basilar-type migraine, sporadic and easily controlled seizures, and severe EEG abnormalities. Seizures followed a migrainous aura without cephalic pain in all of these patients; in 2 of these, an inappropriately severe pounding headache followed the seizures.

In summary, cephalic pain is a definite component of some partial epileptic seizures but it does not indicate the site of seizure origin. However, occipital-posterior temporal foci may be ultimately shown to be more common in partial seizures with this feature.

Mechanism

The mechanism of seizure-associated cephalic pain remains unknown. A causal link may be free fatty acid release. Under some pathophysiological conditions, such as experimental electroconvulsions or chemically induced seizures, there is a rapid accumulation of cortical free fatty acids, especially arachidonic acid which is a precursor for prostaglandin synthesis (Bazan, 1971; Marion and Wolfe, 1978; Chapman, Ingvar, and Siesjö, 1980). Consequently, there is a sharp rise in the cortical levels of prostaglandins $F_{2\alpha}$ and E_2 during such convulsions (Chapman, 1981; Folco, Longiave, and Bosisio, 1977; Marion and Wolfe, 1978) and of prostaglandin $F_{2\alpha}$ in the cerebrospinal fluid (CSF) of patients with epilepsy (Wolfe and Coceani, 1979).

Whether plasma free fatty acid or prostaglandin levels increase during clinical seizures is unknown. However, the following sequence of events has been postulated to occur in migraine headache. Free fatty acids initially release serotonin from platelets (Anthony, 1982). Serotonin, a cranial artery vasoconstrictor, is then thought to become absorbed onto the vessel walls, combining with histamine and kinins to increase their sensitivity to pain (Fanchamps, 1982). The later drop in plasma serotonin levels, together with a rise in prostaglandins, would each give painful dilatation of the cranial vasculature (Anthony, 1982). A similar mechanism might occur to produce epileptic cephalic pain.

ABDOMINAL GROUP

Three patients, 0.35% of our epileptic population, had painful abdominal aurae leading immediately to clear signs of epileptic seizures. The same sequence occurred in 1.17% of Gowers' (1901) series.

Clinical and EEG data pointed to a temporal lobe origin for the attacks in each of our three cases. In one of these cases an EEG seizure originating in the right anterior-midtemporal region was associated with abdominal pain followed by loss of consciousness and automatisms.

In both this and Gowers' series, when pain was the initial abdominal sensation, it remained in the epigastrium until consciousness was lost.

Despite the popular term "abdominal epilepsy," well-documented cases of epileptic abdominal pain are rare (Prichard, 1958). Associated interictal "epileptiform" EEG abnormalities fail to establish the diagnosis but are frequently cited as supporting evidence in the literature. Obligatory diagnostic criteria should be: (1) a consistent association of abdominal pain with other undeniable signs and symptoms of a cerebral seizure, or (2) abdominal pain occurring during two or more EEG-recorded seizures.

The mechanism of these attacks remains obscure, but involvement of the paleospinothalamic system with its limbic connections is possible.

CASE HISTORIES

Unilateral Group

CASE 1   A 25-year-old man who had a mild congenital right hemiparesis developed seizures at age 10. Initial paresthesiae in the right palm spread to the fingers, then to the shoulder, then to the face, then to the thorax and leg (all on the right side). This was followed by tonic right-sided posturing, then clonic jerks on the right side of the body associated with pain in the right arm "like a thousand bee stings." Examination showed a dense right homonymous hemianopia, poor fine movements of the right hand, and impaired proprioception and stereognosis in the right hand. EEG showed frequent left occipitalparietal and left frontal spikes and sharp waves. Alpha activity was absent on the left side. A computerized tomogram (CT) showed a porencephalic cyst involving the left parieto-occipital regions. During neurosurgery the postcentral gyrus was found to be shrunken. With electrocorticography, spikes were mainly present above the superior part of the cyst. Subpial resection of the margins of the cyst was followed by relief from seizures. On histologic examination extensive gliosis and intracortical calcification were present as well as heterotopic areas of gray matter.

CASE 2   A 16-year-old boy developed seizures at age 10. These began with paresthesiae in the left shoulder that spread to the left arm and then marched to the face. Then a spread of pain "like white noise" marched in the same manner. This was followed by tonic posturing of the left arm and deviation of the head and eyes to the left side. Mild impairment of left foot movements constituted the only abnormality on examination. An EEG showed occasional central sagittal sharp waves. Recorded seizures began with a 30 to 35 Hz rhythm in the central sagittal-right central region. A CT showed an atrophic area in the right central area near the vertex.

CASE 3   A 28-year-old woman had a 5-year history of intractable seizures that began with an illusion of body movement followed by tightness in the left cheek. She then noted an "achy" left retroauricular pain that spread to the left shoulder. This was followed by subjective left-sided numbness with loss of pinprick sensation in the left arm and leg. Then, left-sided tonic posturing occurred, followed by left-sided clonic movements and a generalized clonic seizure. The recorded seizure began with rhythmic waves in the right parieto-occipital-posterior temporal area that spread to the right anterior-midtemporal region and then spread diffusely over the right hemisphere. Right parietal and posterior temporal epileptiform abnormalities appeared interictally on scalp, subdural, and electrocorticographic recordings.

CASE 4   A 35-year-old woman with metastatic malignant melanoma developed seizures beginning with a throbbing sensation in the right hip, ascending to the trunk. This sensation became more intense until she noticed pain in the right hip and trunk. She then developed clonic movements of the right hip. Neurologic examination was negative. An EEG showed 4 to 7 Hz low-voltage waves in the left parietal region as the only abnormality. The CT revealed a metastatic lesion in the left superior parietal lobe with minimal edema.

Cephalic Group

CASE 5   A 21-year-old woman began having seizures at age 12. The most frequent of her four types of seizures began with a throbbing, left parietal headache immediately followed by hearing a "beeping noise." Her arms trembled and she saw flashing colored lights in the left visual field. After this she lost consciousness and had a generalized tonic-clonic seizure. Neurologic examination and general physical examination were negative. An EEG showed independent biocciptal and posterior temporal spikes, maximal on the right side. Electrographic seizures, unaccompanied by clinical symptoms, began with rhythmic saw-toothed 5 Hz waves in the right posterior temporo-occipital region. The cause of the seizures is unknown.

CASE 6   A 46-year-old man had a 1 year history of seizures. A "sharp, severe" headache in the right supraorbital area was followed by loss of consciousness with deviation of head and eyes to the left and then a generalized tonic-clonic seizure. Postictal examination was normal. The EEG showed medium voltage 2 to 3 Hz arhythmic waves in the right occipital-posterior temporal region. An electrographic seizure without clinical accompaniment consisted of 15 Hz medium-voltage rhythmic waves in the right occipital region, with some spread to the posterior temporal and right parietal area lasting 30 seconds and followed by 4 to 5 Hz medium-voltage waves in the same region. A CT showed increased density in the right posterior temporo-occipital region. The histologic nature of the lesion is not yet known.

CASE 7   This 20-year-old woman had generalized tonic-clonic seizures from her early childhood until age 16, when she had seizures that began with a sharp pain in the left temple that then spread to both temporal regions. She then experienced a sensation of "needles picking the scalp," especially in the vertex region. She would then lose consciousness, stare blankly, and have automatisms. Examination was negative. The EEG showed occasional sharp waves in the right temporal region.

Abdominal Group

CASE 8   This 21-year-old man had hemiconvulsions in childhood. His seizures subsequently began with a "sharp" abdominal pain, "like someone hitting me with an axe," followed by a loss of consciousness with automatisms. Apart from dull-normal intelligence, there was no neurologic deficit. His EEG showed multiple independent spikes, maximal in the right anterior temporal and superior frontal regions. A recorded clinical and electrographic seizure began in the right anterior-midtemporal region.

SUMMARY

Pain that is part of an epileptic seizure can be any of three types: (1) unilateral pain involving face, arm, leg, or trunk; (2) cephalic pain involving the calvarial region, or (3) abdominal pain. Unilateral pain appears to be due to involvement of the contralateral rolandic region, especially the primary sensory area, SI. Cephalic pain has no consistent localizing value for the site of the cerebral seizure. It likely is due to a vascular mechanism and may share with migraine an increased free fatty acid and prostaglandin production. Abdominal pain reflected temporal lobe seizures in our patients; the mechanism for its production is uncertain, but may involve the paleospinothalamic system.

REFERENCES

Andersson SA, Keller O, Vyklicky L. Cortical activity evoked from tooth pulp afferents. Brain Res 1973;50:473–5.

Anthony M. Serotonin and cyclic nucleotides in migraine. In: Critchley M, Friedman A, Gorini S, and Sicuteri F, eds. Advances in neurology. New York: Raven Press, 1982;33:45–8.

Bazan NG Jr. Changes in free fatty acids of brain by drug-induced convulsions, electroshock and anaesthesia. J Neurochem 1971;18:1379–85.

Biedenbach MA, VanHassel HJ, Brown AC. Tooth pulp-driven neurons in somatosensory cortex of primates: role in pain mechanisms including a review of the literature. Pain 1979;7:31–50.

Biemond A. The conduction of pain above the level of the thalamus opticus. AMA Arch Neurol Psychiatry 1956;75:231–44.

Bright R. Reports of medical cases. London, vol. 2, Part 2, 1831. Cited by Jasper HH. In: Penfield W, Jasper H, eds. Epilepsy and the functional anatomy of the human brain. Boston: Little Brown, 1954:15.

Brodal A. Neurological anatomy. 3rd ed. Oxford: Oxford University Press, 1981:99.

Camfield PR, Metrakos K, Andermann F. Basilar migraine, seizures and severe epileptiform EEG abnormalities. Neurology 1978;28:584–8.

Carmon A, Dotan Y, Sarne Y. Correlation of subjective pain experience with cerebral evoked responses to noxious thermal stimulations. Exp Brain Res 1978;33:445–53.

Carmon A, Mor J, Goldberg J. Evoked cerebral responses to noxious thermal stimuli in humans. Exp Brain Res 1976;25:103–7.

Carmon A, Friedman Y, Coger R, Kenton B. Single trial analysis of evoked potentials to noxious thermal stimulation in man. Pain 1980;8:21–32.

Casey KL. Unit analysis of nociceptive mechanisms in the thalamus of the awake squirrel monkey. J Neurophysiol 1966;29:727–50.

Casey KL. Somatic stimuli, spinal pathways and size of cutaneous fibers influencing unit activity in the medial medullary reticular formation. Exp Neurol 1969;25:35–56.

Chapman AG. Free fatty acid release and metabolism of adenosine and cyclic nucleotides during prolonged seizures. In: Morselli PL, Lloyd KG, Löscher W, Meldrum B, Reynolds EH, eds. Neurotransmitters, seizures and epilepsy. New York: Raven Press, 1981:165–73.

Chapman A, Ingvar M, Siesjö BK. Free fatty acids in the brain in bicuculline-induced status epilepticus. Acta Physiol Scand 1980;110:335–6.

Chatrian GE, Canfield, RC, Knauss TA, Lettich E. Cerebral responses to electrical tooth pulp stimulation in man. Neurology 1975;25:745–57.

Chen ACN, Chapman CR, Harkins SW. Brain evoked potentials are functional correlates of induced pain in man. Pain 1979;6:365–74.

Collins WF, Randt CT. Midbrain evoked responses relating to peripheral unmyelinated or "C" fibers in cat. J Neurophysiol 1960;23:47–53.

Collins WF, Randt CT. Evoked central nervous system activity relating to peripheral unmyelinated or "C" fibers in cat. J Neurophysiol 1958;21:345–52.

Curry MJ. The exteroceptive properties of neurones in the somatic part of the posterior group (PO). Brain Res 1972;44:439–62.

Erickson TC, Bleckwenn WJ, Woolsey CN. Observations on the post central gyrus in relation to pain. Trans Am Neurol Assoc 1952;77:57–9.

Fanchamps A. The evolution of thinking about the role and site of action of serotonin in migraine. In: Critchley M, Friedman A, Gorini S, Sicuteri F, eds. Advances in neurology. New York: Raven Press, 1982;33:31–3.

Fields HL, Adams JE. Pain after cortical injury relieved by electrical stimulation of the internal capsule. Brain 1974;97:169–78.

Fine W. Post-hemiplegic epilepsy in the elderly. Br Med J 1967;1:199–201.

Folco, GC, Longiave D, Bosisio E. Relations between prostaglandin E_2, F_{2a} and cyclic nucleotide levels in rat brain and induction of convulsions. Prostaglandins 1977;13:893–900.

Goldman PL, Collins WF, Taub A, Fitzmartin J. Evoked bulbar reticular unit activity following delta fiber stimulation of peripheral somatosensory nerve in cat. Exp Neurol 1972;37:597–606.

Gowers WR. Epilepsy and other convulsive disorders: their causes, symptoms and treatment. London: Churchill, 1901:29–58.

Gutnick MJ, Prince DA. Thalamocortical relay neurons: antidromic invasion of spikes from a cortical epileptogenic focus. Science 1972;176:424–6.

Gutnick MJ, Prince DA. Effects of projected cortical epileptiform discharges on neuronal activities in cat VPL. Interictal discharge. J Neurophysiol 1974;37:1310–27.

Hamby WB. Reversible central pain. Arch Neurol 1961;5:82–6.

Hassler R. Dichotomy of facial pain conduction in the diencephalon. In: Hassler R, Walker AE, eds. Trigeminal neuralgia. Philadelphia: WB Saunders, 1970: 123–38.

Head H, Holmes G. Sensory disturbances from cerebral lesions. Brain 1911;34:102–254.

Jones EG, Powell TPS. The projection of the somatic sensory cortex upon the thalamus in the cat. Brain Res 1968;10:369–91.

Kelly DD. Central representations of pain and analgesia. In: Kandel ER, Schwartz JA, eds. Principles of neural science. New York: Elsevier/North-Holland, 1981:199–212.

Kleist K. Kriegsverletzungen des Gehirns in ihrer Bedeutung für die Hirnlokalisation und Hirnpathologie. In: Handbuch der aerztlichen Erfahrungen in Weltkriege 1914/18, vol. 4, part 2. JA Barth Leipzig, 1922:443–7. Cited by Biedenbach MA.

Kusske JA, Rush JL. Corpus callosum and propagation of afterdischarge to contralateral cortex and thalamus. Neurology 1978;28:905–12.

Lende RA, Kirsch WM, Druckman R. Relief of facial pain after combined removal of precentral and postcentral cortex. J Neurosurg 1971;34:537–43.

Lewin W, Phillips CG. Observations on partial removal of the post-central gyrus for pain. J Neurol Neurosurg Psychiatry 1952;15:143–7.

Marion J, Wolfe LS. Increase in vivo of unesterified fatty acids, prostaglandin $F_{2\alpha}$ but not thromboxane B_2 in rat brain during drug induced convulsions. Prostaglandins 1978;16:99–110.

Marshall J. Sensory disturbances in cortical wounds with special reference to pain. J Neurol Neurosurg Psychiatry 1951;14:187–204.

McLachlan RS, Gloor P, Avoli M. Differential participation of specific and non-specific thalamic nuclei in generalized spike and wave discharges in feline generalized penicillin epilepsy. Brain 1984;307:277–87.

Michelsen JJ. Subjective disturbances of the sense of pain from lesions of the cerebral cortex. Res Publ Assoc Res Nerv Ment Dis 1943;23:86–99.

Morillo LE, Ebner TJ, Bloedel JR. The early involvement of subcortical structures during the development of a cortical seizure focus. Epilepsia 1982;23:571–86.

Mountcastle VB. Medical physiology. 13th ed. St. Louis, CV Mosby, 1974;1:364–7.

Peele TL. Acute and chronic parietal lobe ablations in monkeys. J Neurophysiol 1944;7:269–86.

Poggio GF, Mountcastle VB. A study of the functional contributions of the lemniscal and spinothalamic systems to somatic sensibility. Bull Johns Hopkins Hosp 1960;106:266–316.

Prichard JS. Abdominal pain of cerebral origin in children. Can Med Assoc J 1958;78:665–7.

Rasmussen T, Olszewski J, Lloyd-Smith D. Focal seizures due to chronic localized encephalitis. Neurology 1958;8:435–45.

Russell WR. Transient disturbances following gunshot wounds to the head. Brain 1945;68:79–97.

Russell WR, Whitty CWM. Studies in traumatic epilepsy. J Neurol Neurosurg Psychiatry 1953;16:73–97.

Sano K. Intralaminar thalamotomy (thalamolaminotomy) and postero-medial hypothalamotomy in the treatment of intractable pain. Prog Neurol Surg 1977;8:50–103.

Whitty CWM. Causalgic pain as an epileptic aura. Epilepsia 1953;2:37–41.

Wilder BJ, King RL, Schmidt RP. Cortical and subcortical secondary epileptogenesis. Neurology 1969;19:643–58.

Wilkinson HA. Epileptic pain. Neurology 1973;23:518–20.

Wolfe LS, Coceani F. The role of prostaglandins in the central nervous system. Annu Rev Physiol 1979;41:669–84.

Young GB, Blume WT. Painful epileptic seizures. Brain 1983;106:537–54.

Young DW, Gottschaldt K-M. Neurons in the rostral mesencephalic reticular formation of the cat responding specifically to noxious mechanical stimulation. Exp Neurol 1976;51:628–36.

16

Hemicrania Epileptica: Synchronous Ipsilateral Ictal Headache with Migraine Features

H. Isler
H. G. Wieser
M. Egli

Ictal headaches have been described as more or less separate clinical entities since the middle of the nineteenth century: cephalalgia epileptica (Sieveking, 1854), cephalalgia epileptiformis (Sieveking, 1858), hemicrania epileptica (Flatau, 1912), recurrent paroxysmal headache (Livingston, 1954), epileptic cephalea, (Halpern and Bental, 1958), headaches as seizure equivalents (Jonas, 1966), cefalea paroxística epiléptica (Diaz y Diaz, 1976), epileptischer Kopfschmerz (Hess, 1977), seizure headaches (Swaiman and Frank, 1978), cephalic painful epileptic seizures (Young and Blume, 1983), headache as an epileptic manifestation (Laplante et al., 1983).

Although these sources confirm the existence of headache as the only, or at least, the main symptom of seizures, they report headache as an aura as well as headache representing later phases. The topography of the headache is rarely correlated with electroencephalographic (EEG) localization, and the clinical changes seldom correlate with changes in the EEG during the attack (Laplante et al., 1983, and Young and Blume, 1983 are the main exceptions).

The prevailing lack of clear correlations in space and time adds to the difficulties of distinguishing definite ictal headaches from those more vague entities that have been interpreted as "missing links" (Hughlings Jackson, 1931) between migraine and epilepsy, or in the "borderland of epilepsy" (Gowers, 1907), such as Weil's "dysrhythmic migraine" (1952). It appears necessary to confirm this difference since anticonvulsive management is clearly indicated in definite seizure headache while it may be much less appropriate in headache syndromes with inconclusive EEG abnormalities. Although a special drug combination, Sanredo, was created for the treatment of "dysrhythmic migraine," this compound of phenytoin, caffeine, and dihydroergotamine had to be discontinued for lack of results.

We have found a few cases of ictal headache with clear-cut correlations in space and time with topographic EEG changes documented by intracerebral EEG recordings, and we have found similar cases in other clinical groups of patients who could not be investigated by this radical method. We presented these findings in 1982 (Isler et al., 1984), proposing the term "hemicrania epileptica" for these synchronous ipsilateral ictal headaches in order to distinguish them from migraine—for which they had been mistaken over many years—and from other less clearly defined headaches occurring during or after seizures, and to avoid confusion with "dysrhythmic" and other migraine with less specific EEG abnormalities.

THE CASES

Studies Done at the Stereo EEG Section of the Department of Neurology

In order to map epileptogenic areas for surgical excision, 91 patients with drug-resistant seizures were investigated by depth electrodes that were stereotaxically inserted through burr holes, remaining in place for 4 to 20 days. Several spontaneous seizures were recorded in every case by long-term monitored simultaneous surface and depth EEG on split-screen videotape. Cortex and nuclei were also electrically stimulated by repetitive square-wave pulses.

Of 91 patients, 18 complained of headache or painful or disturbing paresthesias in the head during recorded seizure activity. Fifteen of 18 patients had complex partial seizures, 2 had partial motor seizures, and 1 had mixed seizures. Three patients with complex partial seizures complained of acute hemicranial headache ipsilateral to the epileptogenic area. They said that this was the same headache that had been previously diagnosed and treated, without success, as migraine.

In these 18 patients with "cephalic" (Young and Blume, 1983) symptoms, primary epileptogenic areas were mostly in the amygdala and the hippocampal formation, and in the temporoparietal area (Table 16.1). In most cases, the history of seizures was preceded by that of headache (Table 16.2). Altogether, 6 of the 18 "cephalic" patients had at some time been treated for migraine, but only the 3 mentioned above had frequent migraine-like headache coinciding with recorded seizure activity. Their headache was described as more violent and more clearly defined than that of the other patients (Table 16.3).

The histories and findings of these 3 most typical cases are summarized in Table 16.4. Two more patients with histories of "migraine" had ipsilateral hemicranial headache with nausea and vomiting on stimulation of the epileptic

Table 16.1 Primary Epileptogenic Areas

	Number of Patients Affected			
Characteristic	Right	Left	Bilateral	Total
Amygdala, and hippocampal formation	3	1	1	5
And spreading laterally to temporoparietal region	4	1		5
Temporoparietal, and amygdala and hippocampal formation	2*	2		4
Frontal		1*	1	2
Multifocal		1	1	2

*Localization in the three most typical cases (see Table 16.4).

Table 16.2 Sex, Age, and History of Seizures and Headache, in Years

	Female (9)		Male (9)		Total (18)	
Characteristic*	$\overline{x}$	s	$\overline{x}$	s	$\overline{x}$	s
Investigated at age	21	4	28	10	25	8
Headache history	12	4	15	8	13	6
Seizure history	6	4	14	7	10	7
Headache history before seizures	6	5	0.5	5	3	5

*Two males had seizures 10 and 2 years before headache. One male, and one female, had onset of both conditions at the same time. The history of headache was not known in two males. In one of the three most typical cases (see Table 16.4) the history of seizures preceded that of headache; in the remaining two, the history of headache preceded that of seizures by many years.

Table 16.3 The Quality of Headaches and "Cephalic" Symptoms

Characteristic	Number of Patients (n = 18)
a. Paresthesia, or a feeling beyond description, after epigastric aura	13
b. Vague feeling of pressure	9
c. Acute violent local hemicranial pain: "knife, fire, knocking"	3
d. Constricting band around (part of the) head	2
e. "Empty head"	2

Note: Combinations of symptoms were present in 11 of 18 patients:
6 patients experienced symptoms a & b; 3 patients experienced symptoms a & c; 2 patients experienced symptoms a & d.

Table 16.4 The Three Most Typical Cases—Stereo EEG Department

History	Main Symptoms	Aura Symptoms	Stereo EEG Findings
Case 1 Female, investigated age 22; from age 12 "migraine" headache, unsuccessful migraine interval treatment, and psychotherapy for "neurotic disorder"; epilepsy suspected for many years, diagnosed at age 20	Migraine-like headache: right occipital, temporal, parietal pressure-like pain with nausea, vomiting, lasting many hours; confusional twilight states, fugues; psychotic, "neurotic" behavior; no neurological deficit	Nausea, vertigo, retrosternal pain; visual, auditory (musical, thematic) hallucinations, dreamy states	Primary epileptogenic area: right temporal, limbic, Heschl's gyrus; psychomotor status; ipsilateral headache, synchronous with status discharge; after surgery: no seizure, no headaches, 3 yr; no gross neurologic deficit
Case 2 Male, investigated age 29; at age 25 traumatic thrombosis of superior sagittal sinus with left medial frontobasal ischemic lesion; from age 25 seizures; from age 28 migraine-like headache: frequent use of ergot compounds, little success	Focal motor, "psychomotor," and adversive seizures; migraine-like left frontal headache, stinging, constricting "like a band around left side of head," with nausea, lasting hours; no neurological deficit	"Strange feeling"; dyspnea with anxiety; arrest of speech	Primary epileptogenic area: left supplementary motor; ipsilateral headache synchronous with seizure discharge; after surgery: no seizure, no headaches, 2½ yr; initial Broca type aphasia, then no neurologic deficit; lasting pain in craniotomy scar
Case 3 Male, investigated age 52; from age 14 "migraine" attacks, from age 24 seizures, at 28 surgical removal of astrocytoma from right trigone (temporoparietal); moderate relief by ergot compounds and pizotifen	"Classical migraine," then scintillating scotoma, stinging and throbbing right parietal parasagittal headache with nausea and vomiting, seldom with paresthesias of left hand; sensorymotor, "psychomotor" seizures involving left upper extremity; no gross neurologic deficit	Visual (scotoma); epigastric; dysesthesia, left upper extremity; déjà vécu	Primary epileptogenic area: right temporal, neocortical posterior, propagating into right central region and hippocampal formation; ipsilateral headache synchronous with spontaneous and stimulated seizure discharge; after surgery for epilepsy: no seizure, no headache for four years; no gross neurologic deficit

area. In all of the hemicranial attacks recorded in these 5 patients the headache was synchronous with the onset and end of recorded seizure activity. This was true for both spontaneous seizures and for those that were triggered by electrical stimulation (Figs. 16.1, 16.2). In the 3 most typical cases, hemicranial or migraine-like attacks ceased after surgical excision of the epileptogenic area.

The attacks of hemicrania coinciding with seizure activity recorded in this series lasted only for seconds, rarely for over a minute. However, in a subsequent series of similar cases of drug-resistant epilepsies investigated in the same way, one attack with ipsilateral headache that began together with recorded seizure activity lasted for 23.6 minutes, but the duration of the headache could not be verified because communication was soon impeded by increased aphasia, anxiety, dyspnea, and tachycardia.

Patients from an Epilepsy Hospital

Over 4500 patients are seen at the Swiss Epilepsy Hospital every year for known or suspected seizures. Within 3 years, 2 patients with attacks of headache coinciding with recorded epileptic activity were found. One had homolateral hemicranial headache with nausea accurately coinciding with temporal seizure activity; the other had nonhemicranial headache with nausea and diarrhea coinciding with epileptic activity of the type found in "atypical petit mal status." Their histories and findings are summarized below in Table 16.5, and their EEG findings are shown in Figures 16.3 and 16.4.

Patients from a Headache Clinic

Among 235 relatively drug-resistant migraine cases seen at the Zurich Headache Dispensary there were only 2 with obvious epileptic patterns in the EEG recorded between attacks. One had migraine and complex partial seizures. Both conditions had to be managed separately because the migraine attacks did not respond to carbamazepine even though this drug controlled the seizures. The other patient had only "migraine" but no epileptic symptoms beside this. For some time she had been able to keep most attacks at bay with the help of ergotamine combinations containing barbiturates, but she asked for help because this treatment had led to increasing overuse of these compounds, with toxic side effects. Her condition improved on phenytoin alone (see Table 16.5).

RESULTS

"Cephalic" symptoms, including headache are rather common (20%) in a group of patients with severe drug-resistant focal epilepsies. In this group, monosymptomatic or oligosymptomatic seizure headache resembling mi-

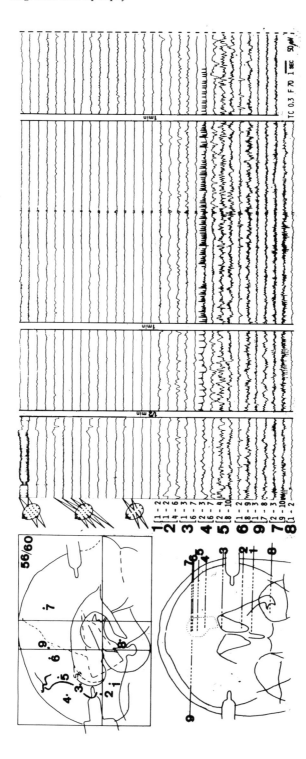

Figure 16.1   Case 2, Table 16.4. Spontaneous seizure discharge at the site of an ischemic lesion (4/2 – 3) from traumatic sinus thrombosis provokes ipsilateral left frontal throbbing and stinging headache which ceases abruptly at the end of the discharge. The discharge does not appear in the surface EEG.

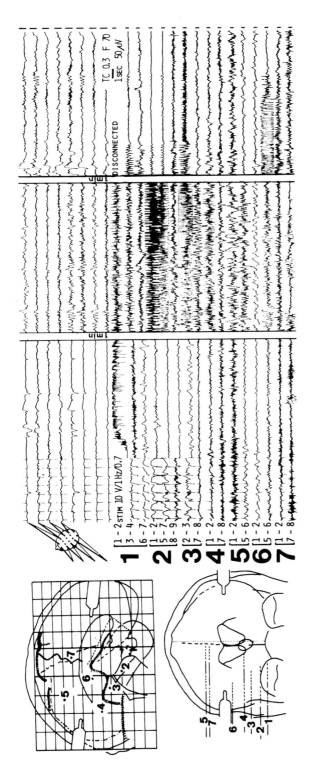

Figure 16.2   Case 3, Table 16.4. Stimulation of right amygdala (1/1–2) by repetitive electrical single-shocks provokes a seizure discharge in the right amygdala spreading to the right hippocampal formation (2/1–2), and then to the right temporoparietal neocortical region (6/5–6). The seizure activity is accompanied by headache described as "tension" behind the right ear.

Table 16.5 Similar Cases from Clinical Practice

History	Clinical Appearance	EEG Findings	Course
Case 4 (Swiss Epilepsy Hospital) Male, age 17; familial migraine; birth injury; from age 7, attacks of headache with anxiety and motor unrest; alternating hemicrania, more often left-sided, worsened by physical or mental strain; during holidays, and from ages 7 to 9, replaced by pain in the region of the heart; EEG had been normal from age 7 to 9; at age 16–17: 3–4 hemicranial attacks per week	Lefthander, minimal right hemiparesis; neuropsychology: slight left frontal dysfunction, verbal and motor; tends to overconform, to dissimulate, to rationalize; CT scan: slight widening left frontal horn, left sylvian fissure; after admission: two slight attacks of headache not noticed by others, third attack with "heart-pain," had to sit down, hardly spoke at all, monosyllabic; reported confusion in the head, incomprehension of speech, difficulty speaking, nausea, and bifrontotemporal headache with left temporal accentuation; all symptoms ceased at the same time	Continuous telemetric monitoring for 7 hours: headache attack; patient becomes pale, muttering "headache," keeps silent 2 min, recovers within ½ min, reports usual symptoms, left-sided headache, nausea; EEG shows critical left temporal activity synchronous with onset and end of ipsilateral headache	On carbamazepine during 2 years: no seizure, and no hemicranial attack, only occasional slight diffuse headache without associated symptoms

Case 5 (Swiss Epilepsy Hospital)
Male, age 39; "screaming fits" in childhood; grand mal seizures from age 15, at intervals of 12, then 2–6 months; received phenobarbital, Prominal, suxinutin; EEG: bifrontal sharp waves; from age 26, seizures replaced by attacks of headache; obtained degree in economics despite severe anxiety problems treated by psychotherapy for 15 years

Bifrontal headache begins in the morning "as if switched on," often with bilaterally scintillating vision, inability to concentrate, nausea, diarrhea; duration 1–2 hours to 1–2 days; aborted by 5 mg diazepam orally; able to work during attacks but "rather mechanically"; behavior during headache sometimes as in very mild clouding of consciousness; no neurological deficit

During one episode irregularly spaced groups of spike and wave discharges were seen, as in so-called atypical petit mal status

Combining therapy with suxinutin, phenytoin, and Maliasin ad libitum despite instructions, he reduced the frequency of the attacks to 2–3 per yr instead of 2–3 per mo

Case 6 (Headache dispensary)
Female, age 39; familial headache; headache from early childhood; from age 13, throbbing in left temple on mental exertion; from 20 to 29, no headache; from 29, daily attacks of hemicrania, free intervals of many months, bouts of abuse of ergot combinations (with butabarbital)

Violent hemicrania, right paravertical, temporal and suboccipital, often with nausea, flushing of face and arms, often so painful that she cried; looks ill during attacks, flushed, or pale, without impairment of consciousness; no neurologic deficit, normal CT scan

Repeated interictal EEGs: bitemporal paroxysmal sharp waves

Improved on phenytoin: despite frequent over-and underdosage (refused blood sampling) 1 yr free of attacks, and of ergot combinations

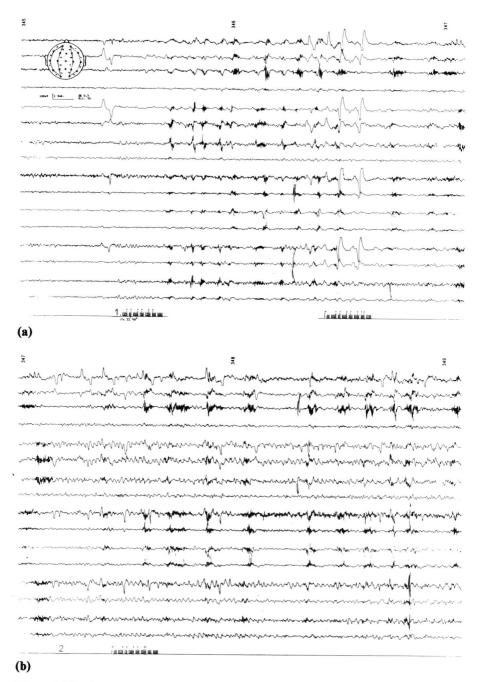

(a)

(b)

Figure 16.3 Case 4, Table 16.5. (a) Complex partial seizure originating from the left fronto temporal region. Onset indicated by slight flattening of the surface EEG, followed by left frontotemporal irregular paroxysmal theta waves. (1): The patient feels left-sided headache accompanied by nausea, arrest of speech, and is pale. (b) Same attack, 18 seconds later: mild oral automatisms. The EEG shows a left frontotemporal ictal discharge of rhythmic theta activity.

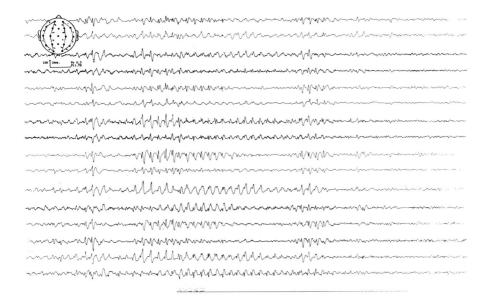

Figure 16.4 Case 5, Table 16.5. Surface EEG recorded during paroxysmal nonhemicranial headache with nausea: pattern of an "atypical petit-mal status" with generalized epileptogenic activity in the form of rhythmical spike and wave.

graine is not very rare (5%), but it is rare among patients selected for special management of drug-resistant migraine and even more rare in a population selected for general management of suspected or known epilepsy without further specification.

Ictal headache as the main symptom may occasionally occur in patients who have not had any other seizure symptoms, but usually there is a history of both ictal headache and other seizure manifestations. In patients with a history of ictal headaches and other seizures, the history of headache usually precedes that of other seizure patterns.

Migraine-like hemicranial ictal headache begins and ends simultaneously with ipsilateral spontaneous or provoked seizure discharges. These seizure discharges do not always appear in the surface EEG, although they appear in EEG recordings from depth electrodes.

This condition, which we have described as *hemicrania epileptica,* responds very well to the medical or surgical treatment that would be indicated in other equally severe seizure disorders with the same electrophysiological characteristics.

The previous history of "migraine" usually refers to attacks of headache lasting many hours. In the cases from the stereo EEG service, hemicranial attacks coinciding with seizure activity lasted only for seconds or minutes, with two exceptions: in one case with complex partial status epilepticus the headache lasted for hours, and in another, originally not included in this series, in which the recorded seizure activity lasted over 20 minutes, the headache may have lasted for the full duration but this could not be determined because of aphasia and partial amnesia.

In one case from clinical practice, ipsilateral headache coinciding with seizure activity lasted for some minutes, while in another with bilateral interictal epileptic surface EEG discharges, and in the case with atypical petit mal status, headache lasted for hours.

DISCUSSION

The concept of headache as an equivalent or as a symptom of seizures is as old as neurology. In the seventeenth century, Thomas Willis, the founder of neurology, thought that "nerve spasms" arriving in the brain caused seizures, whereas those same "spasms" arriving in the meninges caused headache. He explained the voiding of copious clear urine after attacks of both kinds as excretion of serous liquid previously accumulated in the meninges, in the case of headache, or in the brain, in seizures (Willis, 1668, 1672).

The topic surfaced again in the second half of the nineteenth century, and once again in the second half of the twentieth century, when the main results of the general use of electroencephalography had already been assimilated by the medical public, leaving the field open for more special interests.

E.H. Sieveking (1854), who was the first to coin the term *cephalalgia epileptica* for ictal headache and who was involved in the introduction of iodides and bromides as anticonvulsants a few years later, found that 66% of his epileptic patients had headache associated with their seizures (Sieveking, 1858). In our century, only Diaz y Diaz (1976) found a sizable percentage of ictal headache among epileptic patients, 32 of 125, in Mexico, where we may infer that many of his patients had been without adequate treatment before he attended to them. When Gowers (1907) published his statistics of 1450 epileptic patients in 1885, after over 20 years of effective antiepileptic treatment, he found only 50 patients with "cephalic" symptoms, half of which had no painful sensations. A similarly small incidence is reported in most papers on ictal headache published in our century, including that by Young and Blume (1983), who found only 11 cases of "cephalic painful epileptic seizures" among 858 unselected epileptic patients attending their clinic.

This small incidence fits in with the general trend resulting from our own three series: the higher incidence in the intensively monitored group of drug-resistant focal epilepsies is explained by their preselection, their lack of response to anticonvulsants, and the well-known propensity of complex partial seizures to be associated with headache (Lipman and Hughes, 1969; Hughes and Olson, 1981). On the other hand, the particularly small incidence in patients from the epilepsy hospital is explained by negative preselection: focal epilepsies are often directed to the neurologic department for study. As to the incidence of less than 0.5% in the headache clinic group, even Sieveking (1855) had found only 2 cases of what he interpreted as ictal headaches in his group of 100 headache patients, and more recent authors have not found higher incidences of epileptic or ictal headache among unselected headache groups.

We observed ipsilateral focal seizure activity in most of our cases of hemicrania epileptica. Only in 2 cases where invasive exploration was not justified did we find no evidence of lateralization of critical activity. We have shown that the surface EEG is not always sufficient for localization of unilateral seizure activity (Figure 16.2, Case 2). This divergence was confirmed by Laplante et al. (1983). R. Hess (1977) noted that epileptic headache was most often ipsilateral. Young and Blume (1983) found that ictal pain in other parts of the body was consistent with contralateral rolandic seizure activity, whereas ictal pain in the head was not consistent with this pattern. They described contralateral localization in 4, ipsilateral in 3, and lack of correspondent lateralization of headache and seizure activity in the remaining 4 of their 11 cases with "cephalic painful seizures." Of the 3 ipsilateral cases, 2 had reported throbbing, and 1 reported sharp and severe pain, that is, such pain as is usually reported in migraine headache, as in our most typical cases of hemicrania epileptica, while their other cases did not exhibit this symptom.

We must conclude that most typical ictal headaches are ipsilateral to the focal seizure activity. This is difficult to accept because we have been trained or conditioned to accept only the usual contralateral somesthetic representation in all kinds of pain, following Hughlings Jackson's doctrine. But we simply do not know enough about central pain pathways to justify this dogma, and then, we have also been trained to believe that the brain itself is insensitive to pain. However, Penfield and Jasper (1954a), in their investigations of the exposed human brain, found that while mechanical stimulation of the larger cerebral vessels provoked ipsilateral headache, response of the vessels within the sylvian fissure to electrical stimulation was very variable and that these vessels sometimes failed to respond, while "in other individuals stimulation of the brain near these arteries produced ipsilateral headache." Is the brain, then, insensitive to pain, or does it possess mechanisms representing pain localized to the vicinity of the affected or injured part?

Additional examples of ipsilateral manifestations of disorders affecting one hemisphere include those of Penfield and Jasper (1954), who described sensation in the ipsilateral hand on electrical stimulation of the island of Reil; Baldwin et al. (1954) observed ipsilateral lifting of the upper lip on direct stimulation of the amygdala in monkeys and in man; and Schwartz (1937), Luria and Homskaya (1963), and Sourek (1965) found ipsilateral loss or suppression of electrodermal response after various frontal and temporal lesions. Thus sensory, vegetative, and motor manifestations have been found with ipsilateral involvement of the same brain regions that we found capable of producing ipsilateral ictal headache: additional evidence in favor of ipsilateral perception of typical ictal headache, probably not within the traditional somesthetic pattern, and possibly not even of the same sensory category or quality as ordinary peripheral pain.

In five cases investigated with intracerebral electrodes, simultaneous onset and end of both headache and ipsilateral seizure activity was recorded in both spontaneous and electrically induced attacks. This could hardly be interpreted as a vascular response, since the changes of regional cerebral blood flow observed in migraine take many minutes to develop and even more time to disappear (Olesen et al, 1981), while both the abrupt onset and end of these hemicranial headache attacks occurred approximately within the same second as the onset and end of the seizure activity. For the same reason, the mechanism of spreading depression that is often assumed in the pathogenesis of classical migraine (Olesen et al, 1981) must be excluded in our cases with short duration of pain. This means that, at least in the most typical cases of hemicrania epileptica, where attacks last only seconds or a few minutes, the mechanism is most probably neither vascular nor humoral, but directly neural.

However, in the attacks of several hours' duration, secondary vascular pathogenesis, or even spreading depression, may be postulated. This could derive from the well-known (Bonte et al, 1983) reactive hyperemia of the epileptogenic area which, again, takes more than some seconds to develop and much more time to disappear. In focal migraine, the changes of regional cerebral blood flow interpreted as spreading depression sometimes begin with a very short phase of focal hyperemia (Olesen et al, 1981). We have to infer ipsilateral central perception of seizure headache by a mechanism yet unknown but possibly related to ipsilateral vegetative and motor manifestations originating from the same brain regions, and a primary neurogenic process implying an unknown mechanism. We cannot exclude hidden contralateral representation of the headache: the method of recording the headache — the patients' remarks are recorded on the videotape — allows for errors in the range of about one second, which is enough for contralateral transmission, processing, and retransmission.

Despite the observation by Penfield and Jasper (1954) quoted above, Thomas Willis' dogma that the brain is insensitive to pain (Isler, 1968) is usually maintained, and, curiously enough, maintained on the basis of Penfield's other observations on the same pages. One tends to forget the simple facts: the perception of pain is a function of the brain, and in all other parts of the body, pain obviously serves as a signal of distress of the affected part. In our cases with intracerebral recording, as in one of our cases from clinical practice, the ipsilateral headache coincided with ictal activity affecting the function of that hemisphere. We hold that in these cases the pain did indeed serve as a signal of distress of the affected part, as in any other injured part of the body.

Hemicrania epileptica is not a variety of migraine, or one of Hughlings Jackson's "missing links" between migraine and epilepsy. We have proposed Flatau's (1912) term as a separate name for this most typical ictal headache in order to keep it from being confused with migraine or "dysrhythmic migraine," and in order to keep it out of migraine classifications.

Hemicrania epileptica is an electrophysiological and clinical model that shows some traits that are also found in migraine. Further observations of this disorder may allow us to gain some insights into the mechanisms of migraine and its lateralization.

REFERENCES

Baldwin M, Frost LL, Wood CD. Investigation of the primate amygdala. Movement of the face and jaws. Neurology 1954, 4:586–98.

Bonte F, Stokely E, Devous M, Homan R. Single-photon tomographic study of regional cerebral blood flow in epilepsy. Arch Neurol 1983;40:267–70.

Diaz y Diaz H. Cefalea paroxistica epileptica. Neurol Neurocir Psiquiatr (Mexico) 1976;17(2):85–94.

Flatau E. Die Migräne. Berlin: Julius Springer, 1912:76ff.

Gowers WR. Borderland of epilepsy. London: Churchill, 1907.

Halpern L, Bental E. Epileptic cephalea. Neurology 1958;8:615–20.

Hess R. Epilepsie und Kopfschmerzen. Z EEG EMG 1977;8:125–36.

Hughes JR, Olson S. An investigation of eight different types of temporal lobe discharges. Epilepsia 1981;22:421–35.

Isler H. Thomas Willis 1621–1675. New York: Hafner, 1968:90.

Isler H, Wieser HG, Egli M. Hemicrania epileptica. In: Rose FC, ed. Progress in migraine research 2. London: Pitman, 1984:69–82.

Jackson JH. (Taylor J, ed.): Selected writings of John Hughlings Jackson, vol. 1. On epilepsy and epileptiform convulsions. London: Hodder and Stoughton, 1931.

Jonas AD. Headaches as seizure equivalents. Headache 1966;6:78–87.

Laplante P, Saint-Hilaire JM, Bouvier G. Headache as an epileptic manifestation. Neurology 1983;33:1493–5.

Lipman A, Hughes JR. Rhythmic mid-temporal discharges. An electro clinical study. Electroencephalogr Clin Neurophysiol 1969;27:43–7.

Livingston S. The diagnosis and treatment of convulsive disorders in children. Springfield, Ill: Charles C Thomas, 1954.

Luria AR, Homskaya ED. The human brain and psychological processes. Academy of Psychological Sciences of the RSFSR, 1963:450–3.

Olesen J, Larsen B, Lauritzen M. Focal hyperemia followed by spreading oligemia and impaired activation of RCBF in classic migraine. Ann Neurol 1981;9:344–52.

Penfield W, Jasper H. Epilepsy and the functional anatomy of the human brain. Boston: Little, Brown, 1954; 85, 749.

Schwartz HG. Effect of experimental lesions of the cortex on the "psychogalvanic reflex" in the cat. Arch Neurol Psychiatry 1937;38:308–20.

Sieveking EH. On chronic and periodical headache. Medical Times and Gazette (London) August 12th, 19th, 26th, 1854.

Sieveking EH. Tables of analysis of one hundred cases of headache. Association Medical Journal (London) Nov. 9th, Nov. 16th, 1855.

Sieveking EH. On epilepsy and epileptiform seizures. London: John Churchill, 1858.

Sourek K. The nervous control of skin potentials in man. Prague: Rozpravy Ceskoslovenské Akademie ved. Nakladatelstvi Ceskoslovenské Akademie ved, 1965.

Swaiman KF, Frank Y. Seizure headaches in children. Dev Med Child Neurol 1978;20:580–5.

Weil AA. EEG findings in a certain type of psychosomatic headache: dysrhythmic migraine. Electroencephalogr Clin Neurophysiol 1952;4:181–6.

Willis Th. Pathologiae cerebri, et nervosi generis specimen in quo agitur de morbis convulsivis, et de scorbuto. London: 1667; Amsterdam: Elsevier, 1668:125.

Willis Th. De anima brutorum quae hominis vitalis ac sensitiva est . . . Vol. 2. London: Wells and Scott, 1672, 271.

Young GB, Blume WT. Painful epileptic seizures. Brain 1983;106:537–54.

17

Epileptic Headache: Study with Depth Electrodes

J.-M. Saint-Hilaire
P. Laplante
G. Bouvier

It is well known that migraine and epilepsy may be related conditions in the same patient. The exact relationship between the two is not clear and has been the subject of many discussions. We had the opportunity to study two cases in which headache was the main ictal manifestation. Furthermore, they were investigated with depth electrode recordings as well as continuous audio and video monitoring (Saint-Hilaire et al., 1976; Bouvier et al., 1976; Laplante et al., 1983). This provided us with reliable documentation of ictal headache, its relation to migraine, and its localizing value as a symptom.

CASE REPORTS

CASE 1 This 17-year-old right-handed woman had epilepsy since age 16 months; the cause was not known. She had two types of seizures. One began with headache at the vertex and a sensation of shortness of breath occurring many times a day. This was accompanied by light-headedness for minutes or hours. Sometimes, she could not talk, although consciousness was preserved. Some of these episodes were interpreted as evidence of hyperventilation but the patient's mother maintained that the pattern was about the same since the age of 16 months. A second type of seizure was more severe but occurred only about two or three times a year. It consisted of a drop attack with loss of consciousness but no convulsive movement. There was no history of other headache.

Drug treatment failed to control these seizures. Computerized tomography (CT), bilateral carotid angiography, and ventriculography showed no abnormality. Depth electrode studies recorded many seizures. Most began with the patient warning that something was wrong. Then, moving her hands to her head (Figure 17.1), she complained of headache, sometimes screaming. This lasted about a minute without any postictal deficit. In all episodes she remained conscious and could answer questions or name objects. She could always recall what had happened. She described a sensation of "painful emptiness of the head" that was

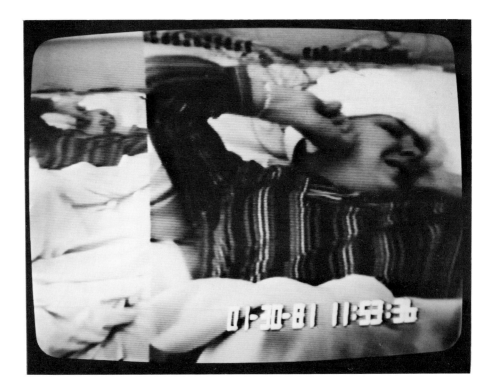

Figure 17.1   Case 1. The patient was screaming just after telling the observer she had headache.

unlike "ordinary" headache. This sensation occurred only in brief paroxysms. She also said that more severe paroxysmal headaches frequently heralded a "severe attack" with loss of consciousness. These headaches always occurred with the beginning of the epileptic electroencephalographic (EEG) activity and never as a postictal symptom. Some of the episodes could be followed by gestural automatisms accompanied by slight confusion and agitation.

Scalp EEG.   Seizures simultaneously began in both temporal regions.

Depth electrode studies.   In most attacks, ictal activity was confined to the right hippocampus and amygdala which discharged almost simultaneously. The contralateral temporal lobe, the ipsilateral temporal cortex, and both frontal lobes did not show any ictal activity.

A right temporal cortectomy was performed, including the amygdala and hippocampus. With minimal medication, there had been no recurrence of headaches or drop attacks 5 years later.

CASE 2   This patient had seizures of unknown etiology since age 5 but his medical history and an examination at age 28 were otherwise negative. His attacks were described as a feeling of dizziness with tinnitus. Despite anticonvulsive therapy, he had about 40 attacks a month. In the laboratory, he had many episodes of headache without any alteration in consciousness. These were always of sudden onset and short duration (30 to 60 seconds). The sensation was a painful feeling of pressure, or a shiver, over both temporal regions, more marked on the right, and the intensity at the beginning of an attack permitted the patient to predict the severity of the seizure. Some of these headaches could be followed by chewing movements, agitation, and head deviation to the left, rarely terminating in a generalized seizure. There was no history of any other type of headache. Bilateral carotid angiography and ventriculography were both normal.

Scalp EEG. Most of the time, clinical events were not accompanied by any change in the scalp EEG. Sometimes 3–4 Hz or rapid rythmic activity in the right frontotemporal region was followed after 10 to 15 seconds by slow activity interspersed with slow spikes.

Depth electrode studies. Many episodes of paroxysmal headache were observed with concomitant ictal activity in the right hippocampus and rapid spread to the right amygdala (Figures 17.2 and 17.3). Ictal activity was restricted to these areas. The contralateral temporal lobe, the ipsilateral temporal cortex, and the right frontal and right parietal lobe were free of ictal activity.

A right temporal lobectomy included the amygdala and hippocampus. There was no recurrence of seizures over an 8-year follow-up.

DISCUSSION

Postictal headache is usually generalized and accompanied by lassitude and myalgia (Forster and Booker, 1980). Ictal headache is not easily described by patients, who note sensations of "swelling, fullness, pressure, heat, pounding, or flush." Frequently, these are not painful sensations. Rarely, headache can be the sole or one of few manifestations of epileptic activity, as in our patients, but definitive diagnosis may be difficult. Many hypotheses have been put forward to explain the relation of epilepsy and headache, for example, that the discharges may be caused by hypoxia after the vasoconstriction of a vascular headache (Barolin, 1966; Ninck, 1970), or that vascular headaches may be induced by focal epileptic activity. Herberg (1975) suggested that increased neuronal activity in the hypothalamus may be responsible for migraine. Headaches caused by excessive discharges in sensory representation areas are rare. They should have the usual character of somatosensory symptoms (paresthetic or dysesthetic) that usually involve one limb or one side of the face (Wilkinson, 1973; Mauguière and Courjon, 1978). Therefore, epileptic headache, being more diffuse, has usually been considered an autonomic manifestation of seizures, like visceral sensations (Schmidt and Wilder, 1968).

We could find only one reported case in which the association between time of headache and ictal activity was demonstrated (Grossman et al., 1971). Usually, authors reported "interictal" EEG abnormalities in patients complaining of epilepsy and/or recurrent headaches (Riley and Massey, 1980;

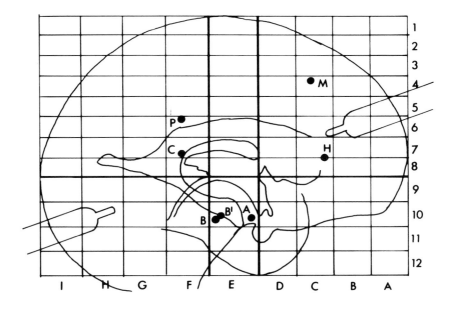

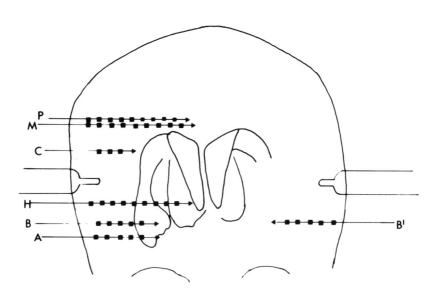

Figure 17.2   Case 2. Sites of depth electrode recording. **B′** Left hippocampus and left temporal T2; **A** Right amygdala and right anterior temporal T2; **B** Right hippocampus and right temporal T2; **C** Right posterior temporal and T1; **P** Right posterior cingular gyrus and right supramarginal gyrus; **M** Right supplementary motor area and right frontal F2; **H** Right anterior cingular gyrus and right frontal F3.

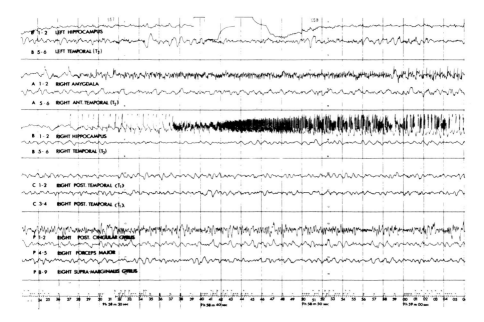

Figure 17.3   Case 2. Depth electrode EEG at the onset of a headache.

Nymgard, 1956; Karlsson, 1960; Jonas, 1966; Geets, 1976; Heyck and Hess, 1955). The success of anticonvulsant therapy in preventing or improving headaches has been considered an argument to prove that these headaches were epileptic manifestations (Heyck and Hess, 1955; Nymgard, 1956; Karlsson, 1960; Viparelli et al., 1967; Geets, 1976; Riley and Massey, 1980). Grossman et al. (1971) discussed a 9-year-old patient; in three episodes of headache, the EEG showed rhythmic sharp waves in the right cerebral hemisphere (with predominance in the occipital region).

In our cases, clinical and EEG abnormalities were observed in the laboratory. The association of headache and ictal activity was demonstrated many times. In both patients, headache was paroxysmal (usually the first manifestation of a seizure), of short duration (less than one minute), of nonspecific nature and description ("not like any other headache before") and sparing consciousness except when a generalized seizure followed. Although both patients told us that their headache was not severe, their behavior suggested acute pain (Figure 17.1).

In both cases, depth electrode studies localized ictal activity in the right amygdala and hippocampus. Surgical treatment stopped their seizures and their headaches.

Differentiation of epileptic headache from migrainous headaches is not a problem (Saint-Hilaire et al., 1984). The epileptic headache is brief (less than 1 minute in our cases), not "vascular" in character, and without the classic accompaniments of migraine. In these aspects, epileptic headache more closely resembles psychogenic headache. Wieser (1983) described a study with depth electrodes and came to simlar conclusions about localization of the primary epileptic focus in the temporal limbic system. He described cases with "migrainoid attacks" that correspond to the "epigastric aura" spreading to the head. Although he did not explicitly mention the duration of these headaches, it seems that they lasted a matter of minutes.

In summary, the diagnosis of epileptic headache must be based mainly on other clearly epileptic manifestations accompanying the headache. Differentiation between migraine and epileptic headache is usually easy because of the duration (less than 1 minute) and the character of the pain.

There may be a relationship between migraine and epilepsy but it is unlikely that migraine headache itself is epileptic in nature.

REFERENCES

Barolin GS. Migraine and epilepsy—a relationship? Epilepsia 1966;7:53–66.

Bouvier G, Saint-Hilaire JM, Vézina JL et al. La chirurgie fonctionnelle de l'épilepsie. Union Med Can 1976;105:1483–5.

Forster FM, Booker HE. The epilepsies and convulsive disorders. In Baker AB, ed: Clinical neurology, vol. 2. Hagerstown Md.: Harper & Row, 1980:17.

Geets W. Céphalée épileptique. Acta Neurol Belg 1976;76:10–15.

Grossman RM, Abramovich I, Lefebvre AB. Epileptic headache: report of a case with EEG recorded during the crisis. Arq Neuropsiquiatr (S. Paulo) 1971;29:198–206.

Herberg LJ. The hypothalamus and aminergic pathways in migraine. In: Pearce J, ed. Modern topics in migraine. London: William Heinemann, 1975:85–95.

Heyck VH, Hess R. Vasomotorische Kopfschmerzen als Symptom larvierter Epilepsien. J Suisse Méd 1955;85:(24)573–5.

Jonas AD. Headaches as seizure equivalents. Headache 1966;6:78–87.

Karlsson B. Headache of epileptogenic nature. A clinical and electroencephalographic study of 23 children. Acta Paediatr Scand 1960;49:17–27.

Laplante, P, Saint-Hilaire JM, Bouvier G. Headache as an epileptic manifestation. Neurology 1983;33:1493–5.

Mauguière F, Courjon J. Somatosensory epilepsy: a review of 127 cases. Brain 1978;101:307–32.

Ninck B. Migraine and epilepsy. Eur Neurol 1970;3:168–78.

Nymgard K. Epileptic headache. Acta Psychiatr Scand 1956;31:291–300.

Riley TL, Massey EW. The syndrome of aphasia, headaches and left temporal spikes. Headache 1980;21:90–2.

Saint-Hilaire JM, Bouvier G, Lymburner J et al. La stéréoélectroencéphalographie synchronisée avec l'enregistrement visuel et sonore dans l'exploration chronique de l'épilepsie. Union Med Can 1976;105:1538–41.

Saint-Hilaire JM, Laplante P, Bouvier G. Epileptic headache. Neurology 1984; 34:988.

Schmidt RP, Wilder BJ. The seizure: variations on a theme. In: Schmidt RP, Wilder BJ, eds. Contemporary neurology series, vol. 2 (Epilepsy). Philadelphia: FA Davis, 1968:33.

Viparelli U, Crispi G, Di Lorenzo R. An unusual case of epilepsy and paroxysmal headache. Ann Neuropsichiatr Psichoanal (Naples) 1967;14:554–8.

Wieser HG, Isler H. Headache as epileptic manifestation. Schweiz Rundschau Med. 1983;24:844–8.

Wilkinson HA. Epileptic pain. An uncommon manifestation with localizing value. Neurology 1973;23;518–20.

18

Headache after Partial Complex Seizures

Roberto D'Alessandro
Tommaso Sacquegna
Paolo Pazzaglia
Elio Lugaresi

The headache that follows generalized convulsions is a well-known phenomenon that may be caused by general metabolic changes and an increase in cerebral blood flow of up to 300% to 400%, as shown in animals (Plum et al., 1968). On the contrary, it is unlikely that a focal reactive hyperemia accounts for headache following seizures without generalized convulsions (Penfield and Jasper, 1954; Ingvar, 1975; Hangaard et al., 1976; Kuhl et al., 1980). Gastaut (1982) reported the occurrence of postictal headache (PIH) in about one-third of all children who have occipital spike and wave epilepsy. However, no reports have been published on PIH in partial seizures and nonconvulsive generalized seizures. The present study was performed in order to define clinical features, semeiological value, and incidence of headache that follows these nonconvulsive seizures (NCS).

METHODS

The study was performed at the Epilepsy Center of Bologna on 240 consecutive epileptic patients who were over 16 years of age. We included patients presenting NCS with or without generalized tonic-clonic seizures. We excluded patients whose seizures were symptomatic of space occupying lesions or vascular malformations and those with moderate or severe mental disturbances. Seizures were classified according to ILAE (Proposal for revised clinical and electroencephalographic classification of epileptic seizures, 1981) on the basis of clinical-anamnestic, electroencephalographic (EEG) and computerized tomography (CT) scan findings. In several cases, EEG sleep recordings were performed. We excluded patients from the study when clinical and EEG information did not allow accurate classification of their seizures.

Table 18.1 Features of Headache Following Partial Complex Seizures

Sex	Age (yrs)	Side	Quality	Duration	Severity	Associated Symptoms	Appearance After Seizures	Interictal Headache	Ictal Symptoms
F	33	Bilateral	Dull	6 h	Severe	—	Always	Yes	Loss of consc. and gestural automatisms
M	33	Bilateral	Dull	3 h	Severe	Nausea	Always	Yes	Epigastric aura, feeling of sadness, confusion
F	33	Unilateral	Dull	2 h	Moderate	—	Sometimes	No	Feeling of anxiety, loss of consc. and oral automatisms
M	34	Bilateral	Throbbing	2 h	Mild	—	Sometimes	Yes	Feeling that objects in right visual field are rotating, loss of consc. and gestural automatisms
F	34	Bilateral	Dull	6 h	Moderate	—	Sometimes	Yes	Loss of consc. and gestural automatisms
F	38	Bilateral	Throbbing	4 h	Moderate	Dizziness Pallor	Sometimes	Yes	Loss of consc. and gestural automatisms

M	38	Bilateral	Dull	1 h	Mild	Drowsiness	Sometimes	Yes	Feeling of dizziness, dimness, loss of consc. and vocal automatisms
F	40	Unilateral	Throbbing	12 h	Severe	Pallor Nausea Vomiting	Sometimes	Yes	Feeling of anxiety, inability to speak, feeling that people nearby are inside her, loss of consc. and slow torsion of head toward left, gestural automatisms
M	46	Bilateral	Throbbing	3 h	Moderate	—	Sometimes	Yes	Loss of consc. and gestural automatisms
M	47	Bilateral	Dull	12 h	Moderate	Drowsiness	Sometimes	Yes	Sudden fear, loss of consc., and oral automatisms
M	51	Unilateral	Throbbing	24 h	Moderate	Pallor Photophobia	Always	No	Epigastric aura, loss of consc., oral and gestural automatisms
M	56	Bilateral	Dull	12 h	Moderate	—	Always	No	Loss of consciousness

The patients were directly interviewed regarding the occurrence of headache, both in the interictal period and following seizures. Clinical features of headache were recorded and severity was graded as follows: mild, not disturbing normal activity; moderate, disturbing normal activity, but not totally disabling; severe, totally disabling. Particular attention was paid to the temporal relationship between seizure and headache, and we considered only those patients who noted onset of their headache "immediately after the seizures" to have PIH.

RESULTS

Of 174 patients with NCS alone or combined with primary or secondarily generalized tonic-clonic seizures, 49 had simple partial seizures, 94 had complex partial seizures, 9 had both simple and complex partial seizures, and 22 had generalized seizures (19 typical absence and 3 myoclonic absence).

We found 23 patients who suffered postictal headaches. In all cases the headache followed complex partial seizures (including 1 patient presenting both simple partial and complex partial seizures).

The association of PIH with complex partial seizures reached statistical significance (chi square tests, Yates correction, $p < 0.001$). PIH was unilateral in 6 and bilateral in 17 patients. The quality of pain was throbbing in 8 patients and dull in 15. Duration of PIH was equal to or less than 1 hour in 7 patients, equal to or less than 6 hours in 9 patients, and longer than 6 hours in 7 patients. Symptoms such as nausea, vomiting, pallor, dizziness, drowsiness, and photophobia occurred in 10 patients during PIH. Thirteen patients stated that the headache "always" followed their seizures, whereas 10 said that it occurred "sometimes." Interictal headache was present in 12 of 23 patients who experienced PIH; in 34 of 80 patients with complex partial seizures; in 21 of 49 patients with simple partial seizures; and in 11 of 22 patients with generalized NCS. No significant difference was found between patients suffering from PIH and other groups as far as interictal headache was concerned. The wide range of PIH is shown in Table 18.1.

DISCUSSION

In our series PIH seems to be a peculiar clinical feature of complex partial seizures and does not tend to occur following other types of NCS. PIH is quite variable with regard to the side of involvement, quality, duration, intensity of pain, and associated phenomena. In some cases true migraine attacks may be triggered by seizures. Moreover, some patients suffer from long-lasting headaches *only* after seizures. Genetic predisposition to headache does not seem to play a role in the occurrence of PIH, since interictal headache is not more frequent in patients with PIH than in others.

The mechanisms underlying the onset of PIH are uncertain. Focal metabolic and blood flow changes due to neuronal discharge do not account for PIH, since they are also present in partial elementary seizures (Penfield and Jasper, 1954; Ingvar, 1975; Hangaard et al. 1976; Kuhl et al., 1980). As for PIH in benign epilepsy with occipital spikes, Gastaut (1982) suggested that epileptic discharges involve the brain stem, where vegetative centers are located. Our findings agree with the hypothesis that deep vegetative centers are involved, since only seizures in which spread of epileptic discharge provoked disturbance of consciousness were followed by headache. Engel et al. (1983) reported that patients with partial seizures who lost consciousness may have a specific metabolic pattern on positron CT with ^{18}F-labeled fluorodeoxyglucose. This finding suggests that more generalized cerebral involvement accompanies loss of consciousness.

Furthermore, Dana-Haeri et al. (1983) and Pritchard et al. (1983) reported a significant rise in serum prolactin levels after complex partial seizures. Such hormonal changes suggest involvement of hypothalamic nuclei in complex partial seizures. As for PIH, we hypothesize that neuronal discharge involving noradrenergic and serotoninergic pathways originating in the locus ceruleus and brain stem raphe triggers the vascular changes that may be responsible for headache. A similar "central" mechanism has been suggested for migraine (Raskin, 1981), and it is noticeable that some of our patients had typical long-lasting migraine attacks that were triggered by seizures. In patients with generalized NCS, PIH does not occur, whereas impairment of consciousness certainly occurs. However, it is likely that in such seizures impairment of consciousness is caused by a primary widespread or generalized interference with cortical function, as suggested by Gloor (1979), without involvement of the upper brain stem. Therefore, the sparing of hypothalamic and brain stem nuclei in generalized NCS may account for the absence of PIH in these patients. Our findings demonstrate that migraine-like headaches may be "central" in origin, that is, they may be due to an acute disturbance of the central nervous system, inducing changes in the function of the hypothalamus and brain stem nuclei.

REFERENCES

Dana-Haeri J, Trimble MR, Oxley J. Prolactin and gonadotrophin changes following generalized and partial seizures. J Neurol Neurosurg Psychiatry 1983;46:331–5.
Engel J Jr, Kuhl DE, Phelps E et al. Local cerebral metabolism during partial seizures. Neurology 1983;33:400–13.
Gastaut H. L'épilepsie benigne de l'enfant à pointe-ondes occipitales. Rev EEG Neurophysiol 1982;12:179–201.
Gloor P. Generalized epilepsy with spike and wave discharges: a reinterpretation of its electrographic and clinical manifestations. The 1977 William G. Lennox Lecture, American Epilepsy Society. Epilepsia 1979;20:571–88.

Hangaard K, Oikawa T, Sveinsdottir E et al. Regional cerebral blood flow in focal cortical epilepsy. Arch Neurol 1976;33:527–35.

Ingvar DH. rCBF in focal cortical epilepsy. In: Langfitt TW, McHenry LC Jr, Reivich M, Wollan H, eds. Cerebral circulation and metabolism. New York: Springer-Verlag, 1975:361–4.

Kuhl DE, Engel J Jr, Phelps ME, Selin C. Epileptic patterns of local cerebral metabolism and perfusion in humans determined by emission computed tomography of ^{18}FDG and ^{13}NH$_3$. Ann Neurol 1980;8:348–60.

Penfield W, Jasper H. Epilepsy and the functional anatomy of the human brain. Boston: Little, Brown, 1954.

Plum F, Posner JB, Tray B. Cerebral metabolic and circulation responses to induced convulsions in animals. Arch Neurol 1968;18:1–13.

Pritchard PB III, Wannamaker BB, Sagel J, Nair R, De Villier C. Endocrine function following complex partial seizures. Ann Neurol 1983;14:27–32.

Proposal for revised clinical and electroencephalographic classification of epileptic seizures. From the Commission on classification and terminology of the International League Against Epilepsy. Epilepsia 1981;22:489–501.

Raskin NH. Pharmacology of migraine. Annu Rev Pharmacol Toxicol 1981;21:463–78.

III

Genetic and Epidemiological Studies

19

Migraine – Epilepsy Relationships: Epidemiological and Genetic Aspects

Eva Andermann
Frederick Andermann

In the literature on migraine, the variation in findings on the prevalence of this condition is enormous, the range being 1% to 60% (Table 19.1). This reflects the great range in the frequency and severity of this disorder, as well as in the spectrum of opinions on what constitutes migraine.

VARIABILITY IN THE DIAGNOSIS OF MIGRAINE

In the general population, there is considerable variability in conceptualization of headache: people refer to "normal" headaches, headaches occurring only in relation to febrile illness, headaches normally accompanying menstruation, sinus headaches, sick headaches, and tension headaches. Many of these, when described in detail, have obvious features of recurrent vascular headache. Awareness of migraine seems to increase with an individual's level of education and sophistication, and also when such a diagnosis has been made in a family member. On the other hand, initially, parents and relatives of patients seen by a neurologist because of recurrent headaches often insistently deny a personal or family history of migraine.

Frequently, headaches described in other family members are considered to have developed in the recent past, suggesting that earlier headaches may well have been forgotten. Equally important is the recollection by good observers of single or rare migrainous events in their lives, highlighting the extreme variability of the frequency of migrainous events, in addition to the well-known variability of the manifestations over time (Friedman, 1976).

Table 19.1 Prevalence of Migraine in Various Populations

Authors	Population	Percent
Allan, W., 1928	282 men of a general population	57.4
	348 women of a general population	62.6
Grimes, E., 1931	2728 medical personnel, school teachers, and students	9.3
Paskind, H.A., 1934	Patients with non-neurological findings	3.3
Paskind, H.A., 1934	Patients with manic-depressive psychosis	10.0
Paskind, H.A., 1934	Patients with trigeminal neuralgia	23.3
Fitz-Hugh, T. Jr., 1940	4000 consecutive private office case records	22.0
Glasser, G.H. and Golub, L.M., 1955	General population	1.0
Lennox, W.G., Lennox, H.C., 1960	956 medical students and nurses	6.3
Barolin, G.S., 1966	15,000 patients of a neurological service	1.7
Dalsgaard Nielsen, T., 1973	461 Danish doctors	16.0
Waters, W.E., 1975	1129 medical general practitioners—males	13.0
	—females	25.0
Waters, W.E., O'Connor, P.J., 1975	3 general population surveys—males	15.0–20.0
	—females	23.0–29.0
Ekbom, K., Ahlborg, B., Schéle, R., 1978	9803 18-year-old men	1.7
Abramson, J.H., Hopp, C., Epstein, L.M., 1980	General population of 4899—males	5.1
	—females	14.5
Jay, G.W., Tomasi, L.G., 1981	116 children with headache	47.0

There is also a considerable range of opinion on the types of headaches and symptoms that neurologists diagnose as migraine, depending on their training, practice profile, experience, and therapeutic approach. Pediatric neurologists are usually more familiar with migraine-related sympathetic manifestations and disorders of consciousness, whereas adult neurologists tend to see patients who are able to provide a detailed account of the march of an aura or of acephalgic migraine attacks. As a corollary, there is even greater variation in what is diagnosed as tension headaches: some physicians include various forms of vascular headache, whereas others define it as a group of unpleasant cephalic symptoms that are not actually painful.

When taking all these factors into account, one may conclude that the possibility of responding with a migrainous event to some triggering factors may be almost universal in the population, with only a minority of people seeking medical attention because of the frequency or severity of their migrainous symptoms. Attempts at outlining minimal diagnostic criteria tend to include a variable number of major and minor symptoms, and, since these criteria are not generally accepted, such attempts introduce further variability in diagnosis. It is hard to improve on the formulation provided by the World Federation of Neurology study group on headache in 1969: "A familial disorder characterized by recurrent attacks of headache widely variable in intensity, frequency and duration. Attacks are commonly unilateral and are usually associated with anorexia and nausea and vomiting. In some cases they are preceded by, or associated with, neurologic and mood disturbances. All the above characteristics are not necessarily present in each attack or in each patient." Because of its breadth, this definition corresponds most closely to clinical experience, and has withstood the test of time.

There is far more agreement about the diagnosis of the classical, basilar, ophthalmic, and hemiplegic forms of migraine than there is about the common form. Patients with classical migraine constitute a minority, and the prevalence of this form has been estimated as 5% of all patients with migraine. Unlike common migraine, the classical form has an identifiable marker: the clinical features and march of the aura. In most instances, the characteristically slow progression of the migraine aura enables a distinction from epileptic phenomena, despite the occasionally prolonged duration of some, particularly occipital, epileptic manifestations.

There is a strong tendency for inheritance of classical migraine; even particular patterns of aura tend to cluster in families. The infrequent occurrence of classical migrainous events in some family members, and the tendency to forget them, are readily apparent when one obtains a history from several different members of the same family. The current view that the genetic basis for classical and common migraine is the same is based on the clinical experience of finding individuals with classical or common migraine in one family. The patterns of pain and of the sympathetic manifestations in both classical and common migraine are also often similar among affected family members. In addition to the positive family history, a host of other factors, among them, endocrine changes, a characteristic personality profile, stress or relief from stress, sensitivity to dietary or chemical substances, exposure to the sun, exercise, and modification of sleep patterns, trigger or lead to the appearance of the clinical manifestations. Some of these triggering factors may also be found in several affected family members.

RELATIONSHIP BETWEEN MIGRAINE AND EPILEPSY

The question of a possible relationship between migraine and epilepsy has intrigued neurologists from the time these conditions were identified (Whitty,

Table 19.2   Prevalence of Migraine in Epileptic Populations

Authors	Number of Epilepsy Cases	Percent with Migraine
Webber, S.G., 1893	100	8.7
Ely, F.A., 1930	171	15.0
Paskind, H.A., 1934	783	8.4
Lennox, W.G., Lennox, H.C., 1960	1610	11.1

1972). The conclusion that a relationship exists in some patients is inescapable. Attempts at assessing the frequency of such an association in populations of patients with migraine or epilepsy have been much less conclusive, mainly because of differences in methodology, as well as in the criteria for selection and diagnosis. Another major problem in previous studies has been the absence of controls. The prevalence figure for migraine is generally assumed to be 5% to 10% (Appenzeller et al., 1979), whereas that for epilepsy is considered to be 0.5% to 1%. The prevalence of migraine in epileptic populations has been assessed at 8% to 15% (Table 19.2), and the prevalence of epilepsy in migrainous populations at 1% to 17% (Table 19.3).

The difficulties that beset epidemiological studies are also reflected in efforts to determine the frequency of migraine in patients' relatives (Table 19.4). A tenfold variation in prevalence is found when comparing some of the earlier studies. The high incidence of electroencephalographic (EEG) abnor-

Table 19.3   Prevalence of Epilepsy in Migrainous Populations

Authors	Number of Migraine Cases	Percent with Epilepsy
Ely, F.A., 1930	104	8.6
Lennox, W.G., Lennox, H.C., 1960	405	6.5
Selby, G., Lance, J.W., 1960	348	11.0
Ostfeld, A.M., 1963	114	2.63
Dalsgaard Nielsen, T., 1969	100	1.0
Lance, J.W., Anthony, M., 1966	500	1.6
Basser, L.S., 1969	1830	5.9
Hockaday, J.M., Whitty, C.V.M., 1969	560	16.6
Slatter, K.H., 1968	184	7.6
Ninck, B., 1970	591	3.9
Tanikawa, T. et al., 1980	402	2.5
Terzano, M.G. et al., 1981	450	3.5
Tanikawa, T. et al., 1980	47 (classical)	17.0

Table 19.4 Prevalence of Migraine in Relatives of Patients with Epilepsy and Other Diseases

Authors	Number of Relatives	Diagnosis of Proband	Percent with Migraine
Cobb S., 1932	1896	Normal controls	1.56
	9139	Epilepsy	4.5
Paskind S.A., 1934	331	Non-neurologic disorders	14.4
	783	Epilepsy	35.2
	492	Manic-depressive psychosis	34.0
	342	Trigeminal neuralgia	37.7
	890	Psychasthenia	25.5
	216	Dementia praecox	32.8
	136	Tic	37.3
	73	Constitutional inferiority	49.3
	63	Paranoid state	23.8

malities in patients, particularly children with migraine and their siblings as compared with normal controls (Ziegler and Wong, 1967), has led to the establishment of the concept of dysrhythmic migraine and the hypothesis that there may be a genetic relationship between migraine and epilepsy.

GENETIC BASIS OF MIGRAINE AND EPILEPSY

The presence of an important genetic component in both migraine and epilepsy has long been recognized. The multifactorial inheritance of epilepsy has been previously documented (E. Andermann, 1982, 1985). In addition to the genetic component, which can be calculated and expressed as the heritability of different forms of epilepsy, one or more acquired components contribute to the appearance of the clinical disorder. A similar mode of inheritance may be postulated for migraine (Dalsgaard Nielsen, 1965, Heyck, 1982), although autosomal dominant inheritance with incomplete penetrance may also explain the clinical findings. A genetic basis for the migraine-epilepsy relationship has been investigated (Baier and Doose, Chapter 20, this volume). These authors found an increased prevalence of migraine in mothers of children, particularly of girls, with absence attacks associated with 3 Hz spike and wave. Conclusive studies, however, are lacking (Pratt, 1967).

In an attempt to determine whether migraine and epilepsy are in fact genetically related, Kraus (1978), under the guidance of Julius Metrakos, studied the prevalence of migraine in first degree relatives (parents, siblings, and

Table 19.5 Compendium of Populations Examined (Kraus, 1978)

Series	Probands	1st Degree Relatives			2nd Degree Relatives			3rd Degree Relatives	Total
		Parents	Sibs	Offspring	Aunts & Uncles	Nieces & Nephews	Grandparents	Cousins	
1*	51	101	107	—	378	1	197	596	1380
2†	66	132	91	—	593	1	257	587	1661
3†	92	183	126	6	720	31	340	559	1965

*Group 1: probands with 1 or more convulsions.
†Groups 2 and 3: control families seen in medical genetics.

offspring) of probands who had one or more convulsions, compared to first degree relatives of otherwise similar children who did not have a history of seizures. In such a study the contributions of various acquired or triggering factors would not be apparent. The matched control group would ensure that any bias in establishing a diagnosis of epilepsy or migraine would be common to both groups. This careful, well-designed, and well-executed study has been published as a thesis (Kraus, 1978) and is not widely known. It deserves to be quoted *in extenso*.

Three groups of families were studies: series 1, in which the proband had attended Montreal Children's Hospital (MCH) with a history of one or more convulsions; series 2, in which the proband attended the Medical Genetics Department of MCH for any reason except seizures. A questionnaire specifically inquiring about headaches and seizures in family members was used during the initial interview. This was followed by a second, more detailed questionnaire containing 27 questions relevant to a possible diagnosis of migraine. The completed questionnaires were evaluated by a neurologist, Dr. Peter Humphreys, who was not aware whether any given record was from the control or experimental group. Families in which the proband had migraine were excluded from the analysis. A third group, series 3, consisted of families similar to the controls (series 2) in which the detailed questionnaire regarding headache was not used. The populations studied are shown in Table 19.5.

Table 19.6 illustrates the prevalence of migraine obtained after specific and nonspecific questioning. There was a striking absence of positive responses when specific questions regarding a history of headaches were not asked for. This confirms the clinical observation that people do not consider migraine, especially if it occurs in relatives, to represent a specific disease entity worthy of inclusion in a medical case history.

According to this study, the prevalence of migraine was similar among relatives of epileptic and control probands (1.9% vs. 1.6%) (Table 19.6). It was reported most often in first degree relatives (7.2% vs. 5.8%) (Table 19.7), sug-

Table 19.6 Prevalences of Migraine Obtained after Specific Questioning (1, 2) Versus Nonspecific Questioning about Headaches in the Family (3) (Kraus, 1978)

Series	Total		1st Degree Relatives	
	Number	*Percent Affected*	*Number*	*Percent Affected*
1 Epileptic proband	1380	1.9 ± 0.4	208	7.2 ± 1.8
2 Control + stage 1	1661	1.6 ± 0.3	223	5.8 ± 1.6
3 Control	1965	0.0	315	0.0

Table 19.7   Prevalence of Migraine in Relatives of Epileptic and Control Probands (Kraus, 1978)

Relationship to Proband	Epileptic Proband Series 1		Control Series 2		P
	Number	Percent Affected	Number	Percent Affected	
1st degree	208	7.2 ± 1.8	223	5.8 ± 1.6	>.20
2nd degree	576	1.6 ± 0.5	851	1.6 ± 0.4	>.20
3rd degree	596	0.3 ± 0.2	587	0	<.10
Total	1380	1.9 ± 0.4	1661	1.6 ± 0.3	>.20

gesting that the informants were much more knowledgeable about the history of their immediate family. It was four to five times higher in female relatives, both in the epileptic and control groups (Table 19.8), in keeping with the clinical impression of a higher incidence of migraine in females.

As expected, the prevalence of epilepsy was significantly higher in relatives of epileptic probands than in control relatives (Table 19.9).

Kraus (1978) concluded that since migraine is not seen more often in the near relatives of epileptic patients as compared to control relatives, a genetic factor common to both migraine and epilepsy cannot be postulated. Her thesis was therefore appropriately entitled: "Migraine and epilepsy: a case for divorce." However, only the finding of biological markers for migraine and epilepsy, and further elucidation of the basic mechanisms of these disorders, will permit more definitive studies of this question.

Although there is at present no adequate proof of a genetic link between the two conditions, we now have convincing evidence that in some instances migraine may lead directly to seizures or epilepsy. From the studies of patients with migraine and epilepsy, certain syndromes emerge: some patients with classical migraine have seizures during the aura and a few go on to develop epilepsy independent of migrainous symptoms (Andermann, Chapter 1, this volume). In these patients, the epileptic manifestations appear to be caused by

Table 19.8   Sex Predilection for Migraine and Epilepsy (Kraus, 1978)

Series	Female Relatives		Male Relatives		P
	Number	Percent Affected	Number	Percent Affected	
Migraine					
EP Proband	713	3.1 ± 0.6	676	0.6 ± 0.3	<.001
Control	817	2.7 ± 0.6	851	0.7 ± 0.3	<.001
Epilepsy					
EP Proband	713	4.9 ± 0.8	676	4.4 ± 0.8	>.20
Control	817	1.2 ± 0.4	851	0.8 ± 0.3	>.20

Table 19.9 Prevalence of Epilepsy in Relatives of Epileptic and Control Probands (Kraus, 1978)

Relationship to Proband	Epileptic Proband Series 1		Control Series 2		P
	Number	Percent Affected	Number	Percent Affected	
1st degree	208	11.5 ± 2.2	223	2.7 ± 1.1	<.001
2nd degree	576	4.5 ± 0.9	851	1.0 ± 0.4	<.001
3rd degree	596	2.3 ± 0.6	586	0.3 ± 0.2	<.01
Total	1380	4.6 ± 0.6	1661	1.0 ± 0.2	<.001

the migrainous process itself. Whether a genetically determined increased seizure tendency also exists in these patients remains speculative. As discussed elsewhere in this volume, migraine appears to be a risk factor in occipital lobe epilepsy, and a high incidence of migrainous headaches is found in children with benign epilepsy and occipital spike and wave complexes, and in occipital lobe epilepsy in childhood. Occipital epilepsy seems to be of multifactorial origin, and the presence of migraine or a family history of migraine represents one such risk factor leading to the clinical manifestations. Other factors include acquired cerebral damage, the presence of a lesion, as well as a genetically determined predisposition to epilepsy.

Patients with benign rolandic epilepsy also have a high incidence as well as a striking family history of migraine (Bladin, Chapter 9, this volume; Giovanardi Rossi et al., Chapter 21, this volume; Watters, personal communication, 1984). The significance of this association is still uncertain and, interestingly enough, some experts in this area have not been struck by the coexistence of these phenomena (Loiseau, personal communication, 1983; Lombroso, personal communication, 1984). Giovanardi Rossi et al. conclude that the high incidence of migraine and recurrent headache in patients (49%) and parents (81%) was similar to that of the control children (41%) and their parents (60%) and could be attributed to chance association. Baier and Doose (Chapter 20, this volume) suggest that there may be a genetic relationship between migraine and petit mal absence attacks. Further controlled studies of the association of migraine with these epileptic syndromes are needed.

Migrainous symptoms are a feature of mitochondrial encephalomyopathy (Dvorkin et al., Chapter 14, this volume; Pavlakis et al., 1984; DiMauro et al., 1985), but the relationship between the strong family history of migraine in the patients of Dvorkin et al. and the mitochondrial disease of the probands is still unclear. Perhaps a small reduction in the inherited number of neural mitochondria leading to hereditary inadequacy of calcium-binding ability in these patients (VanGelder, Chapter 24, this volume) could lead to the catastrophic strokes that they suffer. The high prevalence of a positive family history of migraine in children with alternating hemiplegia of infancy also remains unexplained (Dalla Bernardina et al., Chapter 13, this volume; M.H. Saint-Hilaire et al., 1985). Here, too, the possibility of an underlying mitochondrial abnormality should be considered when neuropathological material becomes available.

Thus, in these conditions there is a close, and in some cases a causal relationship between migraine and epilepsy.

Recently, several studies have addressed and clarified the nature of ictal headache (Blume and Young, Chapter 15, this volume; Isler et al., Chapter 16, this volume; J.M. Saint-Hilaire et al., Chapter 17, this volume), and have also shown that partial complex seizures may lead to migraine attacks (D'Alessandro et al., Chapter 18, this volume) as well as to the better known headache that follows a generalized tonic-clonic seizure.

Patients who present with these associations may not be very numerous in comparison to the vast majority of people with migraine. However, these associations serve to draw attention to the presence of relationships between these two conditions that are important far beyond their numerical significance.

Well-studied cases, which suggest that certain forms of migraine may lead to epilepsy and vice versa, make one suspect the possibility of yet other, more subtle, relationships between the two disorders; at present, however, there is no convincing evidence of an overall genetic relationship between these conditions.

REFERENCES

Abramson JH, Hopp C, Epstein LM. Migraine and non-migrainous headaches. A community survey in Jerusalem. J Epidemiol Commun Health 1980;34:188–93.

Allan, W. Inheritance of migraine. Arch Intern Med 1928;42:590–9.

Andermann E. Multifactorial inheritance of generalized and focal epilepsy. In: Anderson VE et al., eds. Genetic basis of the epilepsies. New York: Raven Press, 1982:355–74.

Andermann E. Genetic aspects of the epilepsies. In: Sakai T, Tsuboi T, eds. Genetic aspects of human behaviour. Tokyo: Igaku-Shoin, 1985:129–45.

Appenzeller O, Feldman RG, Friedman AP. Migraine headache and related conditions, panel 7. Arch Neurol 1979;36:784–805.

Barolin GS. Migraine and epilepsy—a relationship? Epilepsia 1966;7:53–6.

Basser LS. The relationship of migraine and epilepsy. Brain 1969;92:285–300.

Cobb S. Causes of epilepsy. Arch Neurol Psychiatry 1932;27:1245.

Dalsgaard Nielsen T. Prevalence and heredity of migraine among 461 Danish doctors. Headache 1973;12:168–72.

Dalsgaard Nielsen T. Some aspects of the epidemiology of migraine in Denmark. In: Background to migraine, Cochrane A, ed. 3rd Migraine Symposium, p. 11, 1969 (Heineman 1970).

Dalsgaard Nielsen T. Migraine and heredity. Acta Neurol Scand 1965;41:287–300.

DiMauro S, Bonilla E, Zeviani M, Nakagawa M, DeVivo DC. Mitochondrial myopathies. Ann Neurol 1985;17:521–38.

Ekbom K, Ahlborg B, Schéle R. Prevalence of migraine and cluster headache in Swedish men of 18. Headache 1978;18:9–19.

Ely FA. Migraine-epilepsy syndrome; statistical study of heredity. Arch Neurol Psychiatry 1930;24:943 – 9.

Fitz-Hugh T Jr. Precordial migraine: important form of "angina innocens." New Internal Clin 1 Ser 1940;3:141 – 7.

Friedman AP. The epidemiology of migraine. Hemicrania 1976;7:2 – 4.

Glasser GH, Golub LM. Electroencephalogram of psychomotor seizures in childhood. Electroencephalogr Clin Neurophysiol 1955;7:329 – 40.

Grimes E. Migraine instability. Med J Rec 1931;134:417 – 32.

Heyck H. Der Kopfschmerz. Stuttgart: Thieme, 1982;89,311.

Hockaday JM, Whitty CWM. Factors determining the electroencephalogram in migraine: a study of 500 patients according to clinical type of migraine. Brain 1969;92:769 – 88.

Jay GW, Tomasi LG. Pediatric headaches: a 1 year retrospecific analysis. Headache 1981;21(1):5 – 9.

Kraus D. Migraine and epilepsy: a case for divorce. MSc Thesis, McGill University, 1978.

Lance JW, Anthony M. Migraine. Arch Neurol 1966;15:356 – 61.

Lennox WG, Lennox MA. Borderlands of epilepsy. In: Epilepsy and related disorders. Boston: Little, Brown, 1960.

Ninck B. Migraine and epilepsy. Eur Neurol 1970;3:168 – 78.

Ostfeld AM. The natural history and epidemiology of migraine and muscle contraction headache. Neurology 13: Special issue, March 1963.

Paskind HA. The relationship of migraine and epilepsy and some other neuropsychiatric disorders. Arch Neurol Psychiatr 1934;32:45 – 50.

Pavlakis SG, Phillips PC, DiMauro S, De Vivo DC, Rowland LP. Mitochondrial myopathy, encephalopathy, lactic acidosis and strokelike episodes. A distinctive clinical syndrome. Ann Neurol 1984;16:481 – 8.

Pratt RC. The genetics of neurological disorders. London: Oxford University Press, 1967.

Saint-Hilaire MH, Andermann F, Silver K, Hakim A, Morris N. Paroxysmal alternating hemiplegia in infancy: treatment with calcium channel blockers (Abstr) Can J Neurol Sci 1985;12:217.

Selby G, Lance JW. Observations of 500 cases of migraine and allied vascular headache. J Neurol Neurosurg Psychiatry 1960;23:23 – 32.

Slatter KH. Some clinical and EEG findings in patients with migraine. Brain 1968; 91:85 – 98.

Tanikawa T, Miyazaki T, Iseki H et al. Migraine and epilepsy. Folia Psychiatr Neurol Jpn 1980;34:405 – 6.

Terzano MG, Moretti G, Manzoni GC et al. Association patterns between epileptic and migraine attacks. Acta Neurol 1981;36(4):587 – 98.

Waters WE. Prevalence of migraine. J Neurol Neurosurg Psychiatry 1975;38:613 – 6.

Waters WE, O'Connor PJ. Prevalence of migraine. J Neurol Neurosurg Psychiatry 1975;38:613 – 6.

Webber SG. Report of 160 cases of epilepsy. Boston Med Surg J 1893;128:491 – 500.

Whitty CWM. Migraine and epilepsy. Hemicrania 1972;4:2 – 4.

World Federation of Neurology Research Group on Migraine and Headache. Editorial comment—Hemicrania 1969;1:3.

Ziegler DK, Wong G. Migraine in children: clinical and electroencephalographic study of families: The possible relation to epilepsy. Epilepsia 1967; 8:171 – 87.

20

Migraine and Petit Mal Absence: Familial Prevalence of Migraine and Seizures

Wolfgang K. Baier
Hermann Doose

The combined occurrence of epileptic seizures and migraine (Hockaday and Whitty, 1969; Slatter, 1968), the high incidence of migraine in the families of epileptics (Lennox, 1960), as well as the frequency of "epileptiform" discharges in the electroencephalogram (EEG) of migraineurs (Hockaday and Whitty, 1969; Smyth and Winter, 1961; Rowan, 1974; Ziegler and Wong, 1967; Heyck and Hess, 1955; Weil, 1952, 1961; Scollo-Lavizzari, 1971) have prompted discussion about a suspected pathogenetic, and particularly of a genetic, relationship between migraine and epilepsy. This hypothesis is supported by reports on the high incidence of photosensitivity in migraineurs. Photosensitivity is known to occur in about 50% of children with spike-wave absence (Doose et al., 1973) as compared with 7% to 9% in controls (Eeg-Olofsson et al., 1971; Doose and Gerken, 1973). As family investigations have shown, photosensitivity is genetically determined (Davidson and Watson, 1956). Its incidence is clearly age-dependent and is higher in females. Moreover, photosensitivity seems to be inherited more frequently in the female line (Doose et al., 1970; Doose and Gerken, 1973). In the study of genetics of epilepsy, photosensitivity is one factor within a polygenic system (Doose, 1982). Similarly, absence attacks in childhood occur more often in girls, and, as earlier family investigations have shown, the relatives of female propositi with petit mal absences are at higher risk to experience seizures compared with the relatives of male patients (Doose et al., 1973, Doose and Baier, in press). To explain these findings, polygenic inheritance with sex-dependent risks of manifestation has been postulated (Ottman et al., 1985).

The migraine attack is considered to be a symptom of increased cerebro-vascular responsiveness that is due to sophisticated humoral mechanisms (Lance, 1978; Fanchamps, 1980). After puberty, migraine is more often diagnosed in females (Bille, 1962). With few exceptions (Ziegler, 1978; Lucas, 1977), there is general agreement concerning the significance of genetic factors in the pathogenesis of migraine. The mode of inheritance, however, is still controversial. Dalsgaard-Nielsen (1965) discusses autosomal dominance with incomplete penetrance, or polygenic inheritance. Raskin and Appenzeller (1982) advocate autosomal dominant inheritance, whereas Goodell et al. (1954), in an earlier study, supported a recessive trait. According to some authors, "familial hemiplegic migraine" represents a separate genetic entity (Bruyn, 1968; Raskin and Appenzeller, 1982). The clinical symptomatology of migraine is inconsistent. Although the classification proposed by the Ad Hoc Committee (Friedman et al., 1962, in Heyck, 1982) considers migraine with focal neurologic signs as "classical migraine," European authors mostly use the term "migraine accompagnée" to describe those variants of migraine, accompanied by transient focal symptoms, not affecting the visual system (e.g., Heyck, 1982; Rossi et al., 1980; Bücking and Baumgartner, 1974).

The purpose of this study was to determine the risks of migraine and epileptic seizures in relatives of patients suffering from petit mal absence or migraine with onset in childhood. If the "genetic backgrounds" of petit mal absence and migraine were related, the risk of migraine in the families of absence patients might "depend" on the sex of the affected child, as does the risk to convulse. Moreover, the prevalence of migraine and seizures in the families of migrainous children may be calculated. We also hoped to obtain data concerning the genetic significance of two different clinical types of migraine.

PATIENTS AND METHODS

The investigation included 77 patients (37 male, 40 female) suffering from primary generalized epilepsy with absence attacks and 181 patients (97 male, 84 female) with migraine starting in childhood, and their families, (specifically, proband, siblings, parents, parents' siblings, and grandparents). Probands were included in the "absence" sample only if the disease started after the fifth year of life with absences as the first epileptic symptom, and if their EEGs showed typical 3/sec spike and wave discharges. Nineteen patients (7 male, 12 female) with absence were investigated in an earlier study (Doose et al., 1973).

The diagnosis of migraine was made according to the following criteria: subjects complained of frontal or parietal episodic headaches, without suspected organic disease, and had a set of associated symptoms. "Strongly suggestive" associated symptoms were: (1) vomiting, (2) scintillating scotomata, (3) diplopia, (4) pareses, (5) paresthesiae, (6) aphasia. "Mildly suggestive" associated symptoms were defined as: (1) nausea, (2) vertigo, (3) photophobia, (4) hyperacusis, (5) onset on awakening, (6) relief after sleep.

To fulfill the criteria for a diagnosis of migraine, one strongly suggestive and/or two mildly suggestive and, in the case of strictly hemicranial pain, one mildly suggestive symptom, had to be reported. If a subject mentioned pareses, paresthesiae, or aphasia, he/she would be allocated to the clinical subtype "migraine accompagnée." The term "common migraine" was used for probands without transient focal neurologic signs.

After reading a written explanation of the aims of the study, families were asked for consent and were visited by an interviewer. The data were obtained during a semistandardized conversation, using a questionnaire that itemized the desired information, including the symptomatology of headaches, if any, in family members. Statistical evaluation used chi-square tests, Fisher's exact test, the tetrachoric correlation, and logistic regression. Statistical significance was assumed if $p < 0.05$.

RESULTS

Figures concerning the absence sample are presented in Tables 20.1 and 20.2, which describe the families of male and female probands separately. Results obtained in migraine patients are presented in Tables 20.3 through 20.7, where the families of male and female patients with common migraine or migraine accompagnée are listed separately. Except in Table 20.3, prevalence regarding combined groups (e.g., including male *and* female, or common *and* migraine accompagnée patients) is not tabulated, but can easily be calculated from the detailed tables.

Probands with Petit Mal Absence

Probands: Both Sexes (Tables 20.1 and 20.2)

Seizures. Seizures were reported by 5% of family members. The highest prevalence was found in siblings (brothers 18.5%, sisters 10.6%; not significant [NS]). The rate seemed to be higher in the maternal than in the paternal line (4.6 vs. 2.4%; $0.05 < p < 0.10$).

Migraine. Migraine was reported by 31.2% of mothers and 15.3% of siblings. The differing rates in mothers and fathers (31.2% vs. 9.1%) as well as in sisters and brothers (22.7% vs. 7.7%) were highly significant ($p < 0.05$). Maternal as compared with paternal siblings did not show significant differences.

Male Probands (Table 20.1)

Seizures. Only fathers' sisters as compared with mothers' sisters (19.4% vs. 0%; $p < 0.05$) reported significantly different rates of seizures; brothers were affected more often than sisters (15.2% vs. 3.9%; NS).

Table 20.1   Probands with Petit Mal Absences—Prevalence of Epileptic Seizures and Migraine in Relatives of 37 Male Patients

Familial Relationship	Total Number	Epileptic Seizures		Migraine	
		Number Affected	Percent Affected	Number Affected	Percent Affected
Brothers	33	5	15.2	1	3.0
Sisters	26	1	3.9	5	19.2
Siblings	59	6	10.2	6	10.2
Fathers	37	0	0	4	10.8
Fathers' brothers	39	3	7.7	2	5.1
Fathers' sisters	31	6	19.4	1	3.2
Mothers	37	1	2.7	7	18.9
Mothers' brothers	40	2	5.0	0	0
Mothers' sisters	45	0	0	3	6.7
Fathers' fathers	37	0	0	1	2.7
Fathers' mothers	37	0	0	2	5.4
Paternal line	181	9	5.0	10	5.5
Mothers' fathers	37	1	2.7	0	0
Mothers' mothers	37	1	2.7	0	0
Maternal line	196	5	2.6	10	5.1
Total	436	20	4.6	26	6.0

Table 20.2   Probands with Petit Mal Absences—Prevalence of Epileptic Seizures and Migraine in Relatives of 40 Female Patients

Familial Relationship	Total Number	Epileptic Seizures		Migraine	
		Number Affected	Percent Affected	Number Affected	Percent Affected
Brothers	32	7	21.9	4	12.5
Sisters	40	6	15.0	10	25.0
Siblings	72	13	18.1	14	9.4
Fathers	40	0	0	3	7.5
Fathers' brothers	63	1	1.6	0	0
Fathers' sisters	46	0	0	6	13.0
Mothers	40	3	7.5	17	42.5
Mothers' brothers	63	6	9.5	1	1.6
Mothers' sisters	58	3	5.2	5	8.6
Fathers' fathers	40	0	0	0	0
Fathers' mothers	40	0	0	4	10.0
Paternal line	229	1	0.4	13	5.7
Mothers' fathers	40	1	2.5	1	2.5
Mothers' mothers	40	2	5.0	6	15.0
Maternal line	241	15	6.2	30	12.5
Total	542	29	5.4	57	10.5

Migraine.   Migraine was reported by 19.2% of sisters, but only 3% of brothers ($p < 0.05$); 18.9% of mothers and 10.8% of fathers were affected (NS).

Female Probands (Table 20.2)

Seizures.   Seizures were reported by 6.2% of the members of the maternal and 0.4% of the paternal line ($p < 0.05$). Brothers were affected more often than sisters (21.9% vs. 15.0%; NS).

Sisters of female absence patients experienced seizures in 15.0%, sisters of males (see *Male Probands* above) in only 3.9% ($0.05 < p < 0.10$). There were no significant differences among parents and grandparents in the families of male as compared with female absence patients. The comparison of maternal and paternal lines shows that paternal relatives of males were more often affected, as were the maternal relatives of female patients (0.4% vs. 6.2%, $p < 0.05$%; 5.0% vs. 2.6%, $p < 0.05$; see also *Male Probands* above).

Migraine.   Migraine was reported by 42.5% of mothers, but only 7.5% of fathers ($p < 0.05$). A comparison of other corresponding relatives did not reveal significant differences. Mothers of girls more often had migraine than mothers of boys (42.5% vs. 18.9%, $p < 0.05$; see also *Male Probands* above). The prevalence of migraine was higher in the maternal line of girls than of boys (12.5% vs. 5.1%, $p < 0.05$; see also "Male Probands" above).

Probands with Migraine

In Figure 20.1, patients are plotted according to the age of onset of migraine. Mean age of onset in boys was 8.5 ± 3.5 years (common migraine: 7.3 ± 2.9 years; migraine accompagnée:10.8 ± 3.2 years), and 9.0 ± 3.6 years in girls (common migraine: 7.3 ± 3.4 years; migraine accompagnée: 10.0 ± 3.4 years).

Probands: Both Sexes (Table 20.3)

Seizures.   Seizures were reported by 1.2% of family members. More sisters than brothers (5.7% vs. 1.5%; NS), and more members of the maternal than of the paternal line (1.5% vs. 0.2%; $p < 0.05$), experienced seizures.

Migraine.   Migraine was reported by 17.3% of relatives. More sisters than brothers were affected (23.0% vs. 16.7%; NS). Table 20.3 shows that half of the mothers and one-fifth of the fathers reported migraine (51.4% vs. 20.4%; $p < 0.05$). Comparison of parental lines showed that migraine was diagnosed significantly more often in the maternal than in the paternal line (26.7% vs. 11.5%; $p < 0.05$), with an exceptionally high incidence in females.

The literature repeatedly refers to the number of "positive family histories" in patients with migraine. In this study, only 29 of 181 patients (16.0%; not tabulated) had no family history of migraine.

The incidence of common migraine and of migraine accompagnée has been calculated at 14.8% and 2.5%, respectively. The incidence of migraine

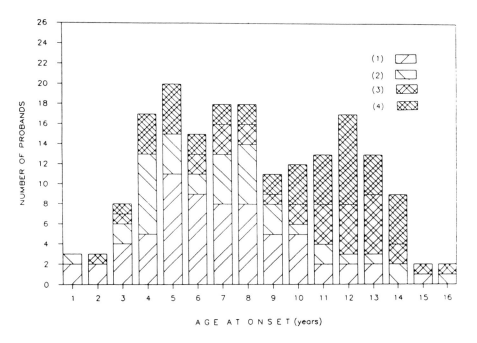

Figure 20.1   Age at onset of common migraine and migraine accompagnée in 181 children. (1) boys, common migraine; (2) girls, common migraine; (3) boys, migraine accompagnée; (4) girls, migraine accompagnée.

accompagnée was similar in fathers and mothers (6.6% vs. 7.2%; NS), whereas common migraine was much more often reported by mothers (44.2% vs. 13.8%; $p < 0.05$). In fathers, the ratio between common migraine and accompagnée was 2.1, whereas it was 6.2 in mothers. Sisters were more often affected by migraine accompagnée than were brothers (5.7% vs. 1.5%; NS). The prevalence of migraine accompagnée was approximately equal in parents' siblings, whereas the prevalence of common migraine was significantly higher in mothers' compared with fathers' brothers (8.5% vs. 3.8%; $p < 0.05$). Prevalence in maternal and paternal sisters showed no statistically significant difference.

Probands: Males and Females Separated (Tables 20.4–20.7)

The prevalence of epileptic seizures was very low when the group was broken down further: the respective figures were therefore omitted from the following tables.

The prevalence of common migraine and migraine accompagnée in the families of male as compared with female probands was not significantly different.

Table 20.3 Probands with Migraine — Prevalence of Epileptic Seizures, Common Migraine, Migraine Accompagnée* and Total Migraine in Relatives of 181 Patients of Both Sexes

Familial Relationship	Total Number	Epileptic Seizures		Common Migraine		Migraine Accompagnée		Total Migraine	
		Number Affected	Percent Affected	Number Affected	Percent Affected	Number Affected	Percent Affected	Number Affected	Percent Affected
Brothers	132	2	1.52	20	15.15	2	1.52	22	16.67
Sisters	122	7	5.74	21	17.21	7	5.74	28	22.95
Siblings	254	9	3.54	41	16.14	9	3.54	50	19.69
Fathers	181	1	0.55	25	13.81	12	6.63	37	20.44
Fathers' brothers	213	0	0.00	8	3.76	0	0.00	8	3.76
Fathers' sisters	184	1	0.54	21	11.41	3	1.63	24	13.04
Mothers	181	4	2.21	80	44.20	13	7.18	93	51.38
Mothers' brothers	212	5	2.36	18	8.49	2	0.94	20	9.43
Mothers' sisters	174	3	1.72	26	14.94	5	2.87	31	17.82
Fathers' fathers	181	0	0.00	3	1.66	1	0.55	4	2.21
Fathers' mothers	181	0	0.00	31	17.13	4	2.21	35	19.34
Paternal line	940	2	0.21	88	9.36	20	2.13	108	11.49
Mothers' fathers	181	2	1.10	10	5.52	1	0.55	11	6.08
Mothers' mothers	181	0	0.00	52	28.73	3	1.66	55	30.39
Maternal line	929	14	1.51	186	20.02	24	2.58	210	22.68
Total	2123	25	1.18	315	14.84	53	2.50	368	17.33

*Migraine accompagnée: classical migraine with pareses, paraesthesia, or aphasia.

Table 20.4 Probands with Migraine — Prevalence of Common Migraine, Migraine Accompagnée* and Total Migraine in Relatives of 66 Male Patients

Familial Relationship	Total Number	Common Migraine		Migraine Accompagnée		Total Migraine	
		Number Affected	Percent Affected	Number Affected	Percent Affected	Number Affected	Percent Affected
Brothers	47	4	8.51	2	4.26	6	12.77
Sisters	40	9	22.50	3	7.50	12	30.00
Siblings	87	13	14.94	5	5.75	18	20.69
Fathers	66	11	16.67	3	4.55	14	21.21
Fathers' brothers	83	5	6.02	0	0.00	5	6.02
Fathers' sisters	66	7	10.61	0	000	7	10.61
Mothers	66	30	45.45	6	9.09	36	54.55
Mothers' brothers	90	7	7.78	1	1.11	8	8.89
Mothers' sisters	73	11	15.07	0	0.00	11	15.07
Fathers' fathers	66	2	3.03	1	1.32	3	4.55
Fathers' mothers	66	16	24.24	0	0.00	16	24.24
Paternal line	347	41	11.82	4	1.13	45	12.97
Mothers' fathers	66	4	6.06	0	0.00	4	6.06
Mothers' mothers	66	19	28.79	1	1.32	20	30.30
Maternal line	361	71	19.67	8	2.22	79	21.88
Total	795	125	13.72	17	2.14	142	17.86

*Migraine accompagnée: classical migraine with pareses, paraesthesia, or aphasia.

Table 20.5 Probands with Common Migraine—Prevalence of Common Migraine, Migraine Accompagnée* and Total Migraine in Relatives of 39 Female Patients

Familial Relationship	Total Number	Common Migraine		Migraine Accompagnée		Total Migraine	
		Number Affected	Percent Affected	Number Affected	Percent Affected	Number Affected	Percent Affected
Brothers	20	4	20.00	0	0.00	4	20.00
Sisters	27	3	11.11	1	3.70	4	14.81
Siblings	47	7	14.89	1	2.13	8	17.02
Fathers	39	4	10.26	3	7.69	7	17.95
Fathers' brothers	45	1	2.22	0	0.00	1	2.22
Fathers' sisters	32	2	6.25	1	3.13	3	9.38
Mothers	39	20	51.28	3	7.69	23	58.97
Mothers' brothers	44	3	6.82	0	0.00	3	6.82
Mothers' sisters	34	6	17.65	1	2.94	7	20.59
Fathers' fathers	39	1	2.56	0	0.00	1	2.56
Fathers' mothers	39	6	15.38	1	2.56	7	17.95
Paternal line	194	14	7.22	5	2.58	19	9.79
Mothers' fathers	39	4	10.26	0	0.00	4	10.26
Mothers' mothers	39	10	25.64	0	0.00	10	25.64
Maternal line	195	43	22.05	4	2.05	47	24.10
Total	436	64	14.68	10	2.29	74	16.97

*Migraine accompagnée: classical migraine with pareses, paraesthesia, or aphasia.

Table 20.6 Probands with Migraine Accompagnée*—Prevalence of Common Migraine in Relatives of 31 Male Patients

Familial Relationship	Total Number	Common Migraine		Migraine Accompagnée		Total Migraine	
		Number Affected	Percent Affected	Number Affected	Percent Affected	Number Affected	Percent Affected
Brothers	23	7	30.43	0	0.00	7	30.43
Sisters	24	4	16.67	1	4.17	5	20.83
Siblings	47	11	23.40	1	2.13	12	25.53
Fathers	31	5	16.13	0	0.00	5	16.13
Fathers' brothers	33	1	2.86	0	0.00	1	2.86
Fathers' sisters	34	2	5.88	1	2.94	3	8.82
Mothers	31	14	45.16	1	3.23	15	48.39
Mothers' brothers	29	1	3.45	1	3.45	2	6.90
Mothers' sisters	19	3	15.79	0	0.00	3	15.79
Fathers' fathers	31	0	0.00	0	0.00	0	0.00
Fathers' mothers	31	5	16.13	0	0.00	5	16.13
Paternal line	162	13	8.02	1	0.62	14	8.64
Mothers' fathers	31	1	3.23	0	0.00	1	3.23
Mothers' mothers	31	10	32.26	0	0.00	10	32.26
Maternal line	141	29	20.57	2	1.42	31	21.99
Total	350	53	15.14	4	1.14	57	16.29

*Migraine accompagnée: classical migraine with pareses, paraesthesia, or aphasia.

Table 20.7　Probands with Migraine Accompagnée*—Prevalence of Common Migraine, Migraine Accompagnée and Total Migraine in Relatives of 45 Female Patients

Familial Relationship	Total Number	Common Migraine		Migraine Accompagnée		Total Migraine	
		Number Affected	Percent Affected	Number Affected	Percent Affected	Number Affected	Percent Affected
Brothers	42	5	11.90	0	0.00	5	11.90
Sisters	31	5	16.13	2	6.45	7	22.58
Siblings	73	10	13.70	2	2.74	12	16.44
Fathers	45	5	11.11	6	13.33	11	24.44
Fathers' brothers	50	1	2.00	0	0.00	1	2.00
Fathers' sisters	52	10	19.23	1	1.92	11	21.15
Mothers	45	16	35.56	3	6.67	19	42.22
Mothers' brothers	49	7	14.29	0	0.00	7	14.29
Mothers' sisters	48	6	12.50	4	8.33	10	20.83
Fathers' fathers	45	0	0.00	0	0.00	0	0.00
Fathers' mothers	45	4	8.89	3	6.67	7	15.56
Paternal line	237	20	8.44	10	4.22	30	12.66
Mothers' fathers	45	1	2.22	1	2.22	2	4.44
Mothers' mothers	45	13	28.89	2	4.44	15	33.33
Maternal line	232	43	18.33	10	4.31	53	22.84
Total	542	73	13.47	22	4.06	95	17.33

*Migraine accompagnée: classical migraine with pareses, paraesthesia, or aphasia.

Probands: Common Migraine and Migraine Accompagnée
Separated (Tables 20.4 – 20.7)

In both groups, the incidence of migraine accompagnée was low (2.2% and 2.9%). The incidence of both types of migraine, however, was higher in the mothers of patients with common migraine (56.2% vs. 41.7%; NS). The comparison of further corresponding relatives did not provide additional information.

Probands: Males and Females Separated/Common Migraine
and Migraine Accompagnée Separated (Tables 20.4 – 20.7)

Males (Tables 20.4 and 20.6).   Comparison of the families of boys with common migraine and those with migraine accompagnée showed that the total familial prevalences of migraine were about equal. In the families of boys with migraine accompagnée the incidence of migraine accompagnée was even somewhat lower than in the sample of comparison (2.1% vs. 1.1%; NS). The comparisons did not indicate significant differences; there was no systematic correlation between the diagnosis in the index case and the prevalence of the two types of migraine in the pertinent relatives.

Females (Tables 20.5 and 20.7).   Prevalence of migraine was equal when families of girls with common migraine and with migraine accompagnée were compared (17.0% vs. 17.5%). However, mothers of girls with common migraine reported the highest, whereas those of girls with migraine accompagnée had the lowest prevalence of migraine (59.0% vs. 42.2%; NS). Fathers reported the highest incidence of migraine in the female migraine accompagnée sample. This is due to the high proportion of paternal migraine accompagnée (13.3%).

Age at Onset of Migraine in the Probands and
Familial Prevalence

In another evaluation, the index cases were subdivided into 4 different groups with respect to the age at onset. Figure 20.2 shows the total incidences of common migraine and migraine accompagnée in the families with respect to the age of onset in the index case. Table 20.8 summarizes the numerical values. Figure 20.2 suggests that the familial impact of migraine might be higher in the families of patients with early-onset migraine. Table 20.8 can be tested by means of the binomial homogeneity test. Its inhomogeneity is highly significant. ($\chi^2 = 31.3$; degrees of freedom [DF] = 3; $p < 0.05$). If the sample is subdivided into an "early-onset" group and a "late-onset" group (manifesting up to age 8, or later, respectively), a tetrachoric correlation of -0.20 can be calculated.

By means of logistic regression, different supposed "risk factors" were tested with respect to their effect on the risk of siblings to be migrainous. These factors were (1) onset up to age 8 years in the index case, (2) paternal migraine, and (3) maternal migraine. The "relative risk" is 1.7 in the siblings of probands with early-onset migraine. In the siblings of patients with an affected mother it is 2.3, in those with an affected father it is 2.5.

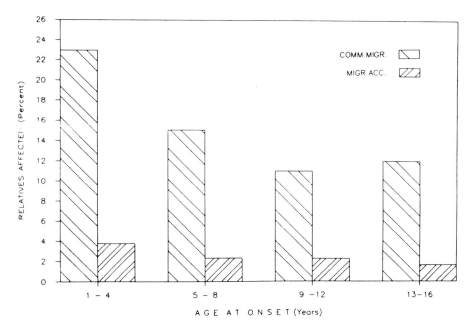

Figure 20.2 Age at onset of (total) migraine in 181 children, arranged in 4 classes. Familial prevalences of common migraine and migraine accompagnée.

DISCUSSION

Petit Mal Absence and Migraine

One of the aims of this study was to determine the familial prevalence of migraine and seizures in a strictly defined sample of children with petit mal absence that started in childhood. In a study of the genetic relationship between migraine and epilepsy, one must keep in mind that the epilepsies comprise a heterogeneous variety of disorders with different genetic backgrounds. Therefore, genetic studies in epileptic patients must aim at clinically — and probably

Table 20.8 Probands with Migraine: Family Members Affected by Proband's Age of Onset

	Proband's Age of Onset (years)			
	1–4	*5–8*	*9–12*	*13–16*
Family Members Affected (number)	92	150	81	42
Family Members Unaffected (number)	252	712	528	266

genetically — homogeneous groups. Here, patients suffering from a prototype of primary generalized or "corticoreticular" epilepsy — spike-wave absences with onset after the fifth year of life — were deliberately selected. The restriction regarding age of onset was considered to be justified, since infantile epilepsies with absence seem to have a worse prognosis when compared with absence of later onset (Doose et al., 1965). Moreover, recent family studies have shown different sex ratios among affected relatives of patients with early- and late-onset spike-wave epilepsies (Doose and Baier, in press). These data indicate different genetic entities or different sex-dependent threshold factors. We did not intend to classify epileptic seizures in family members, since the EEG information essential for such electroclinical correlation was lacking.

In the families of both male and female patients, the incidence of migraine is highest in maternal and in female relatives. This is not astonishing, and is not necessarily related to the epileptic disorder of the probands. The preponderance of migraine in females is well-known. In a review of a series of twelve epidemiological studies, the prevalence was 8% for men and 16% for women (Goldstein and Chen, 1980). Although a migraine prevalence of 30% in mothers of patients with absence is remarkably high, it cannot be readily compared with the generally lower figures quoted in the literature on incidence of migraine in the general population. Factors related to case selection and ascertainment rather than to the epileptic disorder have to be considered. However, the differing incidence of migraine in mothers of male and female patients with absence cannot be explained in this way. Obviously, a reporting bias which might induce fathers to deny symptoms of pathology more often than mothers is not significant in this context. Such a bias, however, must be watched for if maternal and paternal risks are to be compared.

The presence in mothers of paroxysmal EEG patterns, such as spike and wave (Gerken and Doose, 1973), and probably photosensitivity (Doose et al., 1970), and its dependence on the sex of the affected subject, is remarkably similar to the maternal affliction with migraine and its difference between mothers of boys and mothers of girls. As mentioned, girls are more often affected with absence epilepsy of childhood when compared with boys. If a sex-dependent threshold were to explain the preponderance of female subjects, such a threshold should be lower in girls. Judging from present data, maternal migraine might reduce the "threshold of manifestation" or facilitate the occurrence of absence epilepsy of childhood in female subjects. A familial predisposition to migraine probably deserves as much attention as genetic characteristics that are recorded by EEGs and that are more overtly related to epilepsy.

Migraine and Epileptic Seizures

In the ascertainment of migraine, our diagnostic criteria were similiar to those used by other authors (Vahlquist, 1955; Bille, 1962) except for the item "positive family history," which they evidently could not include. The definition of migraine published by the Ad Hoc Committee (Friedman et al., 1962, in Heyck, 1982) was not applicable, since it is descriptive and inappropriate for the purpose of standardized decisions. In our migraine sample, the familial prevalence of epileptic seizures does not exceed the generally accepted epidemiological risk to experience convulsions (e.g., Doose and Sitepu, 1983). These low figures, however, cannot be compared to epidemiological data. In many cases, family members may not have recalled convulsive episodes, especially those benign conditions of infancy and childhood that are of no significance regarding the psychosocial prognosis of the individual. Furthermore, "epilepsy" is subject to social prejudices, which may contribute to a considerable reporting gap.

If genetic relationships between migraine and epilepsy are assumed (see "Petit Mal Absence and Migraine," above), the low familial prevalence of seizures in migrainous children needs an explanation in addition to the possible sources of bias noted above. Findings in the families of nonepileptic photosensitive children should be recalled (Doose et al., 1969): In these families, a seizure frequency of only 1.55% (as opposed to 4.38% in photosensitive epileptics) was obtained. It shows that photosensitivity alone, without the contribution of additional threshold-lowering factors, produces no striking change in the incidence of seizures. Recent studies, however, have shown (Gundel and Doose, 1986; Baier and Doose, in press) that photosensitivity is an important "risk factor" with respect to spikes and waves, but only if it coexists with "parietal theta rhythms," which are another genetic marker of an increased liability to seizures. Photosensitivity and parietal theta rhythms are distinctly age-dependent, and, most likely, polygenically determined (see Doose and Baier, in press). Genetically, these traits are independent, obviously reflecting expressions of different subsets of genes. In girls, a maternal disposition to migraine might play an analogous role in reducing the "threshold of manifestation" of spike and wave discharges or absences as their clinical correlate. It cannot be decided on the basis of the present data whether such an effect is less important or even absent in boys. It might, in part, explain the peculiar "gynecotropism" of absence epilepsy of school-age. Therefore, a genetic predisposition to migraine might only marginally influence the clinical threshold of epilepsy, unless it interacts with other factors in a multifactorial pathogenetic system.

Common Migraine and Migraine Accompagnée

Both common migraine and migraine accompagnée are considered to be largely inherited in the maternal line. About half of the mothers, but only one-fifth of the fathers, gave a history of migraine. This is in keeping with the finding of other authors (Goldstein and Chen, 1980). Bille (1962), in his exhaustive study, stated that two-thirds of the mothers in his sample were affected. However, he accepted the item "positive family history" for proband ascertainment, which inevitably leads to genetically skewed samples. The distinction of probands presenting focal neurologic signs from those who do not, does not reflect an increased incidence of focal findings in the families.

Obviously, the maternal excess of migraine is only due to common migraine. The "relative risk" of fathers, as compared to mothers, to suffer from common migraine is 0.3, while it is 0.9 (not significantly different from 1.0) for migraine accompagnée. This might suggest that the "core" of the migraine syndrome including the classical cases is about equally frequent in men and women, while the often borderline symptomatology of common migraine is much more frequent in females. If the female preponderance of migraine in adults were due to a sex-dependent threshold of manifestation, this should be *higher* in males (i.e. the less frequently affected sex). Hence it would be predicted that male probands would have more affected relatives than female probands. Likewise, the offspring of migrainous fathers should be affected more often than the offspring of affected mothers. However, as reported above, the effects of paternal and maternal migraine are equal with respect to the siblings' risk. It follows that the different incidences of migraine by sex are very likely not due to genetic factors. As could be shown in twin studies (Ziegler et al., 1975; Lucas, 1977), the symptomatology of migraine also does not have genetic significance. We feel that this is in keeping with the findings of the present study.

Age at Onset of Migraine and Familial Prevalence

In children with early-onset migraine, the familial prevalence was higher than in families of probands with later onset. These statistically significant data strongly support the assumption of polygenic inheritance. This phenomenon or "anticipation" describes a postulated earlier onset of genetic disease in offspring of affected parents. In monogenic diseases, such as Huntington's chorea or myotonic dystrophy, it could be ascribed to ascertainment bias (Vogel and Motulsky, 1979), related to the selection of parents with a more benign form who are likely to reproduce. This objection, however, is not plausible in migraine, which does not influence reproductive expectation. Though the findings are highly significant statistically according to the binomial homogeneity test, this does not imply a high correlation between age of onset and familial prevalence. The low value of $r = -0.20$ indicates that much of the variability in manifestations and onset must be explained either by inherited traits, not detectable as migraine in relatives, or by an important contribution of exogenous factors.

CONCLUSION

The findings support the hypothesis of a genetic relationship between migraine and petit mal absences. This is supported particularly by different maternal risks of migraine, depending on the sex of the proband. Polygenic inheritance seems to be the most plausible model to explain the findings in the families of children with migraine. A single mendelian trait cannot be identified, and its advocates have to refer to badly defined marginal terms like "incomplete penetrance," sometimes colloquially referred to as "genetic background" or "modifying genes." This, however, is only a semantic and not a fundamental alternative to polygenic inheritance. We would like to reiterate the warning expressed by Vogel and Motulsky (1979) that the assumption of multifactorial inheritance deserves priority as long as a simple mendelian trait has not been positively demonstrated. The two major clinical variants of migraine, common migraine and migraine accompagnée, do not seem to be inherited as genetic entities. They probably represent different degrees of expression of the same underlying disorder. The generally accepted female preponderance in adult migraine is most likely due to non-genetic factors.

REFERENCES

Baier WK, Doose H. Interdependence of different genetic EEG patterns in siblings of epileptic patients. J Electroencephalogr. Clin Neurophysiol (in press).

Bille B. Migraine in school children. Acta Paediatr Scand 1962;51:1(Suppl 136)1–151.

Bruyn GW. Complicated migraine. In: Vinken PJ, Bruyn GW, eds. Handbook of clinical neurology. Vol. 5. Amsterdam: North Holland, 1968:59–95.

Bücking H, Baumgartner B. Klinik und pathophysiologie der initialen neurologischen Symptome bei fokalen Migränen (migraine ophthalmique, migraine accompagnée). Arch Psychiatr Nervenkr 1974;219:37–52.

Dalsgaard-Nielsen T. Migraine and heredity. Acta Neurol Scand 1965;41:287–300.

Davidson S, Watson CW. Hereditary light-sensitive epilepsy. Neurology 1956;6:235–261.

Doose H. Photosensitivity: genetics and the significance in the pathogenesis of epilepsy. In: Anderson VE, Hauser WA, Penry JK, Sing CF, eds. Genetic basis of the epilepsies. New York: Raven Press 1982:113–21.

Doose H, Baier WK. Genetic factors in epilepsies with primarily generalized minor seizures. Neuropaediatrie (Suppl., in press).

Doose H, Baier WK, Reinsberg E. Genetic heterogeneity of spike wave-epilepsy. In: Porter RJ, Ward AA, eds. Advances in epileptology. Vol. XV. Proceedings of the 15th Epilepsy International Symposium, Washington, 1983. New York: Raven Press 1984.

Doose H, Gerken H. On the genetics of EEG anomalies IV: photoconvulsive reaction. Neuropaediatrie 1973;4:162–71.

Doose H, Völzke E, Scheffner D. Verlaufsformen kindlicher Epilepsien mit spike wave-Absencen. Arch Psychiatr Nervenkr 1965;207:394–415.

Doose H, Gerken H, Hien-Völpel KF, Völzke E. Genetics of photosensitive epilepsy. Neuropaediatrie 1969;1:56–73.

Doose H, Gerken H, Horstmann T, Völzke E. Genetic factors in spike-wave-absences. Epilepsia 1973;14:57–75.

Doose H, Gerken H, Leonhard R, Völzke E, Völz C. Centrencephalic myoclonic-astatic petit mal. Neuropaediatrie 1970;2:59–78.

Doose H, Sitepu B. Childhood epilepsy in a German city. Neuropaediatrie 1983;14:220–4.

Eeg-Olofsson O, Petersen J, Seldèn U. The development of the electroencephalogram in normal children from the age of 1 through 15 years. Neuropaediatrie 1971;2:375–404.

Fanchamps A. The evolution of thinking about the role and site of action of serotonin in migraine. In: Critchley M, Friedman AP, Gorini S, Sicuteri F, eds. Advances in neurology. Vol. 30, New York: Raven Press 1980;31ff.

Gerken H, Doose H. On the genetics of EEG anomalies in childhood III. Spikes and waves. Neuropaediatrie 1973;4:88–97.

Goldstein M, Chen TC. The epidemiology of disabling headache. In: Critchley M, Friedman AP, Gorini S, Sicuteri F, eds. Advances in neurology. Vol. 30. New York: Raven Press 1980;377ff.

Goodell H, Lewontin R, Wolff HG. Familial occurrence of migraine headache. A.M.A. Arch. neurol. psychiat. 1954;72:325–34.

Gundel A, Doose H. Genetic EEG patterns in febrile convulsions—a multivariate analysis. Neuropaediatrie 1986;17:3–6.

Heyck H. Der Kopfschmerz. Stuttgart: Thieme 1982;89ff., 311ff.

Heyck H, Hess R. Vasomotorische Kopfschmerzen als Symptom larvierter Epilepsien. Schweiz. Med. Wochenschr 1955;85:573–5.

Hockaday JM, Whitty CWM. Factors determining the electroencephalogram in migraine: a study of 560 patients, according to clinical type of migraine. Brain 1969;93:769–88.

Lance JW. Mechanisms and management of headache. London: Butterworth 1978:165–77.

Lennox WG. Epilepsy and related disorders. Boston: Little, Brown 1960:438ff.

Lucas RN. Migraine in twins. J. Psychosom Res 1977;21:147–56.

Ottman R, Hauser WA, Susser, M. Genetic and maternal influences on susceptibility to seizures. Am J Epidemiol 1985;122:923–939.

Raskin NH, Appenzeller O. Kopfschmerz. Stuttgart: S. Fischer 1982:36ff.

Rossi LN, Mumenthaler M, Vassella F. Complicated migraine (migraine accompagnée) in children. Neuropaediatrie 1980;11:27–35.

Rowan AJ. The electroencephalographic characteristics of migraine. Arch Neurobiol (Madrid) 1974;37:95–104.

Scollo-Lavizzari G. Prognostic significance of epileptiform discharges in the EEG of non-epileptic subjects during photic stimulation. Electroencephalogr Clin Neurophysiol 1971;31:174.

Slatter KH. Some clinical and EEG findings in patients with migraine. Brain 1968;91:85–98.

Smyth VOG, Winter AL. The EEG in migraine. Excerpta Medica International Congress Series 1961;37:136–7.

Vahlquist B. Migraine in children. Int Arch Allergy 1955;7:348–55.

Vogel F, Motulsky AG. Human genetics. Problems and approaches. Berlin: Springer 1979:97–158ff.

Weil AA. EEG findings in a certain type of psychosomatic headache. Electroencephalogr Clin Neurophysiol 1952;4:181–6.

Weil AA. Observations on 'dysrhythmic' migraine. Excerpta Medica International Congress Series 1961;37:144.

Ziegler DK. The epidemiology and genetics of migraine. Res Clin Stud Headache 1978;5:21–33.

Ziegler DK, Hassanein RS, Harris D, Stewart R. Headache in a non-clinic twin population. Headache 1975;14:213–8.

Ziegler DK, Wong G. Migraine in children: clinical and electroencephalographic study of families. The possible relation to epilepsy. Epilepsia 1967;8:171–87.

21

Epidemiological Study of Migraine in Epileptic Patients

Paola Giovanardi Rossi
Margherita Santucci
Giuseppe Gobbi
Roberto D'Alessandro
Tommaso Sacquegna

Since 1908, when Gowers included migraine in the "borderland of epilepsy," the possible relationship between migraine and epilepsy has been debated, but no final answers have been reached. Some authors (Lennox and Lennox, 1960; Barolin, 1966; Slatter, 1968; Basser, 1969; Prensky and Sommer, 1976) reported an incidence of epilepsy of between 5.7% and 8% in migraine patients. Such an incidence is far higher than the 0.5% figure usually accepted for the general population. Moreover, Lennox and Lennox (1960) found a higher incidence of migraine in epileptic patients compared with a normal control group (11.1% and 6.3%, respectively). Other authors (Froelich et al., 1960; Ziegler and Wong, 1967: Hockaday and Whitty, 1969; Millichap, 1978; Kinast et al. 1982) found a high incidence of electroencephalographic (EEG) abnormalities in migrainous children, although the definitions for the EEG abnormalities differed in each of these studies. Other studies (Friedman and Pampiglione, 1976; Giovanardi Rossi et al., 1981) failed to confirm an increased incidence of EEG abnormalities in children with migraine.

Because of these EEG abnormalities, Weil (1962), Chao et al. (1964), and Swaiman and Frank (1978) suggested that certain types of headache were epileptic in nature. Despite the fact that some of the EEG abnormalities are paroxysmal, a diagnosis of "epileptic disorder" seems inappropriate for migraine headache with associated EEG abnormalities. The response of headache to antiepileptic drugs is also insufficient to classify such headache as an "epileptic equivalent."

Attention has also been focused on the association of epileptic seizures and migraine attacks. Camfield et al. (1978) reported four patients with basilar migraine associated with epileptic seizures and severe epileptiform EEG abnormalities. A similar case was described by Panayiotopoulos (1980), who was not certain whether the patient suffered from basilar migraine or epilepsy. Gastaut (1982) described a number of similar cases but concluded that the primary phenomenon was epileptic and that postictal headache, reported in 36% of his 36 cases, was an epiphenomenon. Terzano et al. (1980) studied a number of patients who developed seizures during a classical migraine aura, and Beaumanoir (1982) recorded a patient who developed an epileptic seizure during the aura of a classical migraine attack.

We studied the incidence of recurrent headache independent of seizures, postictal headache, and headache closely related to a seizure, in a group of epileptic children. We attempted to determine which kind of epilepsy is most frequently associated with headache.

Because of the high incidence of headache found in patients who have benign epilepsy with rolandic spikes, a case–control study was subsequently done in patients suffering from this epileptic syndrome.

HEADACHE IN EPILEPTIC CHILDREN

Materials and Methods

We observed 104 epileptic patients who were under 16 years of age for a period of 5 months at the Center for the Study and Treatment of Epilepsy and the Child Neurology Department of the University of Bologna. In order to assess the incidence of headache, each patient and family was given a questionnaire in which the following points were investigated:

1. The presence or absence of recurrent headache, and its characteristics (site, type of pain, duration, frequency, associated symptoms both neurologic and other, temporal relationship with epileptic seizures)
2. Family history of headache in first and second degree relatives
3. Any effects of antiepileptic treatment on headache
4. Use of antimigraine drugs

Epileptic patients who, because of retardation or emotional disorders, were unable to supply reliable information (23 cases) as well as patients whose seizures were due to space-occupying lesions or vascular malformation (1 case) were excluded.

The neuroradiological examinations, computerized tomography (CT) and pneumoencephalography (PE), carried out on 20 patients revealed significant alterations in 2 cases: these were porencephaly (right hemisphere) and a marked dilatation of the right lateral ventricle in 2 patients with left hemiparesis.

The study was therefore carried out on 80 epileptic children and adolescents.

Results

The 80 patients examined can be classified according to the following epileptic syndromes:

1. Petit mal with or without grand mal (PM $\pm$ GM) defined as absence seizure with or without occasional generalized tonic-clonic or grand mal seizures: 18 patients
2. Grand mal (GM) defined as generalized tonic-clonic seizures: 5 patients
3. Epilepsy with myoclonic absences (AM): 2 patients
4. Partial epilepsy with complex seizures (CPS) occurring alone or with secondarily generalized seizures: 20 patients
5. Partial epilepsy with elementary partial seizures (EPS) occurring alone or with secondarily generalized seizures: 7 patients
6. Partial epilepsy with secondarily generalized seizures, alone (PSGS): 6 patients
7. Benign epilepsy with rolandic spikes or rolandic epilepsy (RE): 22 patients

A family history of headache was present in 45 cases (56.2%).

Of the 80 patients, 43 (53.7%) did not suffer from headache, 29 (36.2%) suffered from recurrent headache independent of epileptic seizures, 13 (16.2%) suffered from postictal headache, and 2 (2.5%) suffered from brief headache which was immediately followed by a complex partial seizure.

Recurrent Headache Independent of Epileptic Seizures

Recurrent headache independent of epileptic seizures was present in 29 patients, 16 males and 13 females. A family history of headache was reported in 15 of these cases (51.7%).

The frequency of recurrent headache was evaluated in each of the epileptic syndromes studied (Table 21.1). The highest incidence was observed in the patients with benign rolandic epilepsy (11 of 22, or 50%) (Table 21.2).

Table 21.1   Headache Distribution in Different Epileptic Syndromes

Epileptic Syndromes	Number of Patients	Patients with Headache	Percent
PM $\pm$ GM	18	6	33.3
GM + PSGS	11	4	36.4
CPS	20	6	30.0
EPS	7	2	28.5
RE	22	11	50.0

Table 21.2 Percentage of Patients with Headache and without Headache in Rolandic Epilepsy (RE) and in Other Epileptic Syndromes (Non-RE)

Epileptic Syndromes	Percent of Patients with Headache	Percent of Patients without Headache
RE	50	50
Non-RE	31	69

χ^2 Test = 7.49; $p < 0.01$

None of the patients was receiving prophylactic antimigraine treatment. All cases (except 2 with RE) were receiving antiepileptic drugs: in the majority (25, or 86.2%), this did not have any effect on recurrent headache.

Postictal Headache

In 13 cases (16.2%), headache appeared immediately after an epileptic seizure. In 6 patients, recurrent headache was also present, independent of the seizures. A positive family history of headache was reported in 7 cases.

In 6 patients, the headache appeared after a generalized tonic-clonic seizure: the pain was described as bilateral or unilateral, throbbing or dull; in 4 cases it lasted for 2 hours or more, and in the same number of cases it was associated with gastrointestinal symptoms. Postictal headache was described in 14.3% of all cases with generalized tonic-clonic seizures.

More rarely, headache appeared after simple partial seizures (12.4%), complex partial seizures (10%), or numerous absence seizures (5.5%) (Table 21.3). Only 1 patient had hemigeneralized seizures, which were always followed by postictal headache.

Headache before Seizures

In two patients, head pain was the initial ictal symptom. The first was a 14-year-old girl with a family history of migraine. At the age of 12 she began to have

Table 21.3 Postictal Headache (13 Cases)*

Type of Seizure	Number of Patients	Patients with Postictal Headache	Percent
Generalized tonic-clonic seizures	42	6	14.3
Simple partial seizures	24	3	12.4
Complex partial seizures	20	2	10.0
Numerous absence seizures	18	1	5.5

*Including one patient with hemigeneralized seizures.

episodes of malaise, lassitude, pallor and, sometimes, loss of consciousness. No improvement was noted following treatment with phenytoin and phenobarbital. Two months after gradual withdrawal of antiepileptic drugs was begun, epileptic seizures appeared and featured (1) unilateral boring headache and, sometimes, abdominal pain, followed by turning of the head and eyes to the right, and impairment of consciousness; and (2) complex partial seizures with automatisms. Since the age of 8 the patient also suffered from a severe bilateral boring headache, independent of her seizures, occurring 1 to 4 times a month and lasting 1 to 6 hours.

Her physical and mental status examinations were normal, as was her CT scan. The EEG revealed spikes, spike and wave, and polyspike and wave discharges over the left centro-parietotemporal region. Treatment with carbamazepine and phenobarbital led to partial control of her attacks.

The second case was a 16-year-old girl who had complex partial seizures from the age of 5 and secondarily generalized seizures since the age of 11.

Since age 13 her seizures consisted of slight biparietal throbbing headache ("I can feel banging in my head") followed by a confusional state lasting about 1 minute, during which she suddenly sat down, performed motor automatisms, and had blinking of her eyelids.

Her physical examination, CT scan and waking EEG were normal. During sleep, occipital spikes appeared with clear right-sided predominance, first in short sequences, then almost periodically throughout Stage 2 sleep. Treatment with carbamazepine, phenytoin, and phenobarbital did not lead to seizure control, although her attacks were less frequent after clobazam was added to her treatment.

RECURRENT HEADACHE IN PATIENTS WITH BENIGN ROLANDIC EPILEPSY

Epidemiological studies of headache in children have often produced contradictory results. The prevalence of headache found (Bille, 1962; Osler, 1972; Sillanpää, 1976, 1983; Del Bene, 1982) has varied from 20% to 66%. This discrepancy may be due to the lack of a clear or universally accepted classification of idiopathic headaches.

In our series of 80 epileptic patients, which constituted a selected population, the prevalence of recurrent headache (36.2%) agreed with the results of epidemiological studies in the general population. We also found that in benign rolandic epilepsy, the prevalence of recurrent headache was significantly higher than in other forms of epilepsy.

On the basis of these results and in view of reports of a high incidence of benign, focal epileptiform discharges (BFED) in children suffering from migraine (Kinast et al., 1982), a case–control study was carried out to analyze more precisely the relationship between headaches and benign epilepsy with rolandic spikes (RE). The intent of this study was to evaluate the incidence of recurring headache and migraine in this form of epilepsy in comparison with a normal control group.

Materials and Methods

A study was made of 43 patients between ages 6 and 15 who suffered from RE and 129 control subjects, matched for age and sex, randomly chosen from public schools.

From both groups we excluded children who were moderately retarded mentally and those with neurologic abnormalities. We also excluded from the control group subjects with epilepsy or with previous febrile convulsions. All of the children were interviewed about their headaches by the same interviewer. To establish the family history of headache or migraine each subject was given a questionnaire for first and second degree relatives. The questionnaire contained simple and specific questions concerning the features of headaches.

Migraine in children was defined according to the criteria of Prensky and Sommer (1979): recurrent headaches separated by headache-free intervals and accompanied by at least three of the following six symptoms:

1. Gastrointestinal symptoms (nausea, vomiting, or abdominal pain)
2. Localized pain or hemicrania
3. Throbbing quality of headache
4. Relief after brief sleep
5. Visual, sensory, or motor aura
6. Family history of migraine in first or second degree relatives

Recurring headache was considered distinct from migraine. Although it was not substantially different from the latter, it did not correspond to the precise criteria defined above. In the analysis of the family data obtained using the questionnaire, a headache with at least three of the following six features was defined as migraine:

1. Recurring headache with symptom-free periods
2. Symptoms such as change of humor, drowsiness, hunger, or thirst in the hours preceding the attack
3. Neurologic disturbances (visual, sensory, or motor aura) preceding the headache by a few minutes
4. Unilateral headache
5. Throbbing headache
6. Associated gastrointestinal symptoms

Results

There were 43 patients affected by RE, 19 females and 24 males. The age range of the females was between 6 and 14 years (mean, 10.3 ± 2.7) and that of the

Table 21.4 Prevalence of Migraine and Recurrent Headache in Patients with RE and in Normal Controls

Study Group Characteristic	Migraine	Recurrent Headache	No Headache	Total
RE				
Male	3 (12.5%)	11 (45.8%)	10 (41.7%)	24 (100%)
Female	3 (15.7%)	4 (21.1%)	12 (63.1%)	19 (100%)
Total	6 (13.9%)	15 (34.9%)	22 (51.1%)	43 (100%)
Control				
Male	8 (11.1%)	23 (31.9%)	41 (56.9%)	72 (100%)
Female	9 (15.8%)	14 (24.6%)	34 (59.6%)	57 (100%)
Total	17 (13.2%)	37 (28.6%)	75 (58.2%)	129 (100%)

males was between 6 and 15 years (mean, 11.2 ± 2.2). Migraine was present in 6 patients (13.9%) (3 males and 3 females) and recurrent headaches occurred in 15 patients (34.9%) (4 female and 11 male) (Table 21.4).

The age-matched control group consisted of 129 subjects, 57 female and 72 male: 17 (13.2%) suffered from migraine (9 males and 8 females), and 37 (28.6%) suffered from recurrent headache (14 females and 23 males) (Table 21.4).

There was no statistically significant difference in the prevalence of headache between the group of patients with RE and the control group.

A family history of migraine was found in 44.3% of the patients with RE and 45% of the control subjects. The family history was positive for nonmigrainous headache in 37.1% and negative in 16.3% of the patients with RE; in the control subjects this was 15.5% and 29.4%, respectively (Table 21.5).

DISCUSSION

The prevalence of recurrent headache independent of seizures in epileptic subjects found in this study (36.2%) falls within the wide range defined for the

Table 21.5 Family History of Headache and Migraine in Patients with RE and in Normal Controls

Family History	RE	Control
Positive for migraine	19 (44.3%)	58 (45.0%)
Positive for headache	16* (37.1%)	20 (15.5%)
Negative	7 (16.3%)	38 (29.4%)
Unknown	1 (2.3%)	13 (10.1%)

*In one case: cluster headache.

general population of the same age (Bille, 1962; Osler, 1972: Sillanpää, 1976; Del Bene, 1982; Sillanpää, 1983). We found a significantly greater incidence of interictal headache in RE compared with all other epileptic syndromes studied ($p < 0.01$). However, in our case-control study of children with RE, the prevalence of migraine in both patients and controls is similar to that found by others (Sillanpää, 1983) and no significant difference was found between the two groups. A similar result was obtained for recurrent nonmigrainous headache.

In children with migraine, a significantly higher frequency (9%) of benign focal epileptiform discharges (BFED) than would be expected in a nonselected sample (Eeg-Olofsson et al., 1971) was reported by Kinast et al. (1982). One of the possible explanations for the association between BFED and migraine is genetic correlation. Although such a hypothesis could have been reinforced by a high incidence of migraine in RE, our study showed that children with RE do not suffer from recurrent headache (migrainous or nonmigrainous) any more frequently than a normal control group.

The discordance with our findings may be due to the different physio-pathological significance of BFED with or without epilepsy. Children with rolandic epilepsy have a higher incidence of birth anoxia and of family histories of epilepsy compared with children who have rolandic (or midtemporal) spikes but no epilepsy. Furthermore, the electroencephalographic abnormalities in these two groups of subjects behave differently during spontaneous sleep (Ambrosetto et al., 1977). Moreover, the findings of Kinast et al. (1982) may be due to a "Berksonian bias" (Berkson, 1946).

Postictal headache was found in our group of epileptic subjects, most frequently after tonic-clonic seizures (14.3% of cases). This may be due to systemic metabolic changes and to the increase in cerebral blood flow that occurs in a major convulsive seizure. The explanation may be different for postictal headache found after simple partial or complex partial seizures or after numerous typical absence seizures (in, respectively, 12.4%, 10%, and 5.5% of cases). Metabolic or focal blood flow modifications could cause headaches after partial seizures (Penfield and Jasper, 1954; Hangaard et al., 1976; Ingvar, 1975; Kuhl et al., 1980). However, according to Gastaut (1982), the headache that appears after the epileptic seizures of benign occipital epilepsy may be due to the diffusion of the discharge in brain stem structures that regulate cerebral vaso-motor activity and gastrointestinal motility. A similar hypothesis has been suggested for headache following complex partial seizures (D'Alessandro et al., Chapter 18, this volume).

Brief headache immediately followed by a complex partial seizure is reported by two of our patients: in one case the headache preceded loss of consciousness and deviation of the head and eyes to the right; in the other there was loss of consciousness with motor automatisms. Similar patients are reported by Blume and Young (Chapter 15, this volume).

Epileptic seizures in which the only symptom was facial pain have been described and documented by EEG recordings (Giovanardi Rossi et al., 1979). With regard to our two cases, it may be that the headache described as immediately preceding the other manifestations of a complex partial seizure is an epileptic phenomenon. This has been demonstrated in two patients by Saint-Hilaire et al. (Chapter 17, this volume).

CONCLUSION

Nonepidemiological studies that show an association between migraine and epilepsy or epileptiform EEG abnormalities may lead to the erroneous conclusion of a physiopathological correlation between these two conditions. There is no proof for such a correlation, and the presence of recurrent interictal headache in an epileptic patient must still be attributed in most cases to the "random coincidence" of two common diseases.

Postictal headache and head pain closely connected with an epileptic seizure have a different significance. Vascular or metabolic changes or diffusion of the epileptic discharge may be responsible for the former, and it has been shown that a brief headache may be a symptom of an epileptic seizure.

REFERENCES

Ambrosetto G, Gobbi G, Sacquegna T. Rolandic spikes in children with and without epilepsy during sleep. Waking and Sleeping 1977;1:211–5.

Barolin GS. Migraine and epilepsy, a relationship? Epilepsia 1966;7:53–66.

Basser LS. The relation of migraine and epilepsy. Brain 1969;92:285–300.

Berkson, J. Limitations of the application of fourfold table analysis to hospital data. Biometrics 1946;2:47–52.

Bille B. Migraine in school children. Acta Paediatr Scand 1962;136(Suppl):1–151.

Beaumanoir A. Communication in VI Congresso Nazionale della Società Italiana delle Cefalee Bologna 1982.

Camfield P, Metrakos K, Andermann F. Basilar migraine, seizures and severe epileptiform EEG abnormalities. Neurology. 1978;20:584–8.

Chao D, Sexton JA, Davis SD. Convulsive equivalent syndrome of childhood. J Pediatr 1964;64:499–508.

Del Bene E. Multiple aspects of headache risk in children. In: Critchley M, Friedman AP, Gorini S, Sicuteri F, eds. Advances in Neurology. New York: Raven Press, 1982;33;187–98.

Eeg-Olofsson O, Petersen I, Seldèn U. The development of the electroencephalogram in normal children from the age of 1 through 15 years: paroxysmal activity. Neuropaediatrie 1971;2:375–404.

Friedman E, Pampiglione G. Sindrome periodica nei bambini. In: Lugaresi E, Pazzaglia P, Canger R, eds. Le Epilessie. Aulo Gaggi Editore, 1976:53–8.

Froelich WA, Carter CC, O'Leary JL et al. Headache in childhood: electroencephalographic evaluation of 500 cases. Neurology 1960;10:639–42.

Gastaut H. L'épilepsie benigne de l'enfant à pointe-ondes occipitales. Rev EEG Neurophysiol 1982;12:179–201.

Giovanardi Rossi P, Gobbi G, Moschen R, Bresciani A, Brayda HG. Aspetti eziologici, clinici ed evolutivi delle epilessie con crisi parziali a semeiologia elementare nell'età evolutiva. Neuropsichiatr Infant 1979;216:639–58.

Giovanardi Rossi P, Santucci M, Gobbi G, Sacquegna T. Diagnosi differenziale tra emicrania ed epilessia nell'età evolutiva. Boll Lega It Epil 1982;37/38:77–81.

Gowers WR. The borderland of epilepsy. Leipzig, Vienna: Deuticke, 1908.

Hangaard K, Oikawa T, Sveinsdottir E et al. Regional blood flow in focal cortical epilepsy. Arch Neurol 1976;33:527–35.

Hockaday JM, Whitty CWH. Factors determining the electroencephalogram in migraine. Brain 1969;92:769–88.

Ingvar DM. rCBF in focal cortical epilepsy. In: Langfitt TW, Mc Henry LR Jr, Reivich M, Wallan H, eds. Cerebral circulation and metabolism. New York: Springer Verlag, 1975;361–4.

Kinast M, Lueders H, Rothner D, Erenberg G. Benign focal epileptiform discharges in childhood migraine (BFEDC). Neurology 1982;32:1309–11.

Kuhl DE, Engel J Jr, Phelps ME, Selin C. Epileptic patterns of local cerebral metabolism and perfusion in humans determined by emission computed tomography of ^{18}FDG and ^{13}NH$_3$. Ann Neurol 1980;8:348–60.

Lennox WG, Lennox MA. Epilepsy and related disorders. Boston: Little, Brown, 1960.

Millichap JG. Recurrent headaches in 100 children: electroencephalographic abnormalities and response to phenytoin (Dilantin). Childs Brain 1978;4:95–105.

Osler J. Recurrent abdominal pain, headache and limb pain in children and adolescents. Pediatrics 1972;50:429–36.

Panayiotopoulos C. Basilar migraine, seizures and severe epileptic EEG abnormalities? Neurology 1980;30:1122–5.

Penfield W, Jasper H. Epilepsy and the functional anatomy of the human brain. Boston: Little, Brown, 1954.

Prensky AL, Sommer D. Diagnosis and treatment of migraine in children. Neurology 1979;29:506–10.

Sillanpää M. Changes in the prevalence of migraine and other headaches during the first seven school years. Headache 1983;23:15–9.

Sillanpää M. Prevalence of migraine and other headache in Finnish children starting school. Headache 1976;16:288–90.

Slatter KH. Some clinical and EEG findings in patients with migraine. Brain 1968;91:85–98.

Swaiman KF, Frank Y. Seizure headaches in children Dev Med Child Neurol 1978;20:580–5.

Terzano MG, Manzoni GC, Maione R, Mancia D. Epilessia benigna con parossismi occipitali ed emicrania: problema delle crisi intercalate. Atti Congresso SINPI (San Marino) 1980;1:827–32.

Weil AA. Observations on "dysrhytmic" migraine. J Nerv Ment Dis 1962;134:277–81.

Ziegler DK, Wong GJ. Migraine in children: clinical and electroencephalographic study of families. The possible relations to epilepsy. Epilepsia 1967;8:171–87.

IV

Pathophysiological Studies

22

Cerebral Blood Flow in Migraine and Spreading Depression

Martin Lauritzen

The typical migraine aura is a sensory disturbance preceding headache by 20 to 30 minutes. When it involves vision, the aura manifests as a zigzag pattern (scintillations) near the center of vision and propagates to the periphery of the visual field, followed by dimmed acuity within the zigzag area (scotoma). When the symptoms of the aura are referred to an extremity, tingling usually commences in the hand and slowly ascends to the arm, leaving behind a numb and sometimes clumsy extremity. The scintillation-scotoma corresponds to the ascending paresthesia-hypesthesia, reflecting the same pathophysiological event in different regions of the brain (Gowers, 1908).

Several investigators have themselves observed migraine prodromes. On more than one occasion Lashley (1941) mapped his scotomata of classical migraine at brief intervals. The scotomata were symmetrically placed in the visual fields, indicating cortical origin. The character of the aura suggested a wave of intense excitation that moved at the speed of 3 mm/min across the visual cortex. This wave seemed to be followed by complete inhibition of neuronal activity that lasted as long as 30 minutes. Lashley noted that the aura was confined to the primary visual cortex and raised the question of communication between different cytoarchitectonic regions. Did the spread of the migrainous disturbance depend on the number and interactions of different cell types in the cortical tissues? The answer to the question appeared to be affirmative, indicating propagation of the migraine aura along established neuronal connections.

Spreading depression (SD) of electroencephalographic (EEG) activity was identified and intensively studied by Leão (1944a). However, little attention was paid to its possible clinical significance. Leão noted the possible implications of SD in epilepsy and migraine (Leão and Morrison, 1945). The parallel between the wave of intense excitation followed by complete inhibition as described by Lashley (1941) and the phenomenon of SD was addressed by

Milner (1958) and later by a multitude of researchers in the field of migraine. In contrast, Wolff was of the opinion that the migraine aura was the effect of a spasm of brain vessels (Dalessio, 1980). In this review, I would like to propose a synthesis of the two views: the function of the blood vessels and of the cerebral cortex can be perturbed at the same time. The casual relationship, however, seems to be the opposite of what was previously proposed.

The review begins with an introduction to the phenomenon of SD. The changes of cerebral blood flow in migraine and SD are then summarized, and the hypothetical interrelationship between the two phenomena is discussed in the light of recent investigations in this field.

CHARACTERISTICS OF SPREADING DEPRESSION

SD is a common response of the cerebral cortex to different noxious stimuli. Sometimes it develops during the course of an experiment in which the cerebral cortex is exposed. Nicholson and Kraig (1981) divide the course of SD into four phases: conditioning, triggering, event, and recovery.

Conditioning the brain to the initiation of SD can be accomplished by applying to the cortex: (1) saline solutions containing a high level of potassium (20 mM or more); (2) depolarizing amino acids; (3) agents that block the Na-K pump; or (4) solutions containing decreased concentrations of Cl^-. SD may then be elicited by local electrical stimulation. SD can also be initiated without conditioning by local application of concentrated potassium, focal injury (needle stab), mechanical stimulation (Bures et al., 1974), induction of bicuculline seizures (Astrup et al., 1978), or microinjections of homologous blood in the subarachnoid space (Hubschman and Kornhauser, 1982). The increase of extracellular potassium associated with a volley of incoming activity may be sufficient to initiate SD in the metrazol treated animal (Van Harreveld and Stamm, 1955).

The event itself is characterized by depression of spontaneous EEG activity, spreading at a rate of 3mm/min across the cortical surface (Leão, 1944a). Prior to cessation of activity, an intensive burst of action potentials is usually seen (Grafstein, 1956) lasting for 5 to 10 seconds. At each cortical point, the EEG decreases to the level of maximal depression in 20 to 30 seconds. Maximal depression lasts up to 10 minutes, but EEG activity is never completely abolished and returns to predepression amplitudes during the recovery period. Both neurons and glial cells are depolarized during SD (Sugaya et al., 1975). A highly characteristic sign of SD is the change of the extracellular potential accompanying the SD front. It is a triphasic shift consisting of a surface positive wave of 1 to 2 mV amplitude (1–2 minutes), a surface negative wave of 15 to 30 mV (1–2 minutes), and a surface positive wave of 1 to 2 mV (1–2 minutes) (Leão, 1947). Evoked potentials and direct cortical responses are usually impaired during SD and may be reduced in amplitude up to 1 hour after SD.

The SD front is accompanied by transient local changes in the composition of extracellular ions; these last for the duration of the negative wave of the extracellular potential change and move with the same speed (Hansen and Zeuthen, 1981). The extracellular potassium activity increases to 60 mM, sodium and chloride activity decreases to approximately 60 mM, and calcium activity decreases from 1.0 to 0.1 mM. At the same time, the volume fraction of the extracellular space decreases by 50% (Hansen and Olsen, 1980), as is also shown by an increase in tissue resistance. These extracellular ionic changes suggest that cortical membrane function during SD is transiently abolished: ions run along their electrochemical gradients so that concentration differences between intracellular and extracellular compartments disappear (Hansen and Zeuthen, 1982). The slow velocity of SD propagation precludes normal mechanisms of neuronal information transfer and implicates the diffusion of substances in the process. The most probable mediator of SD appears to be potassium, as proposed by Grafstein (1956). Enhanced neuronal activity in a localized region leads to a buildup of potassium in the extracellular space with depolarization of neighboring, inactive neurons, leading to a further increase of potassium activity. Hence, propagation of the SD appears to be accomplished by a combination of electrical conduction of neuronal activity and diffusion of potassium in the extracellular space.

SD is more easily elicited in lower animals, such as rodents, than in primates. This property is probably due to the higher density of neural elements in lower mammals. From a pathophysiological and experimental point of view it is important that SD remain within the cellular architecture of the structure in which it starts: an SD in the neocortex does not spread to the archi- or paleocortex or to subcortical structures in the same hemisphere or to the opposite hemisphere. Within the neocortex, SD stops at the cytoarchitectonic borders of the surface when the number of neural membranes per unit volume of tissue decreases, e.g., at the central sulcus in the primate or at the parasagittal sulcus of the rabbit. These properties of SD propagation constitute important criteria for SD identification in brain-imaging studies in man. Thus, in experimental studies, the SD hemisphere can be compared with the contralateral control hemisphere in the same animal (Bures et al., 1974).

The recovery of extracellular ion concentrations to normal values is an energy-dependent process, since active transport across the cell membranes is needed to restore electrochemical gradients. Glucose consumption increases by 200% (Shinohara et al., 1979; Gjedde et al., 1981), and oxygen tension drops for 1 to 2 minutes, leading to activation of the glycolytic pathway with a consequent rise in lactate production by more than 100%. The accelerated energy metabolism is accompanied by an approximate 20% reduction in the level of nicotinamide adenine dinucleotide, (NADH) (Mayevsky et al., 1974). Concentrations of lactate, glucose, and NADH normalize within the following 10 minutes of recovery, whereas glycogen remains reduced by 40% for 45 minutes (Krivanek, 1962).

Cortical SD may induce a variety of behavioral effects, ranging from long-lasting hemihypesthesia (Carew et al., 1970), impairment of memory and learning, yawning, and abnormal intake of food (Bures et al., 1974). Pain reactions have not been observed.

Susceptibility to seizures is normally decreased by cortical SD (Van Harreveld and Stamm, 1955). However, when repeated episodes of SD are evoked at brief intervals the opposite effect has been observed: paroxysmal activity replaces the EEG depression and propagates at the same rate over the cortical surface as SD ("spreading convulsion") (Bures et al., 1974). Conversion of depression to convulsion also occurs when the brain has been pretreated with acetylcholine or pilocarpine, or if SD is elicited while the animal is in a state of hypercapnia (Bures et al., 1974). The electrophysiological, metabolic, ionic, and behavioral aspects of SD have been reviewed in a book by Bures et al. (1974) and in a paper by Nicholson and Kraig (1981).

BLOOD FLOW CHANGES IN SPREADING DEPRESSION

Most studies of perfusion changes in SD have been conducted in barbiturate-anesthetized animals in which cerebral blood flow is reduced because of the decreased energy metabolism. Therefore, the conspicous pial vasodilatation (Leão, 1944b) and blood flow increase of 100% during the SD event (Hansen et al., 1980) occurred against a background of a low cerebral blood flow (Figure 22.1). In the halothane-anesthetized animal, brain perfusion is close to normal. In these animals there was no evidence of elevated perfusion during SD (Lauritzen, personal observation). Apparently, the absence of hyperperfusion was not due to the anesthesia per se, but to the high level of flow, since the reduction in blood flow after indomethacin administration led to the reappearance of hyperperfusion during SD (Lauritzen, 1986). Thus, the SD event itself is associated with hyperperfusion when basic blood flow is low. The mechanism underlying hyperperfusion, when present, probably relates to increased oxygen demand during the rapidly inserting, increased glucose metabolism.

What happened to perfusion following the SD wave front was unknown until recently. We studied the perfusion changes in SD up to 1 hour after passage of the SD front (Lauritzen et al., 1982; Lauritzen, 1984). The post-SD period was characterized by a protracted, 25% to 35% decrease of cortical blood flow lasting an hour or more (Figure 22.2). This delayed hypoperfusion was strictly confined to the cortex (Lauritzen et al., 1982a). The hypoperfusion occurred whether barbiturate or halothane anesthesia was employed, and was also observed in unanesthetized rats. Blood pressure autoregulation was intact in the post-SD period, indicating intact function of the smooth muscle cells of the arterioles. However, the CO_2 reactivity was markedly decreased in the SD cortex, being only half of control values (Lauritzen, 1983). In summary, SD is followed by persistent, moderate hypoperfusion and abnormal vasoreactivity, strictly confined to the cortex. The metabolic disturbance underlying the flow changes remains to be clarified.

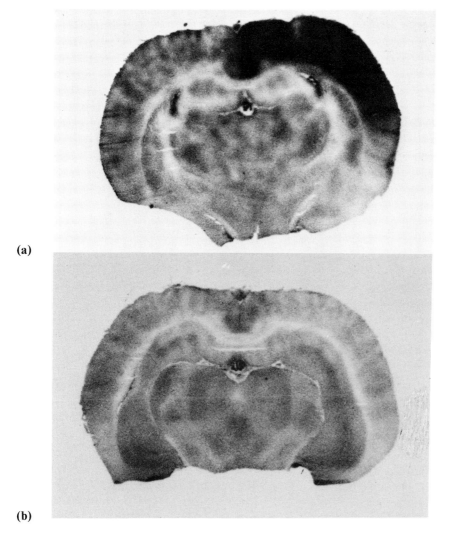

(a)

(b)

Figure 22.1 Cerebral blood flow autoradiograms of rat brain. SD was elicited by 30 second application of 1 M KCl to the cerebral cortex. At selected times after the elicitation of SD, regional CBF was measured by the rapid indicator fractionation method (Gjedde et al., 1980). The rat received 150 μCi/kg of 4–(N–methyl–^{14}C) iodoantipyrine in 200 μ 1 of saline rapidly injected into one femoral vein. The autoradiograms shown are coronal 17.5 m sections through parietal cortex: (a) 1 minute after SD showing the hyperfusion of the SD front in the barbiturate-anesthetized rat; (b) 45 minutes after SD showing the post-SD hypoperfusion. Note that alterations of blood flow are restricted to the neocortex, the region in which the SD was elicited.

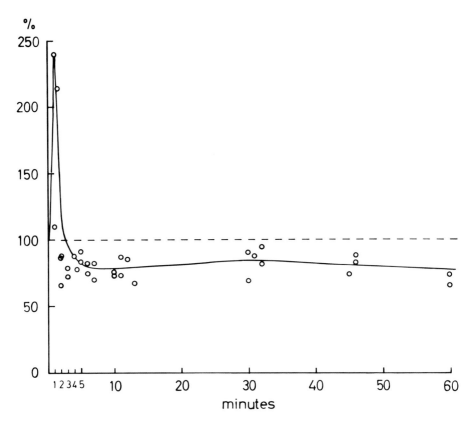

Figure 22.2 Compiled autoradiographic data of rat brains. Change in cortical blood flow at different times after SD, expressed as percentage of cortical blood flow in the control hemisphere. Rats received $150\,\mu$Ci/kg of $4-(N-$methyl$-^{14}$C) iodoantipyrine in $200\,\mu$l of saline rapidly injected into one femoral vein. Frozen brain was cut in 17.5 m slices every 35 mm through the brain and autoradiographed. Cortical blood flow values for approximately ten slices covering 1 minute (at SD speed of 3.5 mm/min^{-1}) were averaged and normalized against averaged cortical blood flow values of control hemisphere. The figure demonstrates the protracted hypoperfusion in the period following SD of approximately 25%, succeeding the hyperperfusion of the SD wave front.

SPREADING DEPRESSION AND THE EEG IN CLASSICAL MIGRAINE

Identification of SD in man by electrophysiological techniques is hampered by its short duration, the non – steady-state character of the condition, and the small area of EEG depression. The wavelength of the severely impaired EEG activity is only 1.5 to 2 cm, and it therefore escapes detection by scalp electrodes; measurement of changes of the direct current (DC) potential is not routine in clinical neurophysiology. These limitations of EEG technique may help to explain the failure to record EEG abnormalities during uncomplicated attacks of classical migraine (Lauritzen et al., 1981). The development of techniques for blood flow measurements in small (1.7 cm²) regions of the human brain has, however, allowed description of vascular phenomena related to SD.

CEREBRAL BLOOD FLOW IN CLASSICAL MIGRAINE

The post-SD period is characterized by a prolonged decrease of cortical perfusion and specific disturbances of cerebral vasomotor reactivity. These experimental results proved useful in the evaluation of our studies of regional cerebral blood flow (rCBF) in migraine patients during an attack. We measured rCBF in 42 patients with common or classical migraine from the onset of an attack and up to 8 hours thereafter. Carotid angiography was carried out as part of the clinical evaluation in 20 patients suffering from classical migraine with hemiplegic manifestations. In 14 of the patients, migraine attacks were induced by the arteriography and were examined during the subsequent, ongoing rCBF study. Xenon–133 was injected into the internal carotid artery and the washout of the isotope was followed by a 254-channel scintillation camera covering the lateral aspect of the hemisphere (Sveinsdottir et al., 1977). Then, during the development of the aura and the headache, rCBF was measured. Subsequently, 22 patients with spontaneous common and classical migraine attacks who applied to the Copenhagen acute headache clinic had rCBF measured with an atraumatic technique, employing Xenon-133 inhalation and single-photon, emission computed tomography (Stokely et al., 1980). The three-dimensional approach circumvented tissue layer superposition and allowed distinction of rCBF in cortical and subcortical regions. The patients in the second study were usually examined during phases of the attacks when measurements were terminated in the first study. By compiling the data of these two series a detailed pattern of the pathophysiological events during the acute migraine attack emerged.

The Concept of "Spreading Oligemia" and Its Relationship to the Development of Premonitory Focal Neurologic Symptoms (Aura) in Classical Migraine

In our first retrospective study of 6 patients with classical migraine it appeared that a specific change of rCBF accompanied the development of symptoms (Olesen et al., 1981). The decrease in blood flow (25% – 30%) usually started in the posterior aspect of the brain and progressed anteriorly in a wave-like fashion, independent of the territorial supply of the large arteries. The term "spreading oligemia" was coined to describe this phenomenon. In a subsequent prospective study of 14 patients, 9 developed classical migraine attacks during the rCBF investigations. In these patients the reduction of rCBF also started posteriorly, in the occipitoparietal region, and progressed anteriorly. By measuring the time between the closely spaced rCBF studies, and simultaneously counting the increasing number of channels included in the oligemia (each covering 1.5 cm^2 of cortical surface), it was possible to estimate the velocity of the "spreading oligemia": it progressed at a rate of 2.2 mm/min over the hemisphere. The calculated rate was probably an underestimate, since we were unable to take the folding of the human cortex into consideration. The "spreading oligemia" did not cross the central or lateral sulcus but appeared in the frontal lobe in areas corresponding to the frontal or orbital operculum, indicating that its progression to the frontal regions occurred through the insula. In other words, the oligemia propagated according to the architecture of the cortex, and not according to the supply territory of major branches of the carotid or vertebral arteries (Lauritzen et al., 1983b).

The oligemia was usually apparent over part of the posterior aspect of the brain before clinical symptoms began. The focal neurologic symptoms in the contralateral side of the body appeared when most of the temporal and parietal lobe exhibited hypoperfusion. The oligemia persisted in the same regions after the symptoms had vanished and sometimes continued to spread to the frontal lobe during the development of headache (Olesen et al., 1981a; Lauritzen et al., 1983a). This dissociation in time between focal symptoms and hypoperfusion indicated that the symptoms were not caused by the hypoperfusion itself but by a disturbance in tissue function underlying the perfusion changes. The hypoperfusion persisted during the development of unilateral pain, while hyperperfusion was not observed. Cerebral hyperperfusion could therefore be disregarded as a source of the migraine headache.

Abnormalities of Blood Flow Regulation of the Partly Hypoperfused Brain

The occurrence of "spreading oligemia" was taken as an opportunity to examine three principles of cerebral blood flow regulation: blood pressure autoregulation, CO_2 reactivity, and metabolic autoregulation. Blood pressure autoregulation was intact in all parts of the partly hypoperfused brain. The CO_2 reactivity of oligemic areas was only half that of the control values obtained in neighboring, normally perfused brain. Metabolic autoregulation, that is, the regional increases of blood flow to physiological activation like hand movement and listening, was markedly impaired in the hypoperfused regions, whereas the adjacent normally perfused tissue reacted normally to activation (Lauritzen et al., 1983b; Olesen et al., 1981a). Between attacks, patients had normal blood flow regulation. The confinement of the regulation abnormalities to small hypoperfused parts of the brain indicated that the abnormal vasoreactivity was caused by dysfunction of the underlying tissue and not abnormality of an unknown and remote center determining vasomotor tone.

**Persistent Cortical Hypoperfusion during Spontaneous
Classical Migraine Attacks, and the Normal Perfusion Pattern
in Common Migraine**

Eleven patients with spontaneous attacks of classical migraine were studied 2 to 3 hours after onset of the aura when their symptomatology was largely stable and consisted of mild neurologic symptoms and headache. Eight of the patients displayed an asymmetrical flow pattern consisting of unilateral hypoperfusion in the hemisphere appropriate to the persistent or just-remitted focal neurologic symptoms. Three patients exhibited a normal flow map. The tomographic approach to rCBF examination permitted localization of the hypoperfusion to superficial or deep brain structures. The area of oligemia was localized to the cortex in all cases, whereas subcortical structures showed a largely normal flow distribution (Figure 22.3). The hypoperfusion remained unchanged in repeated measurements of blood flow at 30 to 45 minute intervals, indicating a steady state of cerebral perfusion. The patients were reexamined after ergotamine treatment or spontaneous recovery, when they were symptom-free. Blood flow had normalized in most patients 4 to 6 hours after onset of the attack. In no case was migraine headache associated with hyperemia. We therefore considered that a hyperperfused state is rare in the uncomplicated, classical migraine attack and is unlikely to be the source of the pain (Lauritzen and Olesen, 1984).

No significant alteration in rCBF was displayed by 12 patients with common migraine who were examined from 7 to 20 hours after onset of an attack. This finding complements the observation of normal blood flow in the initial phases of attacks of common migraine induced by red wine (Olesen et al., 1981b). We concluded that common migraine attacks are rarely associated with intracranial perfusion changes.

CONCLUSION

The compiled cerebral blood flow data in patients with induced and spontaneous classical migraine provide a detailed description of the blood flow changes during the attack. "Spreading oligemia" accompanies the first 1 or 2 hours of the attack, which is when focal neurologic symptoms develop and subside, and the headache ensues. The hypoperfused state persists for the following 4 to 6 hours, until recovery to normal flow values occurs.

The following parallels can be drawn between the rCBF changes of classical migraine and those of spreading depression of Leão:

1. The "spreading oligemia" of migraine starts in the posterior aspect of the hemisphere which contains the highest density of neural elements, this density being maximal at the occipital pole. SD is most easily elicited in animals with a high density of neurons. It is therefore likely that spontane-

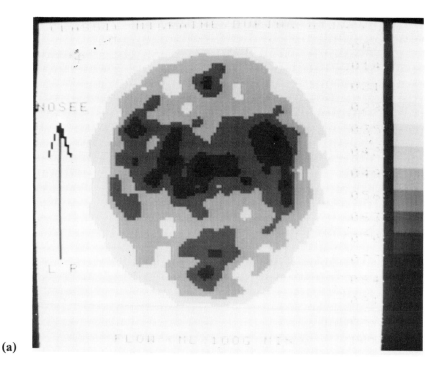

(a)

Figure 22.3 Tomographic cerebral blood flow study of patient with classical migraine. A 24-year-old woman who presented in the Copenhagen Acute Headache Clinic with an attack of classical migraine, 2 hours after the onset of symptoms. Scintillations of both visual fields preceded by ten minutes her right hemihypesthesiae/paresthesiae, light right hemiparesis, difficulty in finding the words, and later headache. (a) During investigation, the patient suffered from slight right hemiparesis and hemihypesthesia, severe bilateral throbbing headache, and a rythmic 10 to 20 Hz tremor of the right hand and fingers. The tomogram shows a moderate hypoperfusion (20%) of the left lateral temporal cortex. No hyperperfused regions were observed during this or the three subsequent rCBF examinations, before treatment, when the headache was maximal; (b) After treatment, when symptom-free. The tomogram shows a hyperperfusion of the previously hypoperfused region.

ous SD in the human brain would be elicited in this region, and that the rCBF reduction would start in this region if it was secondary to SD.

2. The velocity of propagation of "spreading oligemia" is 2 to 3 mm/min. The hypoperfusion does not cross the primary sulci outlining the major macro- and microstructural areas of the cortical surface. SD likewise spreads at 2 to 5 mm/min and is stopped by abrupt architectonic changes of the convexity. The two phenomena thus behave similarly with regard to velocity and mode of spread.

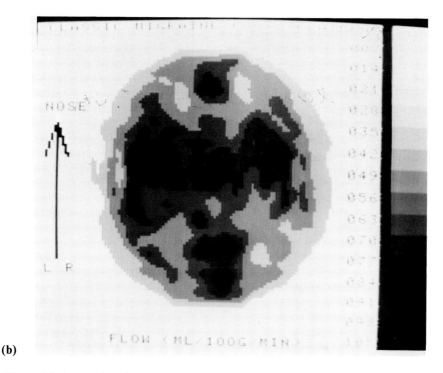

(b)

Figure 22.3 *continued*

3. The reduction of blood flow in migraine is 20% to 25%, comparable to the post-SD hypoperfusion of 25% to 30%.
4. In both conditions abnormalities of blood flow regulation are restricted to the hypoperfused regions. The character of the regulation abnormalities is the same in the two conditions.
5. Blood flow reduction in migraine is cortical in the same manner as the persistent, cortical hypoperfusion after SD. Hypoperfusion in the patients lasts for 4 to 6 hours. The post-SD hypoperfusion lasts for at least 1 hour; perfusion changes during later stages are unknown at the moment.

From the rCBF studies it appears that spreading depression is the most probable mechanism underlying classical migraine, and that SD may serve as an experimental migraine model. Conversely, we may regard classical migraine as an indication of how spreading depression can express itself in man.

The clinical syndromes where migraine and epilepsy occur simultaneously may prove to be conditions in which spreading depression and its potential clinical counterparts can be studied. We are only at the beginning of the exploration of the possible clinical implications of Leão's spreading depression.

REFERENCES

Astrup J, Heuser D, Lassen NA, Nilsson B, Norberg K, Siesjö BK. Evidence against H^+ and K^+ as main factors for the control of cerebral blood flow: a microelectrode study. In: Cerebral vascular smooth muscle and its control. Ciba Foundation Symposium 56 (new series). Amsterdam: Elsevier, 1978:313–37.

Bures J, Buresova O, Krivanek J. The mechanisms and applications of Leão's spreading depression of electroencephalographic activity. New York: Academic Press, 1974.

Carew TJ, Crow TJ, Petrinovich LF. Lack of coincidence between neural and behavioral manifestations of cortical spreading depression. Science 1970;169:1339–41.

Dalessio DJ. Wolff's headache and other head pain. New York, Oxford: Oxford University Press, 1980.

Gjedde A, Hansen AJ, Siemkowicz E. Rapid simultaneous determination of regional cerebral blood flow and blood-brain glucose transfer in brain of rat. Acta Physiol Scand 1980;108:321–30.

Gjedde A, Hansen AJ, Quistorff B. Blood-brain glucose transfer in spreading depression. *J Neurochem* 1981;37:807–12.

Gowers WR. The borderland of epilepsy. London: Churchill, 1907.

Grafstein B. Mechanism of spreading cortical depression. J Neurophysiol 1956;19: 154–71.

Hansen AJ, Olsen CE. Brain extracellular space during spreading depression and ischemia. Acta Physiol Scand 1980;108:355–65.

Hansen AJ, Quistorff B, Gjedde A. Relationship between local changes in cortical blood flow and extracellular K^+ during spreading depression. Acta Physiol Scand 1980;109:1–6.

Hansen AJ, Zeuthen T. Changes of brain extracellular ions during spreading depression and ischemia in rats. Acta Physiol Scand 1981;113:437–45.

Hubschmann OR, Kornhauser D. Effect of subarachnoid hemorrhage on the extracellular microenvironment. J Neurosurg 1982;56:216–21.

Krivanek J. Concerning the dynamics of the metabolic changes accompanying cortical spreading depression. Physiol Bohemoslov 1962;11:383–91.

Lashley KS. Patterns of cerebral integration indicated by the scotomas of migraine. Arch Neurol Psychiatry 1941;46:331–9.

Lauritzen M. Long-lasting reduction of cortical blood flow after spreading depression with preserved autoregulation and impaired CO_2-response. J Cereb Blood Flow Metab 1984;4:546–54.

Lauritzen M. Regional cerebral blood flow during spreading depression in rat brain: Increased reactive hyperemia in low-flow states. Acta Neurol Scand 1986; (in press).

Lauritzen M, Balslev Jørgensen M, Diemer NH, Gjedde A, Hansen AJ. Persistent oligemia of rat cerebral cortex in the wake of spreading depression. Ann Neurol 1982;12:469–74.

Lauritzen M, Olsen J. Regional cerebral blood flow during migraine attacks by xenon-133 inhalation and emission tomography. Brain 1984;107:447–61.

Lauritzen M, Skyhøj Olsen T, Lassen NA, Paulson OB. The changes of regional cerebral blood flow during the course of classical migraine attacks. Ann Neurol 1983a;13:633–41.

Lauritzen M, Skyhøj Olsen T, Lassen NA, Paulson OB. The regulation of regional cerebral blood flow during and between migraine attacks. Ann Neurol 1983b;14:569–72.

Lauritzen M, Trojaborg W, Olesen J. EEG during attacks of common and classical migraine. Cephalalgia 1981;1:63–6.

Leão AAP. Spreading depression of activity in cerebral cortex. J Neurophysiol 1944a;7:359–90.

Leão AAP. Pial circulation and spreading depression of activity in the cerebral cortex. J Neurophysiol 1944b;7:391–6.

Leão AAP. Further observations on the spreading depression of activity in the cerebral cortex. J Neurophysiol 1947;10:409–19.

Leão AAP, Morrison RS. Propagation of spreading cortical depression. J Neurophysiol 1945;8:33–45.

Mayevsky A, Zeuthen T, Chance B. Measurements of extracellular potassium, ECoG and pyridine nucleotide levels during cortical spreading depression in rats. Brain Res 1974;76:347–9.

Milner PM. Note on a possible correspondence between the scotomas of migraine and spreading depression of Leão. Electroencephalogr Clin Neurophysiol 1958;10:705.

Nicholson C, Kraig RP. The behaviors of extracellular ions during spreading depression. In: Zeuthen T, ed. The application of ion-selective microelectrodes. Amsterdam: Elsevier, 1981:217–38.

Olesen J, Larsen B, Lauritzen M. Focal hyperemia followed by spreading oligemia and impaired activation of rCBF in classic migraine. Ann Neurol 1981a;9:344–52.

Olesen J, Tfelt-Hansen P, Henriksen L, Larsen B. The common migraine attack may not be initiated by cerebral ischemia. Lancet 1981b;2:438–40.

Shinohara M, Dollinger B, Brown G, Rapoport S, Sokoloff L. Cerebral glucose utilization: local changes during and after recovery from spreading cortical depression. Science 1979;203:188–90.

Stokely EM, Sveinsdottir E, Lassen NA, Rommer P. A single photon dynamic computer assisted tomograph (DCAT) for imaging brain function in multiple cross sections. J Comput Assist Tomogr 1980;4:230–40.

Sugaya E, Takato M, Noda Y. Neuronal and glial activity during spreading depression in cerebral cortex of cat. J Neurophysiol 1975;38:822–41.

Sveinsdottir E, Larsen B, Rommer P, Lassen NA. A multidetector scintillation camera with 254 channels. J Nucl Med 1977;18:168–74.

Van Harreveld A, Stamm JS. Cortical responses to metrazol and sensory stimulation in the rabbit. Electroencephalogr Clin Neurophysiol 1955;7:363–70.

23

Visual Sensitivity and Hyperexcitability in Epilepsy and Migraine

Arnold J. Wilkins

The eye is not satisfied with seeing.

ECCLESIASTES 1:8

This chapter compares the stimulus and response parameters of visual sensitivity in epilepsy and migraine. It is divided into five sections. In the first section the characteristics of epileptic visual sensitivity are described, with details of the stimulus parameters optimal (more correctly "pessimal"!) for the induction of epileptiform electroencephalographic (EEG) abnormalities. In the second section it is shown that these abnormalities are induced by stimuli with parameters that are almost precisely the same as those that provoke anomalous visual effects in persons without epilepsy. Susceptibility to these visual effects varies considerably from one person to another, depending on the frequency and nature of the headaches they suffer. The similarity between the stimuli that provoke seizures and those that provoke illusions and headaches suggests that the precipitants share common neural mechanisms. This hypothesis is consistent with the electroencephalographic response parameters in epilepsy and migraine which are compared in the third section. The fourth section considers the theoretical implications of the similarity between the stimulus and response parameters of visual sensitivity in the two disorders. The fifth and final section is devoted to some practical ramifications of the two forms of visual sensitivity.

EPILEPTIC VISUAL SENSITIVITY

About 5% of patients with epilepsy are photosensitive and liable to visually induced seizures. These seizures are commonly associated with television viewing or with flicker, as from sunlight reflected in water or interrupted by roadside trees. In patients with a history of such seizures the EEG may show no abnormalities during rest, but when the patient is exposed to intermittent light a photoconvulsive response is usually recorded. The photoconvulsive response differs from a variety of other anomalous EEG responses to intermittent light and is almost invariably associated with epilepsy. It consists of generalized regular or irregular single or multiple spikes interspersed with slow waves. This activity, which typically has a frequency of 2.5 to 3 Hz, is usually fairly symmetrical and is often of maximum amplitude in the frontocentral regions. It is not phase-locked to the train of flashes but can outlast it (Newmark and Penry, 1979; Chapter 5). When patients exhibiting such a photoconvulsive response are asked to look at patterns of stripes, epileptiform EEG abnormalities are often recorded. The abnormalities may consist of one or more spikes with or without associated slow waves. The proportion of photosensitive patients demonstrating such pattern sensitivity depends on the parameters of the pattern. When the spatial parameters are optimal about one-third of such patients are affected by the stationary pattern. If the stripes are vibrated with optimal parameters of amplitude and temporal frequency about 70% of patients are affected. It is rare for patients to be sensitive to pattern and not to diffuse intermittent light.

Stimulus Parameters of Epileptic Visual Sensitivity

The spatial and temporal parameters of visual stimuli optimal for evoking epileptiform EEG abnormalities have been reviewed by Wilkins, Binnie, and Darby (1980) and will now be summarized.

The Shape of the Pattern

Patterns of stripes are more epileptogenic than patterns of checks of equivalent width. If the component checks in a checkerboard pattern are elongated, the probability of paroxysmal EEG activity (as estimated from repeated randomized pattern presentations) increases with the check length/width ratio as shown in Figure 23.1a.

Spatial Frequency of the Pattern

In Figure 23.2a the patient is shown looking at the center of a pattern of stripes, circular in outline, with a visual angle of 20 degrees. A photometer moved across the pattern in a direction orthogonal to the stripes will give a reading that describes the luminance profile of the pattern. In the example shown, two cycles of the pattern subtend a visual angle of one degree; that is, the spatial frequency of the pattern is 2 cycles/degree.

The probability of paroxysmal activity is a curvilinear function of spatial frequency illustrated in Figure 23.3a.

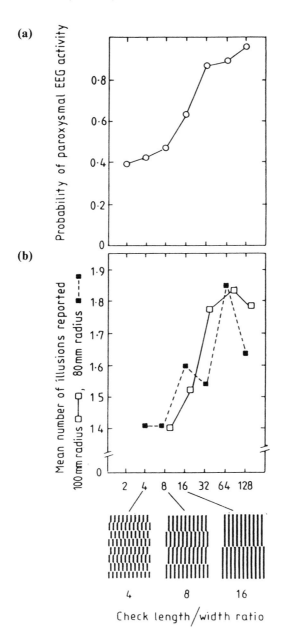

Figure 23.1 (a) Probability of paroxysmal activity in response to a pattern of elongated checks, expressed as a function of the length/width ratio of the checks. Data from a representative pattern-sensitive epileptic patient. After Wilkins, Andermann, and Ives (1975). (b) The corresponding function for the mean number of illusions reported by normal observers. Separate curves for two patterns, each viewed at 0.4 m. Check width 15 minutes of arc. Wilkins et al. (1984).

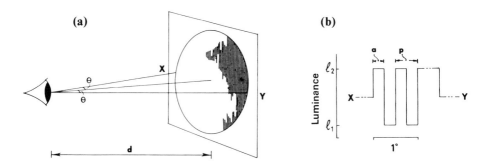

Figure 23.2   (a) Schematic diagram showing the eye of the observer fixating the center of a pattern of stripes circular in outline, subtending 20 degrees visual angle. The viewing distance is d. (b) The luminance profile of the grating in Figure 23.2a with a Michelson contrast of $(L2 - L1)/(L2 + L1)$, a mean luminance of $(L2 + L1)/2$, a period of p degrees, a duty cycle of $a/p - a = 50\%$, and a spatial frequency of $1/p = 2$ cycles/degree.

As can be seen, the spatial frequency optimal for the induction of paroxysmal activity is close to 3 cycles/degree. The pattern shown in Figure 23.4 has a spatial frequency of 3 cycles/degree when viewed at a distance of 40 cm.

Duty Cycle of the Pattern

The luminance profile illustrated in Figure 23.2b has a duty cycle of 50%; that is, the width of the bright parts of the grating (a) is half of the width of one cycle of the grating (p). The probability of paroxysmal activity varies with the duty cycle as illustrated in Figure 23.5a and shows a peak somewhere in the 50% to 70% range. (Wilkins, Darby, and Binnie, unpublished observations). The grating in Figure 23.4 has a duty cycle of 50%.

Contrast of the Pattern

The Michelson contrast is defined as

$$(L2 - L1)/(L2 + L1)$$

where L2 and L1 are the luminance of the light and dark portions of the pattern (see Figure 23.2b). The probability of paroxysmal activity increases precipitously with pattern contrast for contrasts below 30% but for higher values shows relatively little change with contrast. This can be seen in Figure 23.6a which shows the separate functions for seven pattern-sensitive epileptic patients.

Area of the Pattern

The area of a pattern of stripes can be manipulated in a variety of ways. If a pattern of concentric rings is cut into sectors similar to the slices of a cake and

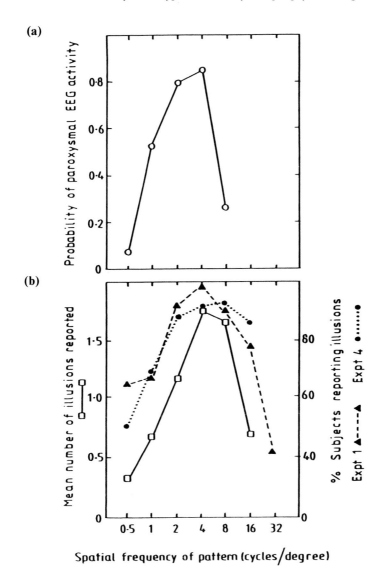

Figure 23.3 (a) Probability of paroxysmal activity expressed as a function of the spatial frequency of a grating, centrally fixated, circular in outline, and subtending 24 degrees at a viewing distance 0.57 m; with square-wave luminance profile, Michelson contrast 0.7, and mean luminance about 300 cd/m² (steady white light). Mean of eight pattern-sensitive epileptic patients. See Wilkins, Binnie, and Darby (1980). (b) The corresponding function for the mean number of illusions seen by normal observers. The pattern parameters were as above with the exception of the viewing distance which was 0.4 m. After Wilkins et al. (1984): experiments 1 and 4.

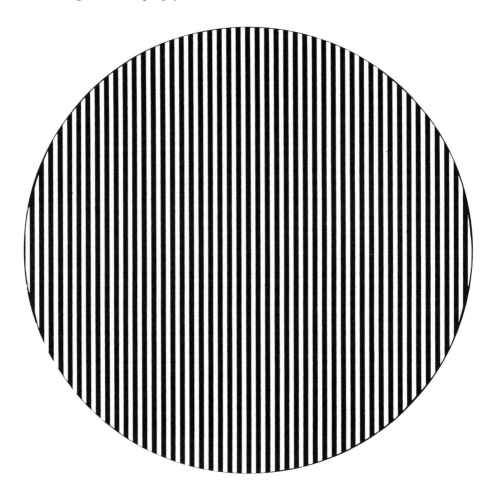

Figure 23.4   An example of a grating with a square-wave luminance profile, and a Michelson contrast of about 0.7. At a viewing distance of 0.4 m this grating subtends 20 degrees and has a spatial frequency of 3 cycles/degree. When illuminated by a 60 W tungsten filament reading lamp at a distance of 1 m the mean luminance is on the order of 10 cd/m².

pairs of sectors are diametrically opposed, as represented schematically in Figure 23.7a, then the probability of paroxysmal activity increases with sector angle. Figure 23.7b shows the data for seven patients plotted as a function of total pattern area. Note that the curves for patterns with two sectors usually overlap with those for four, indicating that the probability of paroxysmal activity is usually a function of the total area of the pattern, regardless of the region of retina stimulated.

When pattern size is manipulated by varying the sector angle, all retinal eccentricities are affected by the change in pattern area. Note that although the

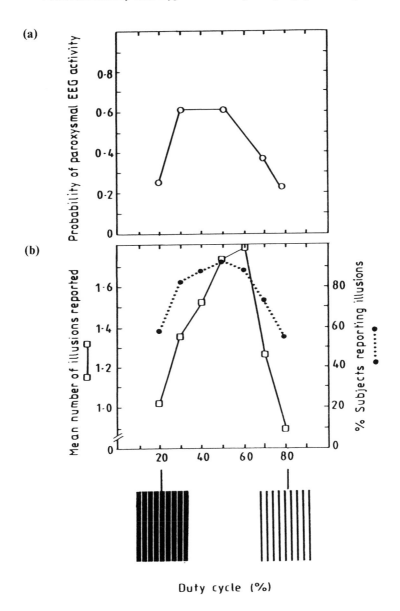

Figure 23.5 (a) Probability of paroxysmal EEG activity as a function of the duty cycle of a grating, centrally fixated, circular in outline, and subtending 20 degrees at a viewing distance of 0.4 m, with Michelson contrast 0.7, and mean luminance about 100 cd/m². Mean of four photosensitive epileptic patients (Wilkins, Binnie, and Darby, unpublished data). (b) The corresponding function for the mean number of illusions seen by normal observers. After Wilkins et al. (1984).

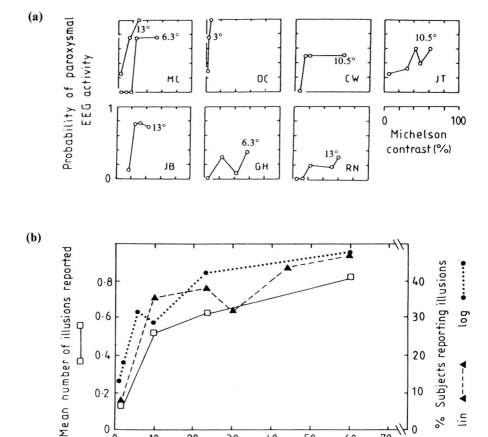

Figure 23.6 (a) Probability of paroxysmal EEG activity as a function of the Michelson contrast of a grating with square-wave luminance profile, spatial frequency 2 cycles/degree, mean luminance about 300 cd/m² (steady white light), centrally fixated at a distance of 0.5 m. The gratings were circular in outline with an angular radius as indicated. Separate panels for seven pattern-sensitive epileptic patients. After Wilkins, Binnie, and Darby (1980). (b) The corresponding function for the mean number of illusions seen by normal observers. Two sets of stimuli were used with contrasts spaced evenly on linear or logarithmic scales. After Wilkins et al. (1984).

x-intercepts differ for each patient, the slopes of the functions are broadly similar from one patient to another, indicating that for different patients the probability of paroxysmal activity increases with the total pattern area at roughly the same rate. This is no longer the case if pattern area is manipulated by increasing the radius of a centrally fixated pattern of stripes (see Figure 23.8a). The functions relating the probability of paroxysmal activity to pattern

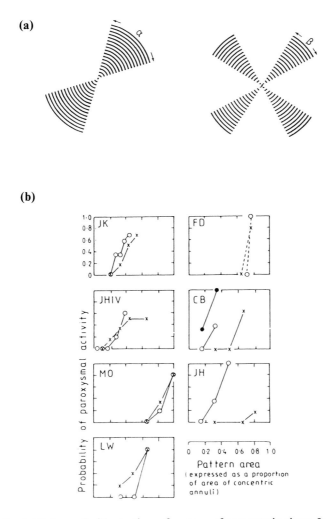

Figure 23.7   (a) Schematic illustration of sectors of concentric rings. In the example shown $\alpha = 2\beta$ and so the total pattern area is the same for both types of pattern. (b) Probability of paroxysmal activity as a function of the total area of the patterns shown in Figure 23.7a. The patterns had a Michelson contrast of 0.7 and a mean luminance of about 300 cd/m² (steady white light). Fixation was central and the viewing distance was 0.5 m. Pattern area was manipulated by varying the sector angle. Patterns with two sectors and a "twenty minutes to two" orientation are represented by open circles and those with a "twenty minutes past ten" orientation by filled circles. Patterns with four sectors are represented by crosses. The spatial frequency (radial measurement) was 2 cycles/degree and the sector radius 24 degrees, except for one patient, FD, who was tested using patterns with a spatial frequency of 3.5 cycles/degree and radius 15 degrees. After Wilkins, Binnie, and Darby (1980).

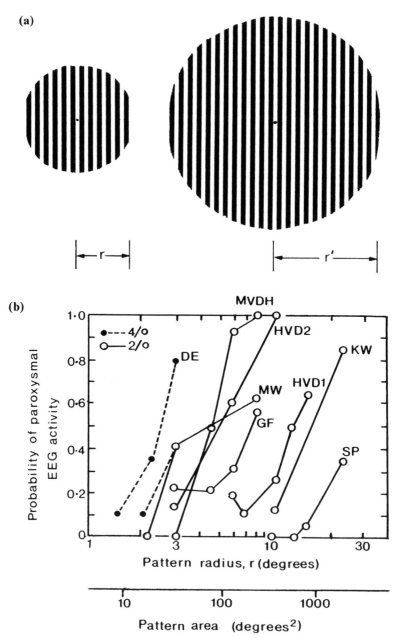

Figure 23.8 (a) Two gratings with square-wave luminance profile, circular in outline and of different radii (r and r′). (b) Probability of paroxysmal EEG activity as a function of the area and radius of gratings with square-wave luminance profile, circular in outline and centrally fixated, with a Michelson contrast of 0.7 and mean luminance of 300 cd/m² (steady white light). The spatial frequency was 2 or 4 cycles/degree, as shown. Each curve represents the data for a different patient. After Wilkins, Binnie, and Darby (1980).

area then have different slopes. The slopes for different patients now resemble one another only when the functions are expressed in terms of the logarithm of pattern area.

As can be seen from Figure 23.8b, the radius of a pattern has to be doubled to increase the probability of paroxysmal activity from near zero to near unity. This finding doubtless reflects the fact that the larger patterns now stimulate proportionately more of the peripheral retina, and the peripheral retina has a smaller cortical representation. Such an interpretation is in line with the effects of selective stimulation of central and peripheral retina that will now be described.

If the central section of a grating is removed, creating an annulus of stripes as shown in Figure 23.9a, the probability of paroxysmal activity is considerably reduced. The probability is then best predicted not by the area of the pattern but by the area of the visual cortex to which the pattern projects. The area of cortex devoted to analyzing the region of visual space occupied by the pattern can be computed from a published estimate of the human cortical magnification factor (Drasdo, 1977). This estimate is surprisingly good at equating the paroxysmal response to discs and annuli, as can be appreciated by comparing the scatterplots shown in Figures 23.9b and 23.9c. In these plots each point represents the data from a single patient and the position of a point is determined by the threshold size of discs and annuli for which the probability of paroxysmal activity is greater than zero but less than one. When the position of the points is determined by the area of cortex to which the disc and the annulus project ("Q" in Figure 23.9b) the correlation between the threshold size for the two types of stimuli is higher than when the points are plotted in terms of the pattern area (Figure 23.9c). These data are somewhat surprising given that no pattern, regardless of its spatial frequency, it likely to stimulate all neurons devoted to analyzing the space that the pattern occupies.

Luminance of the Pattern

As might be expected, the probability of paroxysmal activity increases with the mean luminance of a pattern of constant contrast, but changes in luminance of two log units are usually required to change the probability from near zero to near unity. Different patients have different threshold luminances at which paroxysmal activity first appears, and in some patients this threshold can be in the mesopic range. This is illustrated in Figure 23.10.

Location of the Pattern in the Visual Field

Patterns presented in the lateral fields (Figures 23.11a and 23.11b) are usually more epileptogenic than patterns in the upper or lower visual fields (Figures 23.11c and 23.11d). When one lateral field is stimulated, epileptiform EEG abnormalities usually appear over the contralateral posterior quadrant (usually maximal at the posterior temporal electrode: compare Figures 23.11a and 23.11b) and in some patients these abnormalities can be far more readily induced by stimulation of one field than the other. This evidence for an inequal-

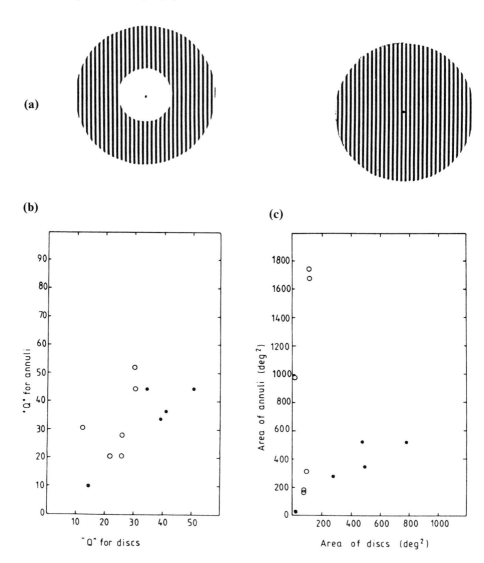

Figure 23.9   (a) An example of an annular grating and a complete disc, (b) and (c). Scatterplots showing the threshold for the size of an annular grating (ordinate) or a complete disc (abscissa) for which the probability of induced paroxysmal EEG activity was greater than zero and less than one. In (b) the size is expressed in terms of the area of the visual cortex to which the pattern projects (Q%; Drasdo, 1977) and in (c) the size is expressed as the area of the pattern. The data for patients tested using annuli with an inner radius of 1.5 degrees are represented by solid points. The open points are for patients tested using annuli with a larger inner radius. The other pattern parameters were similar to those listed in the legend to Figure 23.3. After Wilkins, Binnie, and Darby (1980).

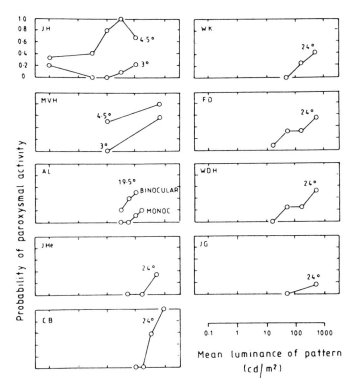

Figure 23.10 The probability of paroxysmal EEG activity expressed as a function of the mean luminance of a grating with square-wave luminance profile, Michelson contrast 0.7, circular in outline and centrally fixated (radius as shown). The presentations were binocular except in the case of one patient whose left eye was occluded on some trials. The natural pupil was used throughout. After Wilkins, Binnie, and Darby (1980).

ity in the hyperexcitability of the cerebral hemispheres is corroborated by responses to diffuse intermittent light which, in these patients, demonstrate a corresponding hemispheric amplitude asymmetry.

In a few patients the response to stimulation of the upper visual field involves lower head regions than the responses to the lower field (compare Figures 23.11c and 23.11d). (See Binnie et al., 1981 and Wilkins et al., 1981).

Presentation of the Pattern to One or Both Eyes

Monocular pattern presentations are less epileptogenic than those that are binocular. If different patterns are presented to the two eyes stereoscopically, patterns that fuse in binocular vision are more epileptogenic than those that induce binocular rivalry.

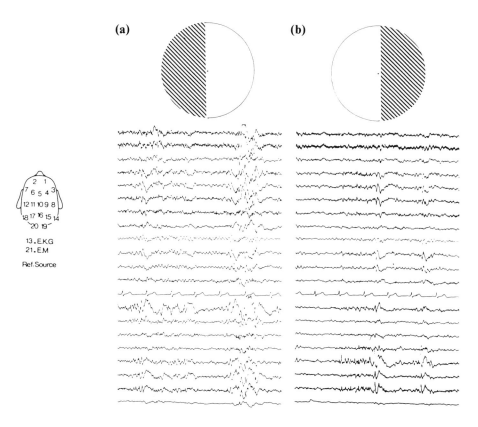

Figure 23.11 (a, b, c, and d) Schematic diagrams of gratings in the left, right, upper, and lower visual hemifields respectively, together with an example of the paroxysmal EEG activity evoked by such patterns. Records are from one patient. In (a) the paroxysmal activity is initially most marked in the right posterior quadrant (particularly the right posterior-temporal electrode: channel 14), whereas in (b) the contralateral quadrant is most affected (particularly the left-posterior temporal electrode: channel 18). In (c) and (d) the activity recorded from the nonstandard midline occipital electrodes show a dissociation: the activity in (c) is initially greater in the lowest electrodes (channels 5 and 6); in (d) higher electrodes (channels 3 and 4) record the most marked activity. After Wilkins, Binnie, and Darby (1981).

Movement of the Pattern

When a pattern of stripes is vibrated in a direction orthogonal to that of the stripes, the temporal frequency of vibration optimal for the induction of paroxysmal activity is about 20 Hz, regardless of the spatial frequency of the grating. The optimal spatial frequency remains the same as that for stationary patterns (about 3 cycles/degree). Variations in the amplitude of oscillation of one-half spatial cycle have little, if any, effect (Binnie et al., 1979). If the left and right halves of a centrally fixated grating are caused to drift continuously toward

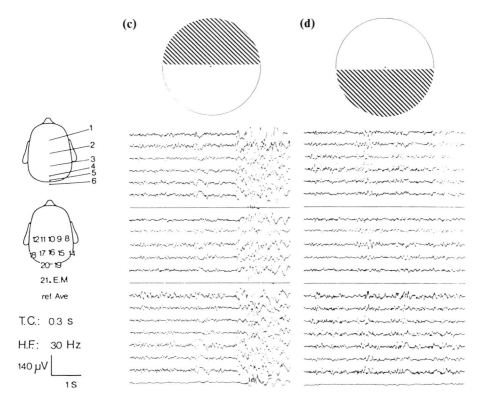

Figure 23.11   *continued*

fixation, the epileptogenic properties are less than those when the same grating is stationary and considerably less than when the movement is oscillatory rather than continuous. This is the case for a wide range of temporal parameters, although at frequencies of vibration in excess of 30 Hz the epileptogenic properties of a vibrating grating are reduced (Binnie et al., 1985).

Temporal Frequency of Modulation of an Unpatterned Field

Paroxysmal activity is more likely to occur if the rate of a succession of brief diffuse flashes is in the region of 15 to 20 Hz but some patients can also be sensitive to isolated flashes and to trains of flashes at frequencies higher than 50 Hz (Jeavons and Harding, 1975).

Inferences About the Nature of the Seizure Trigger

Photosensitive epileptic patients have normal vision, at least interictally, and so it is reasonable to assume that the visual system functions normally up to the point at which a paroxysmal discharge occurs. Our knowledge about the functioning of normal mammalian visual systems (e.g., Hubel and Wiesel, 1979) can therefore be used as the basis for inferences about the nature of the seizure trigger.

Cells in the striate and prestriate cortex have linear receptive fields. The effects of length of line contour would suggest that such cells are implicated in the trigger mechanism. Many cells in the cortex will fire when either eye is stimulated and some fire mainly when the image on the two retinae is similar. The effects of monocular occlusion and binocular rivalry are therefore consistent with a trigger involving these cells. Many of the cells in the striate and prestriate cortex have complex receptive fields and respond selectively to the spatial parameters of the stimulus over a range of retinal positions greater than the size of the stimulus. The independence of spatial and temporal parameters of stimulation by vibrating patterns would be consistent with a trigger mechanism involving such cells (see Wilkins, Binnie, and Darby, 1980). These three considerations point to the role of the visual cortex in the induction of paroxysmal EEG abnormalities. The variation in the topography of the EEG response with the location of the stimulus within the visual field suggests that the visual cortex is indeed the neural substrate responsible.

Cells in the visual cortex increase their rate of firing with the contrast across their receptive fields, but most have saturated or have begun to do so when the contrast exceeds 30%, (Albrecht and Hamilton, 1982). The fact that the probability of paroxysmal activity increases with pattern contrast but reaches a "plateau" at contrasts above 30% suggests that the probability is a function of total cortical excitation. Such an interpretation is supported by the effects of pattern area described previously in this chapter.

The probability of paroxysmal activity in response to a pattern depends on the area of cortex to which the pattern projects, regardless of the region of the visual field stimulated. This would suggest that the particular region of the visual cortex stimulated is less important than the total amount. Some patients may nevertheless show a remarkable difference between the response to stimulation of the two lateral visual fields. Furthermore, the topography of the convulsive response to unilateral stimulation suggests that the hemispheres may act independently in triggering a discharge. This independence would explain the difference between the lateral and upper and lower visual fields. The amount of excitation of one cerebral hemisphere by a pattern in the contralateral field is greater than that resulting when the same pattern stimulates the upper or lower fields.

In layer 4 of the visual cortex there exists a horizontal network of aspinous and sparsely spinous stellate cells. These cells form part of a GABA-ergic (GABA: gamma-aminobutyric acid) inhibitory intracortical system. They appear to control the selectivity of the response of the pyramidal neurons to specific stimuli within the visual field. If this inhibitory system were minimally impaired, excessive excitation of the pyramidal neurons would result in a paroxysmal discharge. This impairment would not necessarily be sufficient to disrupt functioning under normal conditions of excitation. There is considerable pharmacologic evidence for an impairment of GABA-ergic inhibition as the basis of the naturally occurring syndrome of photosensitivity in the baboon *Papio papio.* Meldrum and Wilkins (1984) have combined this pharmacologic evidence with the psychophysical evidence outlined above and have proposed that human photosensitivity may also be the result of a diffuse minimal failure of intracortical inhibition, possibly one that is GABA-ergic or dopaminergic (Quesney, 1981).

VISUAL SENSITIVITY IN PERSONS WITHOUT EPILEPSY

People without epilepsy see illusions of color, shape, and motion in the epileptogenic pattern in Figure 23.4. In this section it will be shown that these illusions are dependent on the same pattern parameters as those that influence the epileptogenic properties in almost precisely the same way.

In a series of studies, Wilkins et al. (1984) attempted to measure the illusions people report using verbal descriptors. Volunteers on the subject panel of the Applied Psychology Unit were asked to look at a grating similar to that in Figure 23.4 for 10 seconds and then to report any effects, visual or otherwise, that the pattern produced. (Subjects with epilepsy were excluded.) The visual effects reported can be paraphrased according to the following list: red, green, blue, yellow, blurring, bending of the stripes, shimmering, flickering, and shadowy shapes. Different groups of subjects were then asked to look at patterns that varied with respect to the parameters of shape, spatial frequency, contrast, duty cycle, area, position in the visual field, and eye of presentation, and to use the check list to describe the effects produced. The mean number of illusions checked on the list varied considerably, although the proportion of illusions of each type showed comparatively little change. For every parameter but one, the value optimal for the induction of paroxysmal EEG activity in epileptic patients was also optimal for the induction of illusions in persons without epilepsy. Figure 23.1b shows how the mean number of illusions reported increases with the length/width ratio of the checks in a checkerboard pattern. Figure 23.3b shows how the mean number of illusions reported varies with the spatial frequency of a square-wave grating, reaching a maximum at 3 cycles/degree. Figure 23.5b shows the corresponding effects of duty cycle. The data in Figure 23.6b indicate that the mean number of illusions increases sharply at low contrasts, although for values in excess of about 30% there is little further increase. In fact, both the mean number of illusions and the average probability of paroxysmal activity show linear increases with log contrast. Table 23.1 shows how the mean number of illusions depends on the total area of a pattern of segmented concentric rings regardless of the region of retina stimulated, and Table 23.2 shows that for gratings in the form of discs and annuli the mean number of illusions depends on the area of cortex to which the gratings project. The illusions increase with vibratory movement of the pattern and are reduced

Table 23.1   Mean Number of Illusions Reported in Sectored Rings

Stimulus		Mean Number of Illusions	t̲ test	p
A		0.56		
			1.09	<0.15
B		0.68		
			0.18	NS
C		0.68		
			2.39	<0.01
D		1.03		

After Wilkins et al. (1984)

by monocular viewing. As in the case of epileptic sensitivity, some individuals report an inequality between the lateral visual fields with regard to the illusions induced.

One point of difference between epileptic sensitivity and illusion susceptibility arises when comparing the effects of stimulation of the upper and lower versus the lateral visual fields. Whereas pattern-sensitive epileptic patients generally show a greater sensitivity to stimulation of a lateral field, no such difference emerges for illusion susceptibility.

Mechanisms for the Illusions

With the one exception referred to above, the pattern parameters listed in the section "Stimulus Parameters of Epileptic Visual Sensitivity" influence the mean number of illusions seen by people without epilepsy in precisely the same way as they do the probability of paroxysmal activity in pattern-sensitive epileptic patients. In the section "Inferences About the Nature of the Seizure Trigger" it has already been shown how the parameters of pattern sensitivity and the topographic characteristics of the EEG activity that the patterns evoke combine to implicate the striate and prestriate cortex in the induction of the

Table 23.2 Mean Number of Illusions Reported in Discs and Annuli

Stimulus	Radii (mm) Inner	Radii (mm) Outer	Area (cm²)	Q (% cortical projection)	Mean Number of Illusions	t test	p
A	—	18	9	14	0.87		
						1.86	NS
B	65	100	181	14	1.00		
						2.49	<0.05
C	—	40	45	28	1.18		
						0.41	NS
D	40	100	269	28	1.20		
						2.69	<0.01
E	—	100	314	55	1.39		

After Wilkins et al. (1984)

discharge. Considerations of parsimony suggest that similar cortical mechanisms are responsible for the visual illusions. Perhaps the illusions are the result of a limited discharge within the striate and prestriate cortex that does not spread but nevertheless causes the activation of neurons inappropriate to the visual stimulus. This is not to deny that some of the illusions have a peripheral ocular origin (cf. Campbell and Robson, 1958); it is simply to argue that peripheral ocular mechanisms are insufficient to account for many of the illusions, a position for which there is already considerable support (Wade, 1977).

The hypothesis outlined above is consistent with the recent finding that deprivation of sleep increases susceptibility to the illusions (Wilkins et al., 1984): loss of sleep is, after all, one of the classic proconvulsants. The hypothesis not only provides a rationale for the similarity between the visual precipitants of illusions and seizures, it can also explain the discrepancy between the effects of stimulation of different visual fields. The greater epileptic sensitivity to stimulation of a lateral field, as compared with the upper and lower fields, was attributed to a recruitment of excitation within one hemisphere. The discharges that sustain illusions are presumably far more localized and extensive recruitment may not occur, in which case no difference between the lateral and the upper and lower fields should be anticipated.

If the illusions represent the failure of inhibitory processes at the cortical level, the extent of such failure may, perhaps, be measured by the number of illusions reported. If so, the large individual differences in susceptibility to the illusions acquire a new significance. They may reflect a continuum of hyperexcitability within the general population, at one extreme of which are patients with primary generalized epilepsy. It is therefore of theoretical significance that there exists a relationship between the illusions people report and the number and nature of the headaches they suffer.

Illusions and Headaches

In four independent samples of normal people a weak positive correlation has been obtained between the number of illusions reported in the epileptogenic pattern shown in Figure 23.4 and the estimates these people make of the annual incidence of their headaches. The correlations (which account for 20% of the variance) are summarized in Figure 23.12.

The samples included nursing and physiotherapy students (Figure 23.12a), members of the Applied Psychology Unit subject panel (Figure 23.12b), and undergraduates in theoretical physics (Figure 23.12c). The relationship shown is mainly for gratings with a spatial frequency of about 3 cycles/degree and is not present for spatial frequencies in the region of 0.5 cycles/degree. This selectivity argues against the correlation being attributable to subject suggestibility, some subjects being more prepared to admit to borderline illusions and borderline headaches. The correlation does not appear if complaints other than headache are investigated, confirming that such suggestibility plays a relatively minor role (Wilkins et al., 1984).

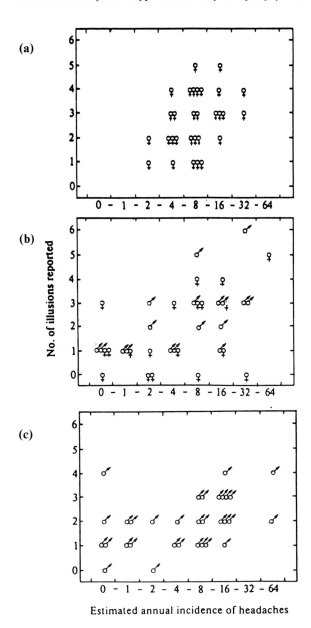

Figure 23.12 Scatterplots showing the relationship between subjects' estimates of the annual incidence of their headaches and the number of illusions they reported in a grating similar to that in Figure 23.4. Each point represents the data from an individual subject. In (a) the subjects were nursing and physiotherapy students (28 women aged between 18 and 23), $r_s = 0.44$; in (b) they were members of the Applied Psychology Unit panel (19 men and 19 women aged between 18 and 76), $r_s = 0.49$; undergraduates in theoretical physics (33 men aged between 19 and 23) contributed the data in (c), $r_s = 0.49$. After Wilkins et al. (1984).

Table 23.3 Association Between Reports of Laterally Asymmetric Illusions and Reports of Unilateral Headache

	Illusions in Visual Hemifields	
	Equal	Unequal
Panel Volunteers		
Bilateral headaches	13	1
Unilateral headaches (consistent side)	6	6*
	$\chi^2 = 6.03\ p < 0.05$	
Neurology patients		
Bilateral headaches	13	3
Unilateral headaches (consistent side)	8	14†
	$\chi^2 = 7.55\ p < 0.01$	

Source: After Wilkins et al. (1984)
*Five maximal in ipsilateral field.
†Seven maximal in ipsilateral field.

There is also a relationship between the location of the illusions within the visual field and the lateralization of head pain. Some people report that the illusions occur predominantly in one lateral visual field. These people tend also to report unilateral headache. The relationship, which is summarized in Table 23.3, is present for the subjects on the Applied Psychology Unit panel and for patients with a primary complaint of headache attending a neurology outpatient clinic. Note that patients with unilateral headache of inconsistent lateralization have been excluded. Note also that the relationship is found in terms of the presence of asymmetry rather than its direction. Such a finding is compatible with the weakness of the relationship between the side of visual aura and the side of head pain in patients with migraine headache (Peatfield et al., 1981). In the sample of neurologic patients, those with a diagnosis of migraine had a slight tendency to report more illusions than other patients, and among those with migraine the illusions are more likely to be lateralized.

In summary, the stimulus parameters of epileptic visual sensitivity have a counterpart in the parameters of stimuli that induce the illusions reported by individuals without epilepsy. These illusions are related to the number and nature of the headaches people suffer. There may be a continuum of cortical hyperexcitability, individuals with a highly excitable cortex being particularly prone to headaches. This hypothesis is very similar to one advanced by Goldensohn (1976) on the basis of the EEG responses to visual stimulation.

RESPONSE PARAMETERS OF VISUAL SENSITIVITY

The photoconvulsive response described at the beginning of this chapter is one of the most extreme EEG reactions to visual stimulation and is usually seen only if the stimulus is maximally epileptogenic (e.g., patterns vibrating at about 20 Hz or diffuse light flickering at a similar frequency). When the stimulus is suboptimal or when a patient's sensitivity is reduced by sodium valproate the response is less extreme: it usually ceases to generalize and instead involves only posterior head regions. It may also decrease in the duration and number of morphological components (it may, for example, be reduced to a single posterotemporal spike, or spike and slow wave complex) (Darby et al., 1986). Ultimately, the response cannot be distinguished from the variety of responses seen in persons without epilepsy. For example, at frequencies of about 7 Hz intermittent light may evoke occipital spikes instead of a photoconvulsive response. These spikes are phase-locked to the stimulus and can appear in individuals without epilepsy, including those with "headaches" (Maheshwari and Jeavons, 1977). Sometimes only an exaggerated "following" response can be discerned. This following response is common in people with no neurologic complaint but is abnormal in patients with migraine who tend to show high amplitude following at flash frequencies greater than 20 Hz (e.g., Goller and Winter, 1959; Jonkman and Lelieveld, 1981). The frequency selectivity of this abnormality is of interest in view of the fact that patients with photosensitive epilepsy who are sensitive to static pattern tend to have a higher upper frequency limit of sensitivity to intermittent diffuse light than patients who are not pattern sensitive (Wilkins, Binnie, and Darby, 1980). (There are no differences with respect to the lower frequency limit.) Perhaps a response to high frequency intermittent light in the form of high-amplitude following is associated with an abnormality broadly similar to that observed in pattern sensitive epilepsy, but not so extreme as to give rise to a photoconvulsive response.

The above response parameters are therefore consistent with the hypothesis advanced earlier that in both migraine and epilepsy visual sensitivity is the result of a hyperexcitability of the visual cortex, but that the degree of hyperexcitability is greater in epilepsy. Of course, the data do not strongly support such a position, they are merely consistent with it. Similar considerations apply with respect to the average evoked potential. The potential evoked by pattern-reversal and flash stimulation is of abnormally high amplitude in both photosensitive epilepsy and migraine. In photosensitive patients the initial limb of the P100 component often shows a negative occipital spike which has a latency of about 90 msec. This response is almost invariably seen when the stimulus is a patterned flash; it is not frequently evoked by less epileptogenic stimuli such as a diffuse flash or a phase-reversing pattern of 20 minute checks (Harding and Dimitrakoudi 1977). The latter simulus evokes no spike in patients with migraine, although the P100 component is delayed (Kennard et al., 1978).

VISUALLY INDUCED DISCOMFORT AND ITS MECHANISMS

Patterns that induce visual illusions of the kind described above are rated as being unpleasant to look at, and if they are viewed for an extended period by persons without epilepsy they may evoke complaints of tired eyes, headache, nausea, or dizziness (Wilkins et al., 1984). In the sample referred to above, some patients with migraine reported that the illusions (particularly those of blurring) resembled their aura. We have recently received an anecdotal report from a colleague (an ophthalmologist) who noted that observation of Figure 23.4 reliably provoked a scintillating scotoma. These adverse consequences of pattern viewing may have common mechanisms, which can, for the purposes of simplification, be divided into those that are peripheral and those that are central.

The central mechanisms might be neural, the direct result of excessive excitation or vascular, a secondary result of excitation. The mechanisms might also be peripheral. We now know that epileptogenic patterns can disrupt occulomotor control, at least insofar as the stability of the eye during the fixation of a small target is decreased when the target is surrounded by a grating such as that in Figure 23.4. There is a weak tendency for persons who see many illusions to have a relatively unstable fixation and to track a moving target spot poorly (Wilkins and Findlay, personal observations). It seems possible that a neuronal disturbance induced by the pattern may disrupt occular motor control. This disruption might be responsible for tired eyes and headache via peripheral mechanisms.

Thus far, the mechanisms whereby visual stimuli induce seizures, illusions, and pain have appeared to have much in common. The stimuli that are most likely to have these adverse consequences are those that induce intense excitation of the visual cortex, or so it may be inferred from the characteristics of these stimuli and the properties of the visual system. However, the excitation necessary for epileptogenesis may differ in at least one critical aspect from that necessary for the induction of illusions and pain. Epileptogenesis may require not only that the excitation of the visual cortex be massive, but that it be temporally organized. This suggestion is derived from inferences that are some of the weakest considered thus far, but they are nevertheless of sufficient importance to deserve mention. The inferences are based on the observation that, over a range of temporal frequencies, drifting gratings are less epileptogenic than static or vibrating gratings. (In order to avoid inducing optokinetic nystagmus, the drifting gratings were divided into two halves, each drifting toward a central fixation point.) The significance of this finding is that the drifting gratings, unlike the static or vibrating gratings, should produce a temporally disorganized pattern of firing. This is because cells will fire when the image of a bar of the grating moves across their receptive field. The receptive fields of neighboring cells overlap and so the drifting grating should produce considerable excitation but not in any temporally organized fashion. This is in sharp contrast with the excitation that a vibrating grating might be expected to induce. In the visual cortex many cells fire maximally when the image of the bar is in motion across their receptive field and some are sensitive only to one direction of motion. Thus, with each alternate movement of vibrating pattern a burst of firing should occur, with relatively quiescent periods when the pattern is stationary, changing direction of motion. To this extent, the firing is temporally organized, and might be expected to result in synchronized volleys. The movements of the eye that occur during fixation mean that a static pattern should also result in synchronization, but perhaps to a lesser extent than a pattern that is vibrating with optimal temporal parameters. The finding that in epileptic patients a drifting grating is very much less likely to induce paroxysmal EEG activity than a static grating or one that is vibrating with frequencies in the region of 20 Hz suggests that synchronization may be contributing to epileptogenesis. The synchronization may contribute at the inception of the discharge and may not simply be a late consequence of the excitation once the discharge is underway. There is no concomitant difference between drifting and static or vibrating patterns with respect to the illusions they produce. The implication would appear to be that temporal organization contributes to epileptogenesis but not to illusions, and, by extrapolation, to those adverse consequences associated with illusions.

The above arguments are speculative and the inferences limited by the fact that there is no way of equating the magnitude of excitation from a drifting grating with that from a static or vibrating grating. Speculative or not, it is plausible that massive cortical excitation can result in headaches, and that seizures arise when this massive excitation is synchronized. The notion is remarkably difficult to quantify, however.

In the next section these theoretical issues will be set aside in favor of a discussion of some practical considerations.

PRACTICAL CONSEQUENCES OF VISUAL SENSITIVITY

There are many striped patterns in the everyday environment but perhaps one of the most common is that formed by the successive lines of printed text. We have measured the average contrast of the lines, their angular height, and their separation and found that the values of these parameters often lie within the epileptogenic range. We asked pattern-sensitive epileptic patients to read and demonstrated an increase in the rate of paroxysmal EEG activity. This activity can be reduced in incidence or eliminated altogether by covering the lines of text above and below those being read, using a simple mask. This consists of two rectangular pieces of darkened plastic with a matt surface, held together at one end on a slide. (The device is now being marketed as the "Cambridge Easy Reader" by Engineering and Design Plastics, 84 High Street, Cherry Hinton, Cambridge CB1 5JG, England.) The gap between the rectangles can be adjusted to allow about three lines of text to be visible, while 5.5 cm above and below are darkened and blurred. Not only does this reading aid prevent the occurrence of paroxysmal abnormalities in pattern-sensitive patients (Wilkins and Lindsay, 1984), it can also reduce the number of headaches suffered by people when they read. We advertized for volunteers who suffered eyestrain or headache from reading and in two placebo-controlled studies demonstrated that about one-third of the volunteers found the reading aid helpful. These volunteers tended to report more illusions in a grating similar to Figure 23.4. This relationship between the effectiveness of the reading aid and susceptibility to illusions was corroborated when a sample of normal subjects on the Applied Psychology Unit panel were shown the reading aid and asked to judge whether it changed their perception of the text. Some of the subjects reported beneficial visual effects such as an apparent increase in the size or contrast of the print, or in the separation of the lines of text. These subjects tended to report more illusions in a grating (Wilkins and Nimmo-Smith, 1984).

Television is a highly epileptogenic stimulus, at least in countries that use a 50 Hz refresh rate. This is only partly because of the flicker generated by the flying spot as it scans down the screen; it is mainly because of the pattern of interlaced lines that the spot creates as it draws the alternate half-frames (Wilkins et al., 1979). Cathode ray tube displays, some with characteristics similar to those of television, are now being used to present text. In view of the findings outlined in this chapter, it is hardly surprising that this use is associated with complaints of eyestrain and headache.

REFERENCES

Albrecht DG, Hamilton DB. Striate cortex of monkey and cat: contrast response function. J Neurophys 1982;48:217–37.

Binnie CD, Findlay J, Wilkins AJ. Mechanisms of epileptogenesis in photosensitive epilepsy implied by the effects of moving patterns. Electroencephalogr Clin Neurophysiol 1985;61:1–6.

Binnie CD, Wilkins AJ, Darby CE. Pattern sensitivity: the role of movement. In Lechner H, Aranibar A, eds. Proceedings of the 2nd European Congress of EEG and Clinical Neurophysiology. Amsterdam: Elsevier, 1979:650–5.

Binnie CD, Wilkins AJ, DeKorte RA. Interhemispheric differences in photosensitivity to intermittent photic stimulation. Electroencephalogr Clin Neurophysiol 1981;52:469–472.

Campbell FW, Robson JG. Moving visual images produced by regular stationary patterns. Nature 1958;181:362.

Darby CE, Park DM, Smith AT, Wilkins. EEG characteristics of epileptic pattern sensitivity and their relation to the nature of pattern stimulation and the effects of sodium valproate. Electroencephalogr Clin Neurophysiol 1986;63:517–25.

Drasdo N. The neural representation of visual space. Nature 1977;226:554–6.

Goldensohn ES. Paroxysmal and other features of the electroencephalogram in migraine. Clin Stud Headache 1976;4:118–28.

Golla FL, Winter AL. Analysis of cerebral responses to flicker in patients complaining of episodic headache. Electroencephalogr Clin Neurophysiol, 1959;2:539–49.

Harding GFA, Dimitrakoudi M. The visual evoked potential in photosensitive epilepsy. In: Desmedt JE, ed. Visual evoked potentials in man: new developments. Oxford: Clarendon Press, 1977:509–73.

Hubel DH, Wiesel TN. Brain mechanisms of vision. Sci Am 1979;241(3):130–44.

Jeavons PM, Harding GFA. Photosensitive epilepsy. London: Heinemann, 1975.

Jonkman EJ, Lelieveld MHJ. EEG computer analysis in patients with migraine. Electroencephalogr Clin Neurophysiol 1981;52:652–5.

Kennard G, Gawel M, de Rudolph N de M, Clifford Rose F. Visual evoked potentials in migraine subjects. Res Clin Stud Headache 1978;6:73–80.

Maheshwari MC, Jeavons PM. The clinical significance of occipital spikes as a sole response to intermittent photic stimulation. Electroencephalogr Clin Neurophysiol 1975;39:93–5.

Meldrum BS, Wilkins AJ. Photosensitive epilepsy in man and the baboon: integration of pharmacological and psychophysical evidence. In: Schwartzkroin PA, Wheal HV, eds. Electrophysiology of epilepsy. London: Academic Press, 1984:51–77.

Newmark ME, Penry JK. Photosensitivity and epilepsy: a review. New York: Raven Press, 1979.

Peatfield RC, Gawel M, Clifford Rose F. Asymmetry of the pain and aura in migraine. Neurol Neurosurg Psychiatry 1981;44:846–8.

Quesney LF. Dopamine and generalized photosensitive epilepsy. In: Morselli PL et al., eds. Neurotransmitters, seizures, and epilepsy. New York: Raven Press, 1981:263–74.

Wade NJ. Distortions and disappearances of geometrical patterns. Perception 1977;6:777–803.

Wilkins AJ, Andermann F, Ives J. Stripes, complex cells, and seizures. Brain 1975;98:365–380.

Wilkins AJ, Binnie CD, Darby CE. Visually-induced seizures. Prog Neurobiol 1980;15:85–117.

Wilkins AJ, Binnie CD, Darby CE. Interhemispheric differences in photosensitive epilepsy. I. Pattern sensitivity thresholds. Electroencephalogr Clin Neurophysiol 1981;52:461–8.

Wilkins AJ, Darby CE, Binnie CD, Stefansson SB, Jeavons PM, Harding GFA. Television epilepsy: the role of pattern. Electroencephalogr Clin Neurophysiol 1979;47:163–71.

Wilkins AJ, Lindsay J. Common forms of reflex epilepsy: physiological mechanisms and techniques for treatment. In: Pedley TA, Meldrum BS, eds. Recent advances in epilepsy II. Edinburgh: Churchill Livingstone, 1984:239–71.

Wilkins AJ, Nimmo-Smith I. On the reduction of eye-strain when reading. Ophthalmic Physiol Optics 1984;4:53–9.

Wilkins AJ, Nimmo-Smith I, Tait A, et al. A neurological basis for visual discomfort. Brain 1984;107:989–1017.

24

Calcium Mobility and Glutamic Acid Release Associated with EEG Abnormalities, Migraine, and Epilepsy

Nico M. van Gelder

A degree of correlation between migraine and abnormal, epileptiform electro-encephalographic (EEG) activity suggests some type of interrelationship between the two phenomena. At the same time, it is also evident that the EEG abnormalities are not directly proportional to either the severity or the frequency of migraine attacks (Hockaday and Whitty, 1969; Lauritzen et al., 1981). The EEG signs are therefore not solely caused by the repeated cerebrovascular dysfunction accompanying migraine, even though this may be a contributing factor. The abnormal central nervous system (CNS) conditions promoting hypersynchronous, high-frequency neural discharges are present as an inherited trait in families of epileptic patients (Metrakos and Metrakos, 1969; Andermann, 1982). Similar discharges may be associated with migraine (Ely, 1930; Critchley et al., 1982). In view of the coincidence between abnormal EEG signs and migraine, the local metabolic environment in the cortex causing the EEG changes may facilitate the triggering of a series of events leading to a migraine attack (Lance, 1981). In one cortical area in particular, namely, the occipital region, the metabolic environment can be further modified by a seizure to predictably produce a migraine attack (see Gastaut and Zifkin, this volume; D'Allesandro et al., this volume). Conversely, the physiological events accompanying a migraine incident may produce in that same cortex area typical epileptic discharge patterns in neurons (Camfield et al., 1978; Van Harreveld and Ochs, 1957). It would appear, therefore, that in one particular cortical region, certain biochemical correlates of hypersynchronous discharge are also associated with physiological events leading to a migraine attack.

Certain criteria can be assigned to postulated metabolic mechanisms that (1) represent an inborn trait; (2) are associated with an increased frequency of hypersynchronous discharges as reflected in the EEG; and (3) create either spreading depression (SD) or hypersynchrony, leading to epileptic manifestations. These criteria are most simply accounted for by postulating that the mechanisms are regulating the accumulation, in varying degrees, of an excitatory, depolarizing substance. That substance in turn might be involved in the pathophysiology of both epilepsy and migraine, depending on concentration, local perfusion, and the assumption that its accumulation will more predictably cause a migraine attack rather than a seizure. The pathophysiology of epilepsy clearly requires factors in addition to the genetic ones that cause hypersynchrony, such as acquired cerebral damage, before a chronic epileptic condition is established.

CLINICAL PATHOLOGY AND THE CHEMICAL ENVIRONMENT

If depolarization blockade — spreading depression (SD) — represents an extension of those conditions that produce hypersynchronous discharges, one must consider that this electrophysiological continuity is represented by a neurochemical continuum: a gradual exaggeration of effect or, simply, an accumulation of a substance (or substances) that first causes EEG abnormalities reflecting synchronous neuronal discharges, and then spreading depression reflecting synchronous cortical depolarization encompassing both neurons and glial cells. It must be assumed that a chemical environment in the cortex promoting EEG abnormalities will only predict an increased probability of migraine. In order for such an environment to become associated with seizures, however, a number of precise modifications of the microenvironment in the cortex must take place.

One requirement for the occurrence of hypersynchronous neuronal discharges is the partial preservation of the membrane potential. This can only be accomplished if glial cells are not depolarized, the extracellular ionic environment remains intact, energy supplies, oxygen provisions and CO_2 removal, pH regulation, and intact, albeit modified, neural microcircuity remain adequate (see various chapters, Jasper and van Gelder, 1983). Thus, the metabolic, physiological, and anatomical prerequisites to create a sustained seizure in the cortex are far more complex than those needed to elicit SD. Because the conditions to create a chronic but periodic tendency for seizures are so precise, and include an adequate energy and oxygen supply, it is equally understood why seizures are not often the cause for migraine or why SD can only be transformed into a seizure phenomenon by manipulation of the cortical circulation (van Harreveld and Ochs, 1957).

It is possible to speculate about the nature of the chemical modifications that predict an electrophysiological continuation between epileptiform EEG activity and SD, with epilepsy as an alternative state on those rare occasions when all the cortical conditions needed for a chronic, periodic seizure state are properly combined owing to hereditary and/or acquired, environmental factors. Evidently, an inborn tendency for synchronous recruitment of neural networks, as indicated by a high ancestral incidence of EEG abnormalities, implies an inherited chemical commonality (Ely, 1930).

BIOCHEMICAL HEREDITY AND PERIODIC DISTURBANCES

A hereditary biochemical disturbance implies that each and every cell of an individual exhibits the same genetic variation from the norm. Even if the anomalies need not be expressed metabolically by all cells or groups of cells and organs, in any location within the individual where the biochemical system is fully expressed and operational, the genetic aberration should be detectable. At the same time, it should be understood that few biochemical systems operating in the CNS are exclusively confined to that body compartment; they more likely find their counterparts in other organs or cell assemblies outside the CNS. Thus, any CNS disorder of partly or predominant genetic origin should be reflected by symptoms or, at least, biochemical aberrations detectable elsewhere, even though the principal, often most dramatic expressions of the disorder can lead to the false conclusion that it represents a unique brain phenomenon. Based on these considerations, many of the neurotransmitter-chemical messenger systems known to date may be eliminated as being directly responsible for causing hypersynchronous activity in the CNS as a consequence of an inborn abnormality in their metabolism.

To take just one example, the acetylcholine system is heavily implicated in muscle function (intestine, heart, motor). Any basic hereditary abnormality in this system should therefore be reflected by functional disturbances in many organ systems besides the CNS. Similarly, the catecholamines function frequently in reciprocal relationship with ACh, and apart from that, disturbances of (nor)epinephrine systems might be expected to differentiate the migraine group from the general population on the basis of chronic differences in blood pressure. Although such a case may be made for the migraine group, this is not tenable for the person with genetically determined EEG abnormalities or epilepsy. With respect to serotonin, histamine, or bradykinin(s), these agents play important roles in maintaining normal blood biochemistry. Substances of this type are found in a number of blood cells such as platelets and leukocytes, from which they are at times released in massive quantities. No precise blood abnormalities are a feature of either epilepsy or migraine. Finally, as to a possible imbalance of hormones or of the multitude of neuropeptides still being discovered, few if any are the exclusive domain of the CNS. Although disturbances of peptide accumulation/elimination/synthesis undoubtedly at times aid in triggering ictal incidents of epilepsy or migraine, this is not an invariable prerequisite for such incidents. Unfortunately, our knowledge is still rudimentary regarding the precise intracranial sites of release of hormones and peptides or their functional role. The possible involvement of one or several proteinaceous classes of substances in epilepsy and/or migraine therefore remains, for the most part, even more speculative than the better investigated chemical messengers.

When one turns to the so-called amino acid transmitters, the situation seems somewhat more favorable for a discussion. Several biochemically related amino acid pairs that may serve in regulating the excitation/inhibition balance are known to exist within the CNS: aspartic acid/beta-alanine; cystein sulfinic acid/taurine; glutamic acid/gamma-aminobutyric acid (GABA). All pairs are composed of an amino acid that produces strong neural excitation when applied iontophoretically or when introduced intraventricularly. A simple decarboxylation transforms the excitatory amino acid into an inhibitory substance, when determined by the identical experimental criteria. Among these pairs, permanent disturbances of glutamate-GABA mediated excitation/inhibition balance are generally conceded to be one likely origin for chronic alterations in cortical excitability.

THE GLUTAMATE–GABA BALANCE

Numerous results from studies of experimental epilepsy, as well as of various types of epilepsy in man, have demonstrated the crucial role of glutamic acid and GABA in the regulation of cortical excitation. Some of the more important findings from which these conclusions were reached are:

1. GABA is the major candidate to serve as the primary inhibitory chemical messenger in the neocortex. Neither glycine nor taurine, the two other widely distributed inhibitory substances, have been demonstrated to be confined to specific anatomical pathways within the cortex, even though they are present in appreciable quantities, especially taurine.
2. The precursor for GABA, glutamic acid, is present in all cells. Whether or not GABA is formed depends entirely on the specific and selective presence in only certain neurons of the GABA synthetizing enzyme, glutamic acid decarboxylase (GAD).
3. Glutamic acid is as excitatory as GABA is inhibitory when iontophoretically applied to neurons.
4. Both GABA and glutamic acid are released under apparently identical physiological conditions: stimulus depolarization, high K^+, Ca^{++} influx dependent. In order to prevent neurons from spontaneously releasing both amino acids, similar conditions must prevail: membrane structure and oxidative metabolism must be intact.
5. GABA and/or glutamic acid levels, with respect to a host of metabolic parameters, have been found to be abnormal in man or animals with either

natural or imposed hyperexcitable conditions: selective deficiencies of the GABA system (synthesis, terminals, etc.); altered GABA receptor sensitivity; excessive glutamate release; altered glial glutamate uptake or enzymatic inactivation.

Although at this time there still exists a strong controversy (see Durelli and Mutani, 1983; van Gelder, 1982 for discussion) as to whether enhanced cortical excitation is a consequence of excessive glutamic acid accumulation or is due to a deficiency of the GABA system, there is general agreement on one issue. In most, if not all, instances in which altered states of cortical excitation have been studied, the condition was shown to be characterized by an imbalance between the biological actions of GABA and glutamic acid. Thus, the increased cortical excitation represents a disturbance of the complex metabolic cycle that interrelates the excitatory precursor glutamic acid with its inhibitory decarboxylation product. Since in the intact CNS both neurons and apposing glial elements are needed for that metabolic interconversion, as well as several transport mechanisms and numerous enzymes, the exact locus for the imbalance may vary from individual to individual according to the precipitating factor — be this hereditary or one that originates from environmental factors, or a combination of both (van Gelder, 1983).

EXCESS GLUTAMIC ACID VERSUS GABA/GLU IMBALANCE

As a number of observations have demonstrated, cortical epileptiform EEG activity may or may not be associated with changes in the metabolic apparatus responsible for GABA mediated inhibitory innervation. However, once seizures do occur in such a cortex, the probability of finding modifications in the GABA system becomes greatly enhanced (Krnjevic, 1983). In contrast to this, even in individuals with a genetic predisposition for epilepsy but who never suffered a seizure, metabolic disturbances have been found that are indicative of excessive extracellular glutamic acid accumulation. Leaving aside for the moment the somewhat contrived GABA versus glutamic acid controversy with respect to seizure generation (van Gelder et al., 1983), there is clear evidence that an enhanced tendency for the cortex to exhibit hypersynchronous neural discharges seems to be invariably associated with tissue conditions that promote extracellular accumulation of glutamic acid.

For example, that an excess tissue release of glutamic acid reflects a hereditary predisposition toward development of epilepsy can be concluded from several separate studies which report abnormal glutamic acid patterns in the blood and urine of epileptic patients (Mutani et al., 1975; van Gelder et al., 1975), besides those consistently found in the epileptic CNS itself (Durelli and Mutani, 1983; van Gelder et al., 1972). It should be noted that GABA deficiencies are not always found within the epileptic brain, nor have genetic abnormalities of GABA outside the CNS been detected in epileptic individuals. This inhibitory neurotransmitter has now been demonstrated in the pancreas, kidney, and intestine. For these reasons, a basic aberration of the GABA system as a cause for epilepsy would not only anticipate the abnormal EEG but also some other clinical signs originating from outside the CNS. On the other hand, abnormal blood glutamate levels found in certain epileptic individuals (Janjua et al., 1982; Huxtable et al., 1983) and their relatives (Janjua et al., 1982), would not introduce noticeable clinical sequelae, since the potentially damaging effects of this phenomenon would be compensated for to a large extent by the excellent buffering capacity of the blood as well as by an increased excretion of glutamate into the urine.

In the light of these considerations, and in view of the sporadic nature of the epileptic attack, one may conclude that a familial predisposition for epilepsy or hypersynchronous EEG activity is most frequently biochemically expressed by an excessive glutamic acid effect rather than being associated with a chronically, inborn deficient GABA function. The electrophysiological correlate of this local glutamic acid accumulation is represented by a greater probability of detecting epileptiform EEG abnormalities; overt seizures may only occur when certain environmental factors modify cortical microcircuits or otherwise interfere with inhibition (Kostopoulos et al., 1983).

The high incidence of EEG abnormalities among migrainous individuals would suggest that this process is also associated with migraine. Since the clinical signs of migraine derive for the most part from the occipital region, excessive glutamic acid accumulation in that region may underlie the initiation of the migraine attack. There is substantive evidence to support this notion.

One of the most reliable methods to create SD is by application of high (mM) concentrations of glutamic acid, usually in combination with potassium or with conditions promoting increased extracellular K^+ concentrations such as physical injury to the cortex (van Harreveld and Ochs, 1957; Nicholson, 1983). The concentrations needed to experimentally elicit SD will certainly influence the osmotic environment of the region and lead to tissue edema. Interestingly, when the CO_2 tension is increased, SD can be transformed into seizures (van Harreveld and Ochs, 1957); increased CO_2 promotes vasodilation and may therefore decrease glutamic acid concentrations and restore the water balance, lowering tissue resistance.

In parallel to the experimental situation, the relationship of altered endogenous glutamic acid metabolism to volume changes within the CNS (van Gelder, 1983), SD or seizures (van Harreveld and Ochs, 1957), and transient anoxia/hypoxia (Bosley et al., 1983), has been well-documented. Many such studies emphasize the importance of the glia in these processes. It is not difficult to conceive how a basic, abnormal, tendency of neurons to "leak" glutamic acid, when combined at the same time with cerebrovascular insufficiency, would rapidly create all conditions required for SD, namely, high extracellular glutamic acid, K^+ mediated glial depolarization and edema, pH changes, and so on. On the other hand, without impairment of cortical circulation that same abnormal leakage would merely create a somewhat enhanced excited state in the cortex, which might be reflected by EEG abnormalities. Hence, based on concentration requirements and, in general, the metabolic needs of the glia, it seems that the association of migraine with EEG abnormalities is primarily determined by the sensitivity of the cerebrovascular system to certain environmental conditions. This is unlike the conditions promoting seizures, which seem intimately associated not only with excessive glutamic acid release from neurons, but also with a series of complex glial and neuronal metabolic processes required to maintain a balance between the action of glutamic acid and GABA (see above).

The combined failure of neuronal-glial metabolic compartmentation, while it can be initiated by cerebrovascular dysfunction, is not immediately restored after the energy status and O_2/CO_2 balance has returned to normal. In this respect, then, migraine may represent a temporary glial failure of, among others, glutamic acid uptake and water regulation. Epilepsy occurs when this process has acquired permanency, so that the primary function of glia to provide adequate synaptic GABA from glutamine remains disturbed and tends to fail periodically. The ultimate difference between migraine and epilepsy may thus be that the former represents simply a periodic stagnation in the interstitial circulation owing to cerebrovascular insufficiency, tissue edema, and total parenchymal depolarization; epilepsy, or at least the ictal phase, may represent an accumulation of glutamic acid owing to excessive release, combined with a periodic deficiency in the GABA system resulting from a glial impairment of glutamine/GABA regulation.

The implicit consequences derived from these presumptions are that:

1. Excessive leakage of glutamic acid from neurons is responsible for epileptiform EEG abnormalities.
2. In combination with cerebrovascular factors, this rapidly culminates in SD, which is accompanied by its own autonomous metabolic changes of the interstitial environment.
3. Epileptiform EEG abnormalities indicate that cerebrovascular dysfunction in a specific part of the cortex may lead to SD, and thus migraine.

The early vascular changes of migraine are opposite to those seen during a seizure. Since a seizure can trigger a typical migraine incident in the occipital cortex (Gastaut and Zifkin, Chapter 3, this volume), it is evident that chemical changes underlying seizure activity will, under appropriate local conditions, cause either vasospasm or vasodilation. At the same time, in this area where neurons are close together with relatively little glial buffering (Lauritzen, Chapter 22, this volume), initial vasospasm will in turn cause rapid accumulation of glutamic acid and glial edema, the latter due to carbonic anhydrase stimulation (Bosley et al., 1983; van Gelder, 1983). Thus, the vasoconstrictor responses of the arterial system, or excessive glutamic acid release from the tissue, when occurring in the occipital region, are both able to create migrainous symptoms.

Since these phenomena, that is, EEG abnormalities and SD-migraine attacks, may be found in the same individual, the possibility must be considered that the excessive arterial responses and glutamic acid leakage may represent two physiological expressions of the same inborn biochemical abnormality.

CYTOPLASMIC FREE (IONIC) CALCIUM

It is well-established that retention and release of the so-called neurally active amino acids are strongly influenced by calcium. Synaptic transmission, as well as practically every secretory process, has now been demonstrated to require the entrance of Ca^{2+} into the cell. The transient increase in Ca^{2+} concentration leads to a depolarizing event. The increase in intracellular free Ca^{2+} is initiated by an influx of extracellular calcium triggered by a voltage-dependent mechanism or certain chemicals, including glutamate itself (Ramsey and McIlwain, 1970; Perkins and Wright, 1969; Baker et al., 1971).

As experimental evidence indicates, the entrance of calcium during a depolarizing event, and the calcium-dependent intracellular events such as muscle contraction and transmitter release, cannot be directly linked. One attractive hypothesis (e.g., Beeler and Reuter, 1970) suggests that the action potential related transmembranal calcium influx ordinarily is offset by the intracellular reserve capacity to bind calcium. As these binding mechanisms become increasingly saturated, the continuation of impulse generation allows a gradual action of ionic cytosolic calcium on numerous calcium sensitive mechanisms. In the small nerve terminals, and other small volume structures, the effect would presumably become apparent earlier. Alternatively, by either first saturating calcium storage "sites" or by damaging such sites, a hypersensitive calcium reaction can be created. Both in nerve and muscle tissue and, among those, especially spontaneously discharging cells (e.g., smooth muscle), the effect will be most apparent: a "hypersensitive" response to normal physiological input.

In summary, therefore, the mobility or ease of displacement of the external membrane-bound Ca^{2+} fraction influences the electrical excitability (threshold) of neurons and muscle fibers. Intracellularly, the balance between Ca^{2+} which is protein bound in some manner or sequestered within mitochondria (as calcium phosphate), and free cytosolic calcium, regulates metabolism (CaATP vs. MgATP), myosin activation (Ca^{2+} ATPase), and transmitter release. The internal free calcium levels can be markedly increased by a series of events.

The intracellular calcium fraction at normal resting potential is not in direct equilibrium with the extracellular ion concentration. Free Ca^{2+} internally can be raised by decreasing the intracellular pH (e.g., increased metabolism, CO_2, etc.), a deficiency of inorganic phosphate, intracellular increases of Mg^{2+} and other divalent ions, or by a depolarizing event that enhances transmembranal calcium mobility. A rise in cytoplasmic free calcium will, among other things, inhibit the ATPase $Na^+ - K^+$ exchange pump and stimulate adenyl cyclase as well as other cyclases, thus promoting an efflux of K^+ and cyclic neucleotide formation. Calcium ionophores, or substances such as caffeine or ergotamine, will also promote an increase in cytoplasmic free calcium. In the context of the present discussion it is worth mentioning that external glutamic acid also acts as a calcium "ionophore" and this property in part explains the excitatory action of glutamic acid.

A SUGGESTED SCENARIO FOR MIGRAINE AND EPILEPSY

Assuming that these two disorders are related by a somewhat increased excitatory state of the cortex, one may begin by examining epilepsy, for which a number of biochemical mechanisms are well-established. Notably, the data appear compatible with the notion that a slightly "excessive" release of glutamate from the tissues creates, within the closed environment of the CNS, a lowered seizure threshold and a greater susceptibility to hypersynchronous neuronal discharge. While in most instances the buffering capacity of the glia can cope with such enhanced release, a damaging event, such as various types of brain injury, may set up a condition in which abnormal glial properties can no longer compensate for the enhanced glutamate release. An excess glutamate excitation, in part mediated via a calcium mechanism, combined with a consequent failure of the GABA system, could then set up conditions propitious for the development of seizures (for discussion, see van Gelder et al., 1983). Excessive glutamate release can be explained by a chronic, somewhat enhanced intracellular Ca^{2+} mobilization, which, moreover, also stimulates glutaminase activity ($GLN \rightarrow GLU + NH_3$; Kvamme et al., 1983) and shifts cellular metabolism toward glutamate formation (Léjhon et al., 1969).

In relation to migraine, rather than the secondary glial damage associated with epilepsy, one may suggest the presence of vascular abnormalities or hypersensitive reactions toward certain nutritional or environmental factors. As a consequence of inadequate calcium sequestration, such an inherent vascular hypersensitivity may be joined to an excessive release of certain vasogenic agents from platelets and other blood cells (see Critchley et al., 1982). Within the CNS, with its extensive and fine vascularization, such a phenomenon would have a more pronounced effect than in other organ systems where compensating reactions by kidney and the cardiovascular mechanisms will more easily dilute and eliminate the action of such agents or of enhanced Ca^{2+} influx (see Siesjö, 1981). Spreading depression may occur as a result of increased glutamate release and accumulation following local hypoxic conditions created by vasospasm (Bosley et al., 1983).

Finally, a factor explaining the increased prevalence of migraine or epilepsy in the young, or in the presence of certain hormonal changes, deserves special consideration. A hereditary inadequacy in cellular calcium binding ability may be due to a number of causes, ranging from a slightly decreased amount of calcium "binding proteins" to a small reduction in the inherited number of neural mitochondria; even a 10% change may be sufficient and would be difficult to detect (see Gregson and Williams, 1969). Furthermore, the amount of inorganic phosphate available to the cell for mitochondrial sequestration of calcium must play an important role under these circumstances. During growth, bone deposition, or under the influence of the hormonal changes of puberty, the concentration of phosphates available for this purpose may reach borderline levels. Any further reduction by diet, further hormonal disturbances, or temporary changes in pH and CO_2-influenced phosphate reabsorption in the kidney might be sufficient to trigger a migraine attack. Since in such individuals brain cells are likely to lose calcium during the attack, lack of phosphates may also impair subsequent reabsorption of this ion during the recovery period. Perhaps prophylactic administration of a phosphate source (e.g., glycerophospates as calcium salts; 100 to 200 mg) might be helpful.

In conclusion, this chapter focuses on possible common mechanisms of migraine and epilepsy. One mechanism proposed is an inadequate cytosolic calcium sequestration. Such an anomaly, inherited or environmentally induced, would give rise to supersensitive chemical messenger responses, platelet reactivity, and subsequent refractoriness to stimuli.

In epilepsy, a superimposed disturbed glial dysfunction may lead to inadequate detoxification of excitatory extracellular glutamate, which eventually must also lead to GABA malfunction. In migraine, a secondary but essential coinciding prerequisite may be a "hypersensitivity" toward environmental factors, including temporary hormonal fluctuations and certain dietary or metabolic conditions. Increasing the availability of inorganic phosphates, together with divalent ions and amino acids, may lead to a therapeutic approach to these conditions.

REFERENCES

Andermann E. Multifactorial inheritance of generalised and focal epilepsy. In: Anderson VE, Hauser WA, Penry JK, Sing CF, eds. Genetic basis of the epilepsies. New York: Raven Press, 1982.

Baker PF, Hodgkin AL, Ridgway EB. Depolarization and calcium entry in squid giant axons. J Physiol 1971;218:709–55.

Beeler GW, Reuter H. The relation between membrane potential, membrane currents and activation of contraction in ventricular myocardial fibres. J Physiol 1970;207:211–29.

Bosley TM, Woodhams PL, Gordon RD, Balàzs R. Effects of anoxia on the stimulated release of amino acid neurotransmitters in the cerebellum in vitro. J Neurochem 1983;40:189–201.

Camfield PR, Metrakos K, Andermann F. Basilar migraine, seizures and severe epileptiform EEG abnormalities. Neurology 1978;28:584–8.

Critchley M, Friedman A, Gorini S, Sicuteri F. Headache. Adv Neurol 1982;33:1–417.

Durelli L, Mutani R. The current status of taurine in epilepsy. Clin Neuropharmacol 1983;6:37–48.

Ely FA. The migraine-epilepsy syndrome: a statistical study of heredity. Arch Neurol Psychiatry 1930;15:943–9.

Gregson NA, Williams PL. A comparative study of brain and liver mitochondria from new-born and adult rats. J Neurochem 1969;16:617–26.

Hockaday JM, Whitty CWM. Factors determining the electroencephalogram in migraine: a study of 560 patients, according to clinical type of migraine. Brain 1969;92:769–88.

Huxtable RJ, Laird H, Lippincott SE, Walson P. Epilepsy and the concentrations of plasma amino acids in humans. Neurochem Int 1983;5:125–35.

Janjua NA, Metrakos JD, van Gelder NM. Plasma amino acids in epilepsy. In: Anderson VE, Hauser WA, Penry JK, Sing CF, eds. Genetic basis of the epilepsies. New York: Raven Press, 1982:181–97.

Jasper HH, van Gelder NM. Basic mechanisms of neuronal hyperexcitability. New York: Alan R. Liss, 1983.

Kostopoulos G, Avoli M, Gloor P. Participation of cortical recurrent inhibition in the genesis of spike and wave discharge in feline generalized penicillin epilepsy. Brain Res 1983;267:101–12.

Krnjevic K. GABA-mediated inhibitory mechanisms in relation to epileptic discharges. In: Jasper HH, van Gelder NM, eds. Basic mechanisms of neuronal hyperexcitability. New York: Alan R. Liss, 1983:249–80.

Kvamme E, Svenneby G, Torgner IA. Calcium stimulation of glutamine hydrolysis in synaptosomes from rat brain. Neurochem Res 1983;8:25–38.

Lance JW. Pathophysiology of the migraine syndrome. In: Current concepts in migraine. Ayerst Laboratories, eds. Ayerst Laboratories 1981:5–9.

Lauritzen M, Trojaborg W, Olesen J. EEG during attacks of common and classical migraine. Cephalalgia 1981;1:63–6.

Léjhon HB, Jackson SG, Klassen GR, Sawula RV. Regulation of mitochondrial glutamic dehydrogenase by divalent metals, nucleotides, and alpha-ketoglutarate. J Biol Chem 1969;244:5346–56.

Metrakos K, Metrakos JD. Genetics of convulsive desorders. II. Genetic and electroencephalographic studies in centrencephalic epilepsy. Neurology 1969;11:474–83.

Mutani R, Monaco F, Durelli L, Delsedime M. Levels of free amino acids in serum and cerebrospinal fluid after administration of taurine to epileptic and normal subjects. Epilepsia 1975;16:765–9.

Nicholson C. Regulation of the ion microenvironment and neuronal excitability. In: Jasper HH, van Gelder NM, eds. Basic mechanisms of neuronal hyperexcitability. New York: Alan R. Liss, 1983:185–216.

Perkins MS, Wright EB. The crustacean axon. I. Metabolic properties: ATPase activity, calcium binding, and bioelectric correlations. J Neurophysiol 1969;32:930–47.

Ramsey RL, McIlwain H. Calcium content and exchange in neocortical tissues during the cation movements induced by glutamates. J Neurochem 1970;17:781–7.

Siesjö BK. Cell damage in the brain: a speculative synthesis. J Cer Blood Flow Metab 1981;1:155–85.

van Gelder NM. Glutamic acid in chronically hyperirritable nervous tissue. In: Akimoto H, Kazamatsuri H, Seino M, Ward A, eds. Adv. Epileptology. XIII Epilepsy International Symposium. New York: Raven Press, 1982.

van Gelder NM. Metabolic interactions between neurons and astroglia: glutamine synthetase, carbonic anhydrase and water balance. In: Jasper HH, van Gelder NM, eds. Basic mechanisms of neuronal excitability. New York: Alan R. Liss, 1983:5–29.

van Gelder NM, Sherwin AL, Rasmussen T. Amino acid content of epileptogenic human brain: focal versus surrounding regions. Brain Res 1972;40:385–93.

van Gelder NM, Sherwin AL, Sacks C, Andermann F. Biochemical observations following administration of taurine to patients with epilepsy. Brain Res 1975;94:297–306.

van Gelder NM, Siatitsas I, Menini C, Gloor P. Feline generalized penicillin epilepsy: changes of glutamic acid and taurine parallel the progressive increase in excitability of the cortex. Epilepsia 1983;24:200–13.

van Harreveld A, Ochs S. Electrical and vascular concomitants of spreading depression. Am J Physiol 1957;189:159–66.

25

Peptides in Migraine and Epilepsy

Elizabeth Matthew
Gary M. Abrams

A transient disturbance of cerebral function occurs in both migraine and epilepsy. However, the triggering mechanisms are not known, and the pathophysiology is poorly understood. Clinical studies have suggested that there may be some similarities between migraine and epilepsy. These observations have provided the major theme of this book, the exploration of possible associations between the two conditions. This chapter focuses upon the opioid peptides, also known as endorphins, and other neuropeptides possibly relevant to migraine and epilepsy. Experimental and clinical evidence pertaining to their role in the pathogenesis of these disorders is reviewed. It must be emphasized, that although brain peptides are involved in neural transmission, these low-molecular-weight, single-chain amino acid compounds have not, so far, been clearly implicated in the pathophysiology of any neurologic disease. In addition, studies of peptide activity in migraine and epilepsy have been limited, perhaps because of the lack of appropriate experimental models. Thus, much of the material to be presented here is, of neccessity, speculative.

THE OPIOID PEPTIDES

Over the last decade, there has been an explosion of interest in the opiate peptides and there has been active speculation about their role in both migraine and epilepsy. While an in-depth discussion of the opioid peptides is beyond the scope of this chapter, it must be mentioned that the biology of the opiates has become increasingly complex since the time of the original characterization of the pentapeptides, methionine and leucine enkephalin, and the larger beta-endorphin (Hughes et al., 1975). It is now recognized that there are several subgroups of opioid peptides, each derived from distinct high-molecular-weight precursor molecules, and that there are several classes of opiate receptors (Paterson et al., 1983). The best-studied opiate subgroup is that derived from pro-opiomelanocortin (POMC) which includes beta-endorphin and adreno-corticotrophin (Eipper and Mains, 1980). Although the sequence of methionine-enkephalin is entirely contained within beta-endorphin, the precursor of brain methionine-enkephalin is thought to be a different molecule, pro-enkephalin (Noda et al., 1982). Leucine-enkephalin and the more recently discovered dynorphin are products of the prodynorphin molecule (Kakidani et al., 1982). Each of these opioid peptide groups has a distinct neuronal localization and varying spectra of biological activity.

Perhaps the most interesting data about the role of the opiates in migraine comes from the work of Sicuteri et al. (1978), who have suggested that migraine as well as other headache disorders are manifestations of deficiencies of the endogenous opioid system. Sicuteri (1982) proposed that migraine was a hypoendorphin syndrome characterized by dysautonomia, anhedonia, and hypernociception and suggested that these clinical symptoms were a reflection of endogenous opioid peptide activity. To support this theory, they provided experimental evidence of the reduction of morphine-like factors in the cerebrospinal fluid sampled during migraine attacks, and showed that vascular responses to serotonin and dopamine were enhanced in both migraine and in morphine withdrawal (Sicuteri et al., 1979). Since the opiates inhibit the neural release of the putative nociceptive transmitter, Substance P, in a variety of experimental paradigms (Jessell and Iversen, 1977; Mudge et al., 1979), they reasoned that "migraineurs" have diminished endorphin activity which may result in the absence of the normal endogenous inhibition of pain (Basbaum and Fields, 1978). This endorphin deficiency may also alter the turnover of central nervous system biogenic amines and subsequently lead to receptor changes in major pathways related to nociception and vascular reactivity. The shared clinical characteristics of the morphine abstinence syndrome and migraine were used as further evidence to implicate the opioid peptides and neural systems modulated by them. Additional support comes from a recent study that has demonstrated reduced beta-endorphin levels in the cerebrospinal fluid of patients with chronic common migraine (Genazzani et al., 1984). Unfortunately, while some aspects of this theory are attractive, convincing experimental evidence is lacking. Most observers would assess the hypothesis as being somewhat simplistic in both its explanation of basic peptide neurobiology and the interpretation of supportive clinical phenomena.

Although migraine has been viewed as a cerebrovascular disorder, it is worth noting that there is growing evidence suggesting that the primary problem in migraine may be a selective change in brain metabolism (Olesen et al., 1981). A suppression of cerebral function similar to the electrophysiological phenomenon of spreading depression (Leão, 1944) has been proposed as a correlate of the migrainous aura, with changes in blood flow occurring as secondary phenomena. What triggers the change in neuronal metabolism is not known, but it is possible that peptidergic substances may play a role. There is some indirect evidence for such a possibility. Enkephalin appears to significantly lower glucose metabolism in many brain regions, including the cortex, while it increases glucose utilization in the limbic system (Chugani et al., 1984). Positron emission tomography has revealed a decline in cerebral hemispheric glucose metabolism during reserpine-induced migraine, although detailed regional changes have not been reported (Sachs et al., 1984). From these data it can be postulated that enkephalin-mediated changes in glucose metabolism may be involved in the pathogenesis of migraine. However, this is an entirely speculative concept. Whether selective peptidergic activation or suppression is involved in the metabolic changes seen in spreading depression or migraine is not known.

The opioid peptides have also been implicated in the pathophysiology of the epilepsies. A convulsant effect was initially postulated, based on the results of high doses administered centrally in rats. Intraventricular injections of beta-endorphin increased muscle tone, decreased motility, and produced convulsive discharges from the hippocampus (Henksen et al., 1978). Methionine-enkephalin also had similar effects when infused intraventricularly (Urca et al., 1977), whereas the effects of leucine-enkephalin were of even longer duration (Frenk et al., 1978). Naloxone, an opiate antagonist, partially reversed these effects. More recently, it has been shown that opiate-induced seizure activity is accompanied by a preferential metabolic activation of the limbic system (Henriksen et al., 1979). In the developing rat brain, Snead and Stephens (1984) showed that leucine-enkephalin-induced seizures were electrographically different from beta-endorphin-induced seizures. They postulated that this represented differences in the rate of development of the enkephalin and endorphin systems.

However, convulsant effects were not observed after opiate administration in several experimental models. For example, pentylenetetrazol-induced seizures and maximal electroshock seizures (MES) in mice were not affected by beta-endorphin (Bajorek et al., 1981). Indeed, there is a body of evidence to suggest that the opioid peptides may have anticonvulsant effects in rodents (Cowan et al., 1981; Berman and Adler, 1981; Schreiber, 1979). Studies in a strain of spontaneously epileptic Mongolian gerbils have shown that intraventricular administration of beta-endorphin diminished the motor and electroencephalographic manifestations of seizures (Bajorek and Lomax, 1982). This "anticonvulsant" effect of beta-endorphin was blocked by naloxone. In primate studies using Senegalese baboons *(Papio papio)* with photosensitive epilepsy, Meldrum et al. (1979) demonstrated that intracranial and systemic injections of morphine, methionine-enkephalin and its synthetic analog FK 33824, leucine-enkephalin, and beta-endorphin had anticonvulsant effects and that this was blocked by low doses of naloxone. They subsequently showed that focal injections of morphine, methionine-enkephalin, and FK 33824 in the hippocampus, amygdala, and centromedian thalamus did not cause local or generalized epileptic activity (Meldrum et al., 1981). Thus, although the opioid peptides have epileptogenic effects when administered in high doses directly into the central nervous system of the rat, they appear to have anticonvulsant effects in experimental models of epilepsy.

Some reports have suggested that endogenous opioids have a role in the generation or suppression of epileptic activity, while other investigators have focused on a potential role for the opiates in postictal changes (Engel et al., 1978). There is some evidence to indicate that the opiates may be involved in the postictal refractory period that occurs after a seizure. Studies in the "kindled" seizure model have shown that pretreatment with naloxone blocked postictal depression whereas morphine administration prolonged it (Frenk et al., 1979). This effect may be caused by a mechanism similar to the "spreading depression" of cerebral activity that has been reported following microinjection of opioid peptides into the hippocampus and neocortex (Sprick et al., 1981). These data raise the interesting possibility that seizure activity may be associated with the release of opiate substances which then act as endogenous anticonvulsants by prolonging the postictal refractory period. Although there is no clear experimental evidence at present to indicate that seizure activity promotes the release of opioid peptides, this is an intriguing hypothesis that has yet to be tested.

OTHER PEPTIDES ASSOCIATED WITH EPILEPSY

Several other neuropeptides have been linked with epilepsy. Perhaps the best known example is adrenocorticotrophin (ACTH). As has been previously stated, the amino acid sequence for ACTH is contained within pro-opiomelanocortin, the precursor molecule from which beta-endorphin is derived. Clinical studies have indicated that, in high doses, it may be effective in the treatment of infantile spasms as well as other intractable seizure disorders (Klein, 1970; Riikonen, 1982). However, the mechanisms that mediate these effects are not clearly understood. Anticonvulsant activity has also been described in some experimental models of epilepsy, notably the "kindled" seizure model (Rose and Bridges, 1982), although in the Mongolian gerbil, high doses of ACTH 1–24 were required to produce this effect (Bajorek et al., 1980).

Other peptides with possible anticonvulsant properties include the cholecystokinin octapeptide (CCK) and the neurohypophyseal peptide, oxytocin. These two substances appear to inhibit the seizures induced by chemical convulsants such as strychnine, picrotoxin, and pentylenetetrazol (Zetler, 1981; Kasting et al., 1983). Interestingly, the other neurohypophyseal peptide, vasopressin, has been associated with convulsant effects. Kasting et al. (1981) reported seizure activity in rats after the intraventricular administration of small doses of vasopressin. The same group showed that vasopressin-treated rats were significantly more susceptible to febrile convulsions than untreated animals. In contrast, Brattleboro rats, genetically deficient in arginine vasopressin, were much more resistant to febrile convulsions than control animals. From these data, it was postulated that arginine vasopressin may play a role in the pathogenesis of febrile convulsions. Whether such a mechanism exists in humans is not known, although the possibility provides some interesting grounds for speculation. The influences of the neurohypophyseal peptides, oxytocin and vasopressin, will be discussed in greater detail in a subsequent portion of this chapter.

Convulsant effects have been attributed to corticotrophin releasing factor (CRF) (Ehlers et al., 1982), a hypothalamic peptide. It is interesting to note that ACTH and its "releasing factor" CRF appear to have antagonistic effects on seizure activity, although it is premature to speculate about the significance of this observation. Another hypothalamic peptide, thyrotrophin releasing hormone (TRH), also appears to have convulsant effects. Studies in the Mongolian gerbil have shown that intraventricular administration of TRH resulted in convulsive activity (Bajorek et al., 1984). An increase in brain TRH levels has been reported following seizure activity in the "kindled" seizure model (Meyerhoff et al., 1982). Interestingly, clinical reports have suggested that TRH may aggravate seizures in patients with epilepsy (Dolva et al., 1983; Maeda and Tanimoto, 1981).

Another interesting area for speculation involves the benzodiazepine receptor. Although not a neuropeptide, it may be the receptor for some yet-to-be-discovered endogenous peptide ligand. Several forms of the benzodiazepine receptor have been described in a variety of tissues. The receptor that is of particular relevance to this discussion is located on the gamma-aminobutyric acid (GABA) receptor-ionophore complex of the neuronal postsynaptic membrane (Squires et al., 1980). Changes in this receptor have been reported following experimental seizures (Paul and Skolnick, 1978; McNamara et al., 1980). It has been suggested that benzodiazepine compounds exert their anticonvulsant effects by acting through this receptor to potentiate GABA-ergic effects. An endogenous peptide ligand for the benzodiazepine receptor would probably act in a similar manner. However, such an "anticonvulsant" peptide has not been identified thus far.

NEUROKININ, SUBSTANCE P, AND MIGRAINE

Classically, migraine has been viewed as a disorder of cranial vasoregulation. The prodromal symptoms occur as the result of vasoconstriction or localized cerebral hypoperfusion, while the headache phase is a manifestation of vasodilatation with localized sterile inflammation. Twenty-five years ago, Harold Wolff and colleagues reported a series of studies characterizing a polypeptide obtained from the extracranial perivascular fluid of "migraineurs" during an attack (Chapman et al., 1960). The peptide increased vascular permeability and lowered pain threshold and could be pharmacologically distinguished from Substance P, bradykinin and oxytocin. The same peptide was found to be released into tissue fluid of skin following antidromic stimulation of dorsal roots in the human and was subsequently known as neurokinin (Chapman et al., 1960a). The concentration of neurokinin in the tissue fluid of "migraineurs" was correlated with the intensity of the headache. Administration of ergotamine tartrate reduced the peptide content coincident with relief of pain.

From these studies, it was concluded that local neurogenic release of neurokinin occurred in response to antecedent migraine-induced cerebral ischemia. The painful vasodilatation of the extracranial circulation was viewed as an unfortunate epiphenomenon that resulted from the excessive operation of a protective physiological mechanism. Recently, this neurokinin theory has been revived, and an excellent and up-to-date account of this concept can be found in a recent review (Moskowitz, 1984).

Although many of Wolff's concepts about migraine are certainly open to question, it is interesting to note that recent studies on the neuropeptide, Substance P, provide indirect support for the role of neurogenic inflammation in vascular headache. This undecapeptide was initially isolated from intestinal tissue by von Euler and Gaddum in 1931 and later "rediscovered" in the hypothalamus (Chang and Leeman, 1970). It was found to be widely distributed in central and peripheral neurons. This distribution included primary sensory neurons in the dorsal root and trigeminal ganglia (Hokfelt et al., 1975). The subpopulation of sensory neurons containing this peptide may be involved in the transmission of pain and it now appears that substance P may be the neurotransmitter for some types of pain (Jessell, 1981). Substance P neurons in the trigeminal ganglion project to intracranial vessels with an innervation pattern loosely overlapping those vascular structures in the brain and meninges that are pain-sensitive (Edvinsson and Uddman, 1982). It is released by antidromic stimulation of the dorsal root and has been proposed as the chemical mediator of neurogenic inflammation (Gamse et al., 1980). The molecular events mediating Substance P-induced inflammation are still unclear, but the similarity to the more crudely defined neurokinin (proposed by Wolff) is striking.

It is also worth noting that a variety of neuropeptides are present in the neurons of the sensory ganglia, including the trigeminal ganglion (Buck et al., 1982). Examples such as vasoactive intestinal polypeptide (VIP) have well-documented vasodilating effects on cerebral blood vessels (Larsson et al., 1976) and may also selectively modulate regional glucose metabolism (McCulloch et al., 1983). Another peptide, neurotensin, demonstrated in autonomic neurons (Lundberg et al., 1979), is also vasoactive, and shares a very similar pharmacological profile to "neurokinin." It is also possible that coordinated effects between peptides and biogenic amines may occur. For example, Substance P and serotonin (a vasoactive amine implicated in migraine) have been shown to coexist in some neurons (Hökfelt et al., 1978), and to independently project to cerebral arteries (Liu-Chen et al., 1981; Edvinsson et al., 1983). One or more of these neurotransmitter substances released from trigeminal nerve terminals may be responsible for the headache phase of migraine (Moskowitz et al., 1979).

CATAMENIAL ASPECTS OF MIGRAINE AND EPILEPSY

It is well known that epileptic seizures and migrainous phenomena may occur more frequently during the premenstrual phase of the menstrual cycle. Increases in epileptic and migrainous activity have also been noted in the ovulatory and menstrual phases of the cycle. Although such cyclical exacerbations suggest that ovarian steroids may be implicated, systematic studies of catamenial influences in migraine and epilepsy have been few. From an exhaustive survey of 126 reports of catamenial epilepsy, Newmark and Penry (1980) concluded that there was a relationship between cyclical seizure activity and plasma levels of estrogen and progesterone. They were, however, unable to correlate exacerbations in seizure activity with well-defined patterns of estrogen – progesterone imbalance.

The mechanism of ovarian steroid action in the pathogenesis of migraine is also not clear. An analysis of 300 female patients with migraine showed that 62% reported menstruation as a precipitating factor (Selby and Lance, 1960). Subsequently, another clinical study demonstrated that premenstrual migraine was related to falling estrogen levels prior to menses (Somerville, 1972). In the same context, a recent report demonstrated that estrogen implants abolished premenstrual migraine in 24 of 25 women followed over 5 years (Magos et al., 1983). Another study has shown that women with migraine have significantly elevated estrogen and progesterone levels throughout their menstrual cycle (Epstein et al., 1975).

These observations suggest that ovarian steroid influences may provide a common neuroendocrine basis for migraine and epilepsy. Since several neuropeptides and their receptors are known to be modulated by ovarian steroids, a general overview of the potential for involvement of neuropeptides in migraine and epilepsy can be obtained by studying some of these relationships. The neurohypophyseal peptides, oxytocin and vasopressin, are well-known examples of such estrogen-peptidergic interactions. Although both peptides are known to be vasoactive, their influence on physiological vasoregulation is poorly understood. Two decades ago, Lloyd and Pickford (1961) performed a series of studies which demonstrated that vascular responses to both oxytocin and vasopressin were dependent upon circulating estrogen levels and that in the case of oxytocin, this dependence could lead to significant reversals in its observed activity. They showed that oxytocin had variable effects on blood pressure and regional blood flow depending on the state of estrogenization. Female rats in natural or induced estrus became hypertensive when given a dose of oxytocin that otherwise produced minimal hypotension or no response. They pursued these studies in both dog and human and demonstrated that oxytocin was typically a vasodilator. However, in the estrogen-treated subject, oxytocin became a vasoconstrictor. In laboratory and clinical experiments, oxytocin-induced vasoconstriction was accompanied by a diminution in local blood flow (Haigh et al., 1963). Coincidentally, and perhaps relevant to migraine, dihydroergotamine and sympathectomy also converted oxytocin from a vasodilator to a vasoconstrictor. This observation was interpreted as indicating that sympathetic tone, perhaps modulated by estrogen, was responsible for the alternative vascular responses to oxytocin. Subsequent work has shown that in addition to any indirect effects, estrogens also increased vascular sensitivity to oxytocin and vasopressin by increasing the number of peptide receptors

(Altura, 1975). Thus, estrogen-related cyclical menstrual changes and autonomic activation, both influential in migraine and to a lesser extent in epilepsy, may influence the functional aspects of neurally released peptides.

It is interesting to speculate about whether an analogous situation can exist within the central nervous system and whether it might be relevant to the neural and vascular activation that has been proposed for migraine and epilepsy. Oxytocin and vasopressin are both known to be widely distributed in the brain and the spinal cord where they may function as neurotransmitters or neurohormones involved in water homeostasis, behavior, or sensory processing (Kozlowski et al., 1983). There is some evidence to suggest that estrogens may partially modify some central actions of oxytocin (Pedersen and Prange, 1979) and it is reasonable to postulate that fluctuations in ovarian steroid levels may modulate the expression of neurohypophyseal peptides in the central nervous system. Sex hormone related changes in the content of opioid peptides, Substance P, and vasoactive intestinal polypeptide in brain tissue have also been documented (Tsuruo et al., 1984), and there is some evidence that receptors for these substances may also be subject to these influences. Selected neuropeptidergic functions are undoubtedly modified by cyclical changes in ovarian steroids. The question then arises as to whether any specific role in the pathophysiology of migraine or epilepsy can be assigned to a neuropeptide, because the expression of this role would undoubtedly be modified by the sex hormones.

As is obvious from the preceding discussion, it is not difficult to establish a superficial relationship between ovarian steroids, neuropeptides, and some of the physiological changes proposed in migraine and epilepsy. The biological effects of the neuropeptides are typically longer in duration than those of other putative neurotransmitters and they may therefore be attractive candidates for precipitating or enhancing such phenomena as the migrainous aura or postictal manifestations of epilepsy. However, from the data reviewed here, it should be readily apparent that there is no convincing evidence to link migraine and epilepsy on the basis of peptidergic dysfunction. Clearly, there are many unanswered questions awaiting the development of more suitable techniques to study these uniquely human problems at a clinical investigative level. Until then, the role of neuropeptides in migraine and epilepsy will probably remain interesting but unclear.

REFERENCES

Altura BM. Sex and estrogens and responsiveness of terminal arterioles to neurohypophyseal hormones and catecholamines. J Pharmacol Exp Ther 1975;193:403–12.

Bajorek JG, Felmar M, Lomax P. Effects of beta-endorphin, ACTH and cortisol on seizures in the mongolian gerbil. Fed Proc 1980;39:981.

Bajorek JG, Lee RG, Carlin DH, Lomax P. Effects of beta-endorphin on experimentally induced seizures in mice. Proc West Pharmacol Soc 1981;24:315–7.

Bajorek JG, Lomax P. Modulation of spontaneous seizures in the mongolian gerbil: effects of beta-endorphin. Peptides 1982;3:83–6.

Bajorek JG, Lee RJ, Lomax P. Neuropeptides: A role as endogenous mediators or modulators of epileptic phenomena. Ann Neurol 1984;16(Suppl):S31–S38.

Basbaum AI, Fields HL. Endogenous pain control mechanism: review and hypothesis. Ann Neurol 1978;4:451–62.

Berman EF, Adler MW. The effects of opioids and beta-endorphin on maximal electro-convulsive seizures in rats. Fed Proc 1981;40:281.

Buck SH, Walsh JH, Yawamura HI, Burks TF. Neuropeptides in sensory neurons. Life Sci 1982;30:1857–66.

Chang MM, Leeman SE. Isolation of a sialogogic peptide from bovine hypothalamic tissue and its characterization as Substance P. J Biol Chem 1970;245:4784–90.

Chapman LF, Ramos A, Goodell H, Silverman G, Wolff HG. A humoral agent implicated in vascular headache of the migraine type. Arch Neurol 1960;3:223–9.

Chapman LF, Ramos A, Goodell H, Wolff HG. Neurokinin—a polypeptide formed during neuronal activity in man. Trans Am Neurol Assoc 1960;42–5.

Chugani HT, Ackerman RI, Chugani DC, Engel J. Opioid-induced epileptogenic phenomena: anatomical, behavioural and electroencephalographic features. Ann Neurol 1984;15:361–8.

Cowan A, Tortella FC, Adler MW. A comparison of the anticonvulsant effects of two systemically active enkephalin analogues in rats. Eur J Pharmacol 1981;71:117–21.

Dolva LO, Riddervold F, Thorsen RK. Side effects of thyrotrophin releasing hormone. Br Med J 1983;287:532.

Edvinsson L, Deguerce A, Duverger D, MacKenzie ET, Seatton S. Central serotonergic nerves project to the pial vessels of the brain. Nature 1983;306:55–7.

Edvinsson I, Uddman R. Immunohistochemical localization and dilatory effect of Substance P on human cerebral vessels. Brain Res 1982;232:466–71.

Ehlers CL, Henriksen SJ, Bloom FE, Rivier J, Wale WJ. Electroencephalographic and epileptogenic effects of corticotrophin releasing factor (CSF) in rats. Neurosci Abstr 1982;8:1013.

Eipper BA, Mains RE. Structure and biosynthesis of pro-adrenocorticotropin/endorphin and related peptides. Endocrinol Rev 1980;1:1–27.

Engel J, Wolfson L, Brown L. Anatomical correlates of electrical and behavioral effects related to amygdaloid kindling. Ann Neurol 1978;3:538–44.

Epstein MT, Hockaday JM, Hockaday TDR. Migraine and reproductive hormones throughout the menstrual cycle. Lancet 1975;1:543–8.

Frenk H, Engel J Jr, Ackerman RF, Shavit Y, Liebeskind JC. Endogenous opioids may mediate post-ictal behavioral depression in amygdaloid kindled rats. Brain Res 1979;167:435–40.

Frenk H, Urca G, Liebeskind JC. Epileptic properties of leucine and methionine-enkephalin: comparison with morphine and reversibility by naloxone. Brain Res 1978;147:327–37.

Gamse R, Holzer P, Lembeck F. Decrease of Substance P in primary afferent neurons and impairment of neurogenic plasma extravasation by capsacin. Br J Pharmacol 1980;68:207–13.

Genazzani AR, Micieli G, Petreglia F, Bono G, Minihola C, Savoldi F. Progressive impairment of CSF β-endorphin levels in migraine sufferers. Pain 1984;18:127–33.

Haigh AL, Kitchin AH, Pickford M. The effect of oxytocin on hand blood flow in man following the administration of an oestrogen and isoprenaline. J Physiol 1963;169:161–6.

Henriksen SJ, Bloom FE, McCoy F. Beta-endorphin induces non-convulsive limbic seizures. Proc Natl Acad Sci USA 1978;75:5221–5.

Henriksen SJ, Morrison F, Bloom F. Beta-endorphin-induced epileptiform activity increases local cerebral metabolism in hippocampus, amygdala and septum. Neurosci Abstr 1979;5:528.

Hökfelt T, Kellerth J-O, Nilsson G, Pernow B. Substance P: localization in the central nervous system and in some primary sensory neurons. Science 1975;190:889–90.

Hökfelt T, Verhofstad A, Nilsson G, Brodin E, Pernow B, Goldstein M. Immunohisto-chemical evidence of Substance P-like immunoreactivity in some 5-hydroxytryp-tamine-containing neurons in the rat central nervous system. Neurosci Abstr 1978;3:517–38.

Hughes J, Smith TW, Kosterlitz HW, Fothergill LA, Morgan BA, Morris HR. Identifi-cation of two related pentapeptides from the brain with potent opiate agonist activity. Nature 1975;258:577–80.

Jessell TM. The role of Substance P in sensory transmission and pain perception. In: Martin J, Reichlin S, Bick K, eds. Neurosecretion and brain peptides: Adv. Bio-chem. Psychopharmacol. Vol. 28. New York: Raven Press, 1981:189–98.

Jessell TJ, Iversen LL. Opiate analgesics inhibit Substance P release from rat trigeminal nucleus. Nature 1977;268:549–51.

Kakidani H, Furutani Y, Takahashi H, Noda M, Morimoto Y, Hirose T, Asai M, Inayoma S, Nakanishi S, Numa S. Cloning and sequence analysis of cDNA for porcine β-neoendorphin/dynorphin precursor. Nature 1982;298:245–9.

Kasting NW, Veale WL, Cooper KG, Lederis K. Vasopressin may mediate febrile convulsions. Brain Res 1981;213:327–33.

Kasting NW, Veale WL, Cooper KE. Vasotocin protects rats against convulsions in-duced by pentylenetetrazol. Experientia 1983;37:1001–2.

Klein R. Effects of ACTH and corticosteroids on epileptiform disorders. Prog Brain Res 1970;32:263–9.

Kozlowski GP, Nilaver G, Zimmerman EA. Distribution of neurohypophyseal hor-mones in the brain. Pharmacol Ther 1983;21:325–49.

Larsson LI, Edvinsson L, Fahrenkrug J et al. Immunohistochemical localization of a vasodilatory polypeptide in cerebrovascular nerves. Brain Res 1976;113:400–4.

Leão AAP. Spreading depression of activity in the cerebral cortex. J Neurophysiol 1944;7:359–90.

Liu-Chen LY, Han DH, Moskowitz MA. Pia-arachnoid contains Substance P originat-ing from trigeminal neurons. Neurosci 1983;9:803–8.

Lloyd S, Pickford M. The action of posterior pituitary hormones and oestrogens on the vascular system of the rat. J Physiol 1961;155:161–74.

Lundberg J, Hokfelt T, Anggard A et al. Peripheral neuropeptide neurons. Distribution, axonal transport and some aspects of possible function. Adv Biochem Psycho-pharmacol 1979;22:25–36.

Maeda K, Tanimoto K. Epileptic seizures induced by thyrotrophin releasing hormone. Lancet 1981;1:1058–9.

Magos AL, Zilkha KJ, Studd JWW. Treatment of menstrual migraine by oestradiol implants. J Neurol Neurosurg Psychiatry 1983;46:1044–6.

McCulloch J, Kelly PAT, Uddman R, Edvinsson L. Functional role for vasoactive intestinal polypeptide in the caudate nucleus: A 2-deoxy (^{14}C) glucose investigation. Proc Natl Acad Sci USA 1983;80:1472–6.

McNamara JO, Peper AM, Patrone V. Repeated seizures induce long term increase in hippocampal benzodiazepine receptors. Proc Natl Acad Sci USA 1980;77:3029–32.

Meldrum BS, Menini C, Stutzmann JM, Naquet R. Effects of opiate-like peptides, morphine and naloxone in the photosensitive baboon, *Papio papio.* Brain Res 1979;170:333–48.

Meldrum BS, Menini C, Naquet R, Riche D, Silva-Comte C. Absence of seizure activity following focal cerebral injection of enkephalin in a primate. Reg Peptides 1981;2:383–90.

Meyerhoff JL, Bates VE, Kubek MJ. Increases in brain thyrotrophin releasing hormone (TRH) following kindled seizures. Neuro sci Abstr 1982;8:457.

Moskowitz MA. The neurobiology of vascular head pain. Ann Neurol 1984;16:157–68.

Moskowitz MA, Reinhard JF Jr, Romero J, Melamed E, Pettibone DJ. Neurotransmitters and the fifth cranial nerve: is there a relation to the headache phase of migraine? Lancet 1979;2:883–5.

Mudge AW, Leeman SE, Fischbach GD. Enkephalin inhibits release of Substance P from sensory neurons in culture and decreases action potential duration. Proc Natl Acad Sci USA 1979;76:526–30.

Newmark ME, Penry JK. Catamenial epilepsy: a review. Epilepsia 1980;21:281–300.

Noda M, Furutani Y, Takahashi M et al. Cloning and sequence analysis of cDNA for bovine adrenal preproenkephalin. Nature 1982;295:202–6.

Olesen J, Larsen B, Lauritzen M. Focal hyperemia followed by spreading oligemia and impaired activation of rCBF in classic migraine. Ann Neurol 1981;9:344–52.

Paterson SJ, Robson LG, Kosterlitz HW. Classification of opiate receptors. Br Med Bull 1983;39:31–6.

Paul SM, Skolnick P. Rapid changes in brain benzodiazepine receptors after experimental seizures. Science 1978;202:892–4.

Pedersen CA, Prange AJ. Induction of maternal behavior in virgin rats after intracerebroventricular administration of oxytocin. Proc Natl Acad Sci USA 1979;76:6661–5.

Riikonen R. A longterm follow up study of 214 children with the syndrome of infantile spasms. Neuropediatrics 1982;13:14–23.

Rose RP, Bridges WH. Hormonal influences on seizure kindling: the effects of post-stimulation ACTH or cortisone injections. Brain Res 1982;231:75–84.

Sachs H, Russell JAG, Christman DR, Fowler JS, Wolf AP. Positron emission tomographic studies on induced migraine. Lancet. 1984;2:465.

Schreiber RA. The effect of naloxone on audiogenic seizures. Psychopharmacology (Berlin) 1979;66:205–6.

Selby G, Lance JW. Observations on 500 cases of migraine and allied vascular headaches. J Neurol Neurosurg Psychiatry 1960;23:23–32.

Sicuteri F. Natural opioids in migraine. In: Critchley M, Friedman AP, Gorini S, Sicuteri F, eds. Advances in neurology. Vol. 33. New York: Raven Press, 1982.

Sicuteri F, Anselmi B, Curradi C, Michelacci S, Sassi A. Morphine-like factors in the CSF of headache patients. In: Costa E, Trabucchi M, eds. Adv. in Biochem. Psychopharm. Vol. 18. New York: Raven Press, 1978:363–6.

Sicuteri F, Del Bianco PL, Anselmi B. Morphine abstinence and sustonin supersensitivity in man: analogies with the mechanism of migraine? Psychopharmacology (Berlin) 1979;65:205–9.

Snead OC, Stephens H. The ontogeny of seizures induced by leucine-enkephalin and beta-endorphin. Ann Neurol 1984;15:594–8.

Somerville BW. The role of estradiol withdrawal in the etiology of menstrual migraine. Neurology 1972;22:355–65.

Sprick U, Oitzl MS, Ornstein K, Huston JP. Spreading depression induced by microinjection of enkephalins into the hippocampus and neocortex. Brain Res 1981;210:243–52.

Squires RF, Klepner CA, Benson DI. Multiple benzodiazepine receptor complexes; some benzodiazepine recognition sites are coupled to GABA receptors and ionophores. Adv Biochem Psychopharmacol 1980;21:285–93.

Tsuruo Y, Hisano S, Okamura Y, Tsukamoto N, Daiokoku S. Hypothalamic Substance P containing neuron sex dependent topographical differences and ultrastructural transformations associated with stage of the estrous cycle. Brain Res 1984;305:331–41.

Urca G, Frenk H, Liebeskind JC, Taylor AN. Morphine and enkephalin: analgesic and epileptic properties. Science 1977;197:83–6.

Zetler G. Anticonvulsant effects of caerulein and cholecystokinin octapeptide, compared with those of diazepam. Eur J Pharmacol 1981;65:297–300.

26

A Dopaminergic Mechanism in Photosensitive Epilepsy and Its Possible Relevance to Migraine

Luis Felipe Quesney
Frederick Andermann

Epileptic photosensitivity is an abnormal electroencephalographic (EEG) and clinical response to flickering environmental light or pattern stimulation, which depends upon a specific genetic mechanism different from that of the generalized spike and wave genetic trait (Doose et al., 1973; Doose, 1980). The EEG hallmark of epileptic photosensitivity is the photoconvulsive response, characterized by photically induced generalized and bilaterally synchronous spike and wave or polyspike and wave activity outlasting the end of photic stimulation (Melsen, 1959; Hughes, 1960; Jeavons and Harding, 1975).

Although early reports in the literature postulated a subcortical origin of epileptic photosensitivity (Gastaut, 1950; Gastaut and Hunter, 1950; Bickford et al., 1952), more recent experimental evidence obtained in the baboon *Papio papio,* an animal with a naturally occurring experimental model of photosensitive epilepsy, supports a cortical origin of photically induced spike and wave activity (Fisher-Williams et al., 1968; Naquet et al., 1975; Ménini, 1976; Wada and Naquet, 1972; Wada et al., 1973).

Substantial electrophysiological evidence indicates that the response to microiontophoretic application of dopamine and norepinephrine to neocortical neurons is mainly inhibitory in nature (Phillis and Tebecis, 1969; Kostopoulos, 1977; Reader, 1978; Reader et al., 1979). Apomorphine, a dopamine agonist, exerts a similar action on cortical neurons (Aghajanian and Bunney, 1973).

Abundant neuropharmacologic evidence supports a blocking effect of dopaminergic agonists upon photically induced seizures in the baboon *Papio*

papio (Meldrum et al., 1975; Ashton et al., 1976; Meldrum et al., 1978; Meldrum and Anlezark, 1981; Anlezark et al., 1981). Conversely, dopaminergic antagonists such as haloperidol and pimozide enhance epileptic photosensitivity in *Papio papio* (Meldrum et al., 1975; Ashton et al., 1976). The pharmacologic action of norepinephrine and serotonin upon photosensitivity in this model is controversial. Although an inhibitory action of these agents upon epileptic photosensitivity has been proposed (Altshuler et al., 1976; Wada et al., 1972), several reports in the literature do not support this view (Brailowsky and Naquet, 1976; Balzano and Naquet, 1970; Meldrum and Balzano, 1971; Meldrum et al., 1972).

We have recently reported that apomorphine, a dopamine receptor agonist (Ernst, 1965; Ernst, 1967; Ernst and Smelik, 1966; Andén et al., 1967; Roos, 1969), abolishes the electrographic and clinical features of epileptic photosensitivity in patients with primary and secondary generalized corticoreticular epilepsy (Figures 26.1, 26.2, 26.3; Table 26.1), without significantly reducing the incidence of spontaneous spike and wave activity (Quesney et al., 1980; Quesney et al., 1981; Quesney, 1981). These observations suggest a rather specific blocking action of apomorphine on epileptic photosensitivity. The apomorphine dose required to induce this phenomenon is small (0.025–0.05 mg/K/I.P.) suggesting pharmacologic action on presynaptic auto receptors (Aghajanian, 1977; Carlsson, 1977; Roth, 1979). However, this does not seem to be the case, since the blockade of epileptic photosensitivity is not associated with the sedation that is a common side effect of apomorphine action on

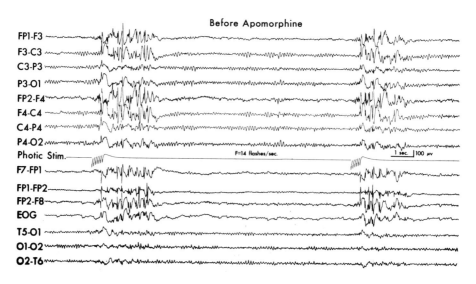

Figure 26.1 An 18-year-old female patient with history of absence seizures since age 10. Intermittent photic stimulation at 14 flashes/sec, consistently triggered bursts of generalized and bilaterally synchronous spike and wave discharge.

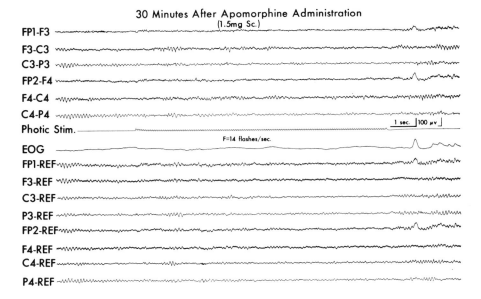

Figure 26.2   Total blockade of epileptic photosensitivity after apomorphine administration. Notice presence of alpha rhythm in both parietal regions prior to and after the photic stimulation train, indicating alertness.

auto-receptors (Di Chiara et al., 1976; Corsini et al., 1977). Furthermore, nausea and/or vomiting was observed in over 50% of patients after apomorphine administration, suggesting action on postsynaptic receptors (Quesney et al., 1981).

Feline generalized penicillin epilepsy (FGPE) is a reliable experimental model of epileptic photosensitivity (Quesney, 1984). Binocular photic stimulation at 4 to 8 flashes/s consistently triggered generalized bilaterally synchronous spike and wave discharges in 12 chronic cats submitted to low dosage (50,000 – 150,000 IU/kg) intramuscular penicillin administration. The photically induced epileptic activity is first and primarily recorded from the cerebral cortex as compared to the lateral geniculate body, therefore supporting a cortical onset of epileptic photosensitivity. At this low penicillin dosage, only minimal spontaneous spike and wave activity is recorded (Figure 26.4a). Approximately one-third of the photically induced epileptic bursts were associated with ictal behavioral manifestations such as eye blinking and myoclonic jerks involving the face and neck muscles.

Intramuscular or intraperitoneal administration of apomorphine at dosages ranging from 0.3 to 0.7 mg/K blocked or significantly reduced epileptic photosensitivity in all chronic cats (Quesney, 1981). This blockade of epileptic photosensitivity (Figure 26.4b) appeared within 0 to 15 minutes after apomorphine administration and persisted for an average of 55 minutes. Side effects to

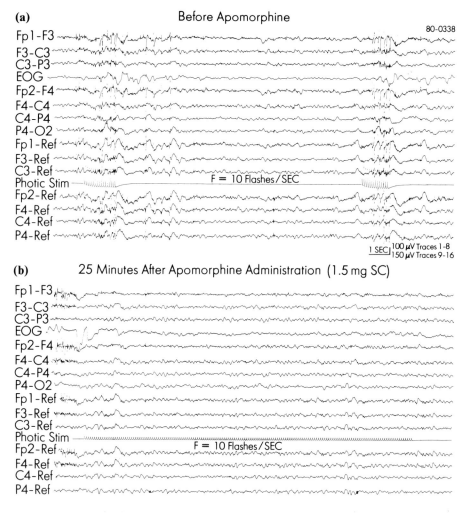

Figure 26.3 (a) Triggering of generalized polyspike and wave activity associated with bilateral myoclonus in a 23-year-old male patient with progressive myoclonus epilepsy. (b) Total blockade of photically induced myoclonus after apomorphine.

apomorphine administration included hypermotility, a stereotyped rotatory motion, sialorrhea, and retching, as reported during the postsynaptic action of apomorphine (Glick et al., 1977; Protais et al., 1976) and lasted anywhere from 5 to 10 minutes. Of 12 cats, 7 experienced such side effects.

The blockade of epileptic photosensitivity by apomorphine in patients with generalized photosensitive epilepsy, as well as in two reliable experimental models of photically induced seizures (the baboon *Papio papio* and FGPE), led us to postulate participation of a common dopaminergic mechanism in the genesis of epileptic photosensitivity in different species. One could postulate

Table 26.1 Epileptic Photosensitivity Blockade by Apomorphine

Before Apomorphine		After Apomorphine						
		Total Blockade			Partial Blockade			
Number of Patients	Percentage Photosensitivity	Number of Patients	Onset (min)	Duration (min)	Number of Patients	Percentage Photosensitivity	Duration (min)
14	92.6 ± 2.1	12	14.2 ± 4.1	37.7 ± 8.5	14	71.3 ± 3.8	26.3 ± 6.7

Total blockade of epileptic photosensitivity was observed in 12 of 14 patients with primary generalized epilepsy after apomorphine administration. Onset of blockade occurred 14 minutes after apomorphine administration and it lasted 37 minutes.

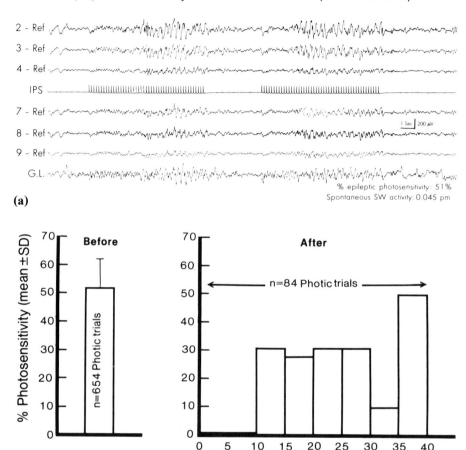

Figure 26.4 (a) Intermittent photic stimulation at 6 flashes/sec induces bursts of generalized and bilaterally synchronous spike and wave discharges 25 minutes after penicillin administration. Referential EEG tracing. Anatomical electrode position is as follows: 2 and 4 = sigmoid area; 3 and 8 = middle lateral gyrus; 4 and 9 = visual cortex; GL = lateral geniculate. Epileptic activity is first recorded from the cortical grey matter before involving GL. Mean of percent photosensitivity = 51%; incidence of spike and wave activity not related to photic stimulations = 0.045 burst/min. (b) Histogram comparing epileptic photosensitivity before and after apomorphine administration in same cat as Figure 26.4a. Mean control epileptic sensitivity was 51% (654 photic trials). 0 to 10 minutes after apomorphine administration, no photosensitive epileptic discharges were elicited. The cat moved around only for 2 to 3 minutes after injection and then remained quiet. A significant reduction of epileptic photosensitivity was observed 10 to 35 minutes after apomorphine administration.

that apomorphine blocks epileptic photosensitivity, inducing neuronal inhibition (Kostopoulos, 1977; Aghajanian and Bunney, 1973). However, this hypothesis does not explain why apomorphine fails to block spontaneous spike and wave discharges, which are entirely similar to discharges induced by photic stimulation, in man. It has been shown that intermittent photic stimulation reduces the endogenous release of dopamine and noradrenaline in the visual and somatosensory cortex in cats (Reader et al., 1976), thereby reducing a source of cortical inhibition. This phenomenon could enhance a preexisting state of cortical hyperexcitability (Quesney and Gloor 1978; Kostopoulos, 1977; Aghajanian and Bunney, 1973), facilitating the genesis of spike and wave discharges in response to photic stimulation (Quesney and Gloor 1978; Kostopoulos et al., 1981). These observations led us to postulate that epileptic photosensitivity is related to a cortical deficit in dopaminergic neurotransmission that can be counteracted by exogenous apomorphine administration.

To further assess this hypothesis, lesions of the mesocortical catecholaminergic pathways and of the cortical dopaminergic and noradrenergic terminals were performed in 12 chronic cats known to be photosensitive. Seven animals became photosensitive only after intramuscular penicillin administration and 5 cats were spontaneously photosensitive (Quesney, 1984). Four cats underwent a unilateral electrolytic lesion of the MFB rostrally to substantia nigra; 4 cats were submitted to unilateral diffuse cortical 6-OHDA topical application (200 μg contained in a soaked filter paper placed directly on the cortical surface for 30 minutes). Using the same technique, four cats underwent bilateral 6-OHDA cortical application (200 μg/hemisphere). Animals subjected to neurochemical lesions were pretreated with desipramine (30 mg/K/ I.P.) to avoid 6-OHDA uptake by noradrenergic terminals in an attempt to achieve a more selective cortical dopaminergic denervation. Serial control of epileptic photosensitivity was performed for up to 68 days after the lesions. The same dose of penicillin as in the pre-lesion studies was administered to animals that were not spontaneously photosensitive. Upon completion of the experiments, the entire brain was surgically removed and frozen in dry ice. Radioenzymatic assay of catecholamine content (DA, NE, E) and 5-HT was performed in cerebral cortex (frontal and occipital lobes) and in subcortical grey matter structures (GL and caudate nuclei) of both cerebral hemispheres in collaboration with Dr. T. Reader (Reader, 1981).

A significant increase in epileptic photosensitivity was observed in all cats submitted to unilateral MFB or unilateral 6-OHDA cortical lesions (Quesney and Reader, 1984), starting 10 to 15 days after the lesions and reaching a maximum within 3 or 4 weeks (Table 26.2). This phenomenon was associated with a marked reduction of DA and NE content in the frontal and occipital lobes (40%–80%) ipsilateral to the lesions. However, only the occipital lobe DA depletion was statistically significant when comparing the lesioned and nonlesioned sides, each animal serving as its own control (Tables 26.3 and 26.4). The catecholamine content in subcortical structures remained virtually unchanged (Quesney and Reader, 1984).

Table 26.2   Effect of Unilateral Cortical 6-OHDA Lesion on Epileptic Photosensitivity in FGPE (Penicillin 50,000 IU/kIM)

	Percent of Photosensitivity (Mean ± SEM)	
Time After Penicillin (Min)	*Before 6-OHDA Lesion 892 Photic Stimulations*	*After 6-OHDA Lesion 535 Photic Stimulations*
0–30	23 ± 4	34 ± 12
30–60	46 ± 5	64 ± 4
60–90	48 ± 7	69 ± 12

Comparison between epileptic photosensitivity before (892 photic trials) and after unilateral 6-OHDA cortical application (535 photic trials) in a chronic cat. Numbers in the left column indicate time interval after intramuscular penicillin.

Table 26.3   Dopamine Content in Cat Cerebral Cortex (ng/mg/prot)

	Frontal Region		*Occipital Region*	
Number of Animals	*Intact*	*Ipsilateral to 6-OHDA Lesion*	*Intact*	*Ipsilateral to 6-OHDA Lesion*
1	1.953	1.518	3.425	1.905
2	2.335	2.068	3.836	2.294
3	1.442	1.087	1.379	0.951
4	3.321	1.730	1.760	1.234
x̄ ± SD	2.262 ± 0.79	1.600 ± 0.41	2.600 ± 1.2	1.596 ± 0.6
p		>0.1		<0.025

Dopamine content in frontal and occipital lobes comparing intact with lesioned side after unilateral 6-OHDA topical application, each animal serving as its own control. x̄ = mean; SD = standard deviation; p = probability as measured by paired sample "t" test. Only dopamine depletion in occipital lobe was significant ($p = 0.025$).

Table 26.4   Norepinephrine Content in Cat Cerebral Cortex (ng/mg/prot)

	Frontal Region		*Occipital Region*	
Number of Animals	*Intact*	*Ipsilateral to 6-OHDA Lesion*	*Intact*	*Ipsilateral to 6-OHDA Lesion*
1	4.611	3.314	2.302	2.546
2	2.531	1.574	3.011	1.160
3	2.210	2.312	1.313	2.015
4	2.360	2.624	1.755	1.972
x̄ ± SD	2.298 ± 1.12	2.456 ± 0.72	2.095 ± 0.73	1.923 ± 0.57
p		>0.2		>0.2

Norepinephrine content in frontal and occipital lobes. Cortical depletion of NE was not significant.

Bilateral diffuse cortical 6-OHDA application induced epileptic photo-sensitivity in three chronic cats without requiring intramuscular penicillin administration (Figure 26.5). The fourth exhibited a mild degree of spontane-ous epileptic photosensitivity during the pre-lesion study (mean of 10%) which was significantly increased after bilateral cortical 6-OHDA application (mean of 6%). The induction of epileptic photosensitivity after bilateral 6-OHDA cortical application was associated with significant cortical DA depletion in the occipital lobes when compared to the frontal regions (Figure 26.6).

Apomorphine administration at high dosage (0.5 – 1 mg/K/I.P.) blocked epileptic photosensitivity before and after bilateral cortical 6-OHDA lesions. However, administration of a low dose of apomorphine (0.025 – 0.05 mg/K/ I.P.) caused opposite effects before and after these lesions. Before bilateral cortical 6-OHDA application, the epileptic photosensitivity was increased and a considerable reduction of this phenomenon was observed after bilateral corti-cal neurochemical lesions (Figure 26.7).

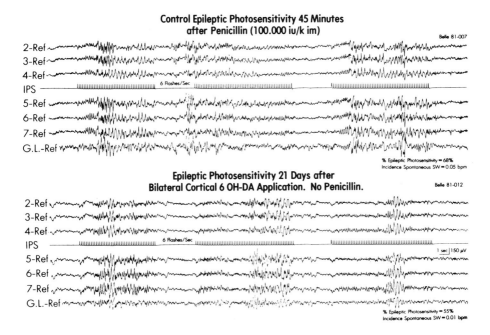

Figure 26.5 Upper tracing: Binocular photic stimulation at 6 flashes/sec triggered generalized and bilaterally synchronous spike and wave discharges in 68% of photic trials in a cat receiving a low dosage of penicillin intramuscularly. The incidence of generalized epileptic discharges occurring independently from photic stimulation was almost negligible (mean = 0.05 burst/min). Lower tracing: Same animal 21 days after bilateral cortical 6-OHDA application. Photic stimulation triggers generalized spike and waves in 55% of photic trials, without requiring intramuscular penicillin administra-tion. Incidence of spike and wave bursts not related to photic stimulation is reduced (0.01 burst/min).

DISCUSSION

Apomorphine, a dopamine receptor agonist (Ernst, 1965, 1967; Ernst and Smelik, 1966; Andén et al., 1967; Roos, 1969), blocks epileptic photosensitivity in experimental models of this condition (Meldrum et al., 1978; Ashton et al., 1976) as well as in patients with generalized photosensitive epilepsy (Quesney et al., 1980; Quesney et al., 1981). This effect cannot be exclusively explained by

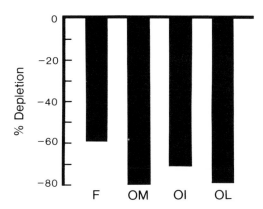

Figure 26.6   Percent depletion of dopamine content in frontal and occipital lobes in the same animal as in Figure 26.5, sacrificed 28 days after bilateral cortical 6-OHDA topical application. The mean cortical dopamine content measured in the same brain regions in five non-lesioned cerebral hemispheres served as control. F = frontal; OM = mesial occipital; OI = intermediate occipital; OL = lateral occipital.

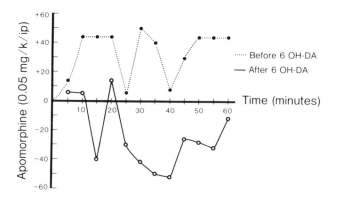

Figure 26.7   Percent variation of epileptic photosensitivity is illustrated in vertical axis ([+] = increase; [−] = decrease). Horizontal axis represents time (minutes) after apomorphine administration. Prior to bilateral cortical 6-OHDA application apomorphine at low dose increases epileptic photosensitivity (dotted line). After bilateral cortical dopaminergic lesion apomorphine reduces photosensitivity. Same animal as in Figures 26.5 and 26.6.

an inhibitory pharmacologic action of apomorphine (Aghajanian and Bunney, 1973) since this drug does not block spontaneous spike and wave discharges, which are identical to those induced by intermittent photic stimulation. These observations and the fact that the brain dopamine content is reduced in homozygous autosomal recessive photosensitive epileptic chickens (Johnson et al., 1981) led us to postulate the participation of a cortical deficit of dopaminergic neurotransmission in the physiopathogenesis of photosensitive epilepsy. Experimental support for this hypothesis derives from recent studies showing that photosensitive epilepsy can be reproduced in nonepileptic cats by bilateral diffuse cortical depletion of catecholamines, particularly dopamine (Quesney and Reader, 1984). Whether the deficit of dopaminergic neurotransmission resides in presynaptic or postsynaptic structures is not well known. However, apomorphine at low dosage (0.025 – 0.05 mg/K) blocks the photosensitive epileptic manifestations in cats submitted to bilateral denervation of cortical catecholaminergic terminals, implying a postsynaptic action and thus indirectly supporting a presynaptic deficit of cortical dopaminergic neurotransmission (Quesney and Reader, 1984) in the genesis of epileptic photosensitivity.

Paroxysmal abnormalities, including photosensitivity, are found with increased frequency in patients with migraine (Smyth and Winter, 1961; Heyck and Hess, 1955; Barolin, 1966; Scollo-Lavizzari, 1971; Rowan, 1974). Such abnormalities are also found in first degree relatives (Ziegler and Wong, 1967).

The clinical significance of the photosensitive EEG abnormalities that may be found in patients with migraine is not clear. The abnormalities are usually not as active nor as characteristic as those found in patients with primary generalized photosensitive corticoreticular epilepsy. Nevertheless, they are more than would be expected on the basis of chance and do not appear to represent a physiological variant. They would also be difficult to explain as genetically determined manifestations of familial epileptic photosensitivity.

Photosensitivity implies involvement of the occipital cortex. The physical parameters of both epileptic and migrainous photosensitivity have been studied by Wilkins (see Chapter 23, this volume) and have been found to be similar.

Photosensitive manifestations in migraine were previously unexplored; Wilkins' findings correlate well with the clinical observation of an unpleasant reaction to certain visual stimuli which many migraineurs describe. Whether patients with subjective visual photosensitivity also have a high incidence of photosensitive EEG abnormalities is not clear presently. In classical migraine, the occipital cortex appears to be involved preferentially and occipital manifestations are far more common in this form of migraine, as opposed to involvement of other cortical areas.

The presence of photosensitivity in both classical migraine and generalized epilepsy and the demonstration of a dopaminergic mechanism in epileptic photosensitivity raise the question of a possible depaminergic mechanism involving the occipital cortex in migraine as well.

Further studies on the effect of dopamine receptor agonists on migrainous photosensitivity and of agents like valproic acid, which are known to be highly effective in the control of photosensitivity in epilepsy as well as studies of antiserotoninergic substances on the photosensitivity associated with migraine, could aid in clarifying this question and could have some therapeutic potential as well.

REFERENCES

Aghajanian, GK, Bunney BS. Pharmacological characterization of dopamine "autoreceptors" by microiontophoretic single-cell recording studies. Adv Biochem Psychopharmacol 1977;16:433–8.

Aghajanian GK, Bunney BS. Central dopaminergic neurons: neurophysiological identification and responses to drugs. Front Catechol Res 1973;643–8.

Altshuler HL, Killam EK, Killam KF. Biogenic amines and the photomyoclonic syndrome in the baboon, *Papio papio.* J Pharmacol Exp Ther 1976;196:156–66.

Andén NE, Rubenson A, Fuxe K, Hökfelt T. Evidence for dopamine receptor stimulation by apomorphine. J Pharm Pharmacol 1967;19:627–9.

Anlezark G, Marrosu F, Meldrum B. Dopamine agonists in reflex epilepsy. In: Neurotransmitters, Seizures and Epilepsy 1981;251–62.

Ashton C, Anlezark G, Meldrum BS. Inhibition of reflex epilepsy by $(\overset{+}{+})$ N-n-propylnorapomorphine. Eur J Pharmacol 1976;39:339–401.

Balzano E, Naquet R. Action de la réserpine chez le *Papio papio* photosensible: modifications comportementales et électroencéphalographiques. Physiol Behav 1970;561–9.

Barolin GS. Migraine and epilepsy—a relationship? Epilepsia 1966;7:53–66.

Bickford RG, Sem-Jacobsen CW, White PT, Daly D. Some observations on mechanisms of photic and photometrazol activation. Electroencephalogr Clin Neurol 1952;4:275–82.

Brailowsky S, Naquet R. Effects of drugs modifying brain levels of catecholamines on photically induced epilepsy in *Papio papio.* Epilepsia 1976;17:271–4.

Carlsson A. Dopaminergic autoreceptors: background and implications. Adv Biochem Psychopharmacol 1977;16:439–41.

Corsini GU, Del Zompo M, Manconi S, Cinachetti C, Mangoni A, Gessa GL. Sedative, hypnotic and antipsychotic effects of low doses of apomorphine in man. Adv Biochem Psychopharmacol 1977;16:645–8.

Dichiara G, Porceddu ML, Vargiu L, Argiolas A, Gessa GL. Evidence for dopamine receptors mediating sedation in the mouse brain. Nature 1976;264:564–7.

Doose H, Gerken H, Horstmann T, Volzke E. Genetic factors in spike and wave absences. Epilepsia 1973;14:57–75.

Doose H. Genetic factors in childhood epilepsy. In: Canger R, Angeleri F, Penry JK, eds. Advances in Epileptology: XIth Epilepsy International Symposium. New York: Raven Press, 1980:289–96.

Ernst AM. Relation between the action of dopamine and apomorphine and their O-methylated derivatives upon the CNS. Psychopharmacologia (Berlin) 1965;7:391–9.

Ernst AM. Mode of action of apomorphine and dexamphetamine on gnawing compulsion in rats. Psychopharmacologia (Berlin) 1967;10:316–23.

Ernst AM, Smelik PG. Site of action of dopamine and apomorphine on compulsive gnawing behaviour in rats. Experientia 1966;22:837–8.

Fisher-Williams M, Poncet M, Riche D, Naquet R. Light-induced epilepsy in the baboon Papio papio: cortical and depth recordings. Electroencephalogr Clin Neurophysiol 1968;25:557–69.

Gastaut H. Combined photic and metrazol activation of the brain. Electroencephalogr Clin Neurophysiol 1950;2:249–61.

Gastaut H, Hunter J. An experimental study of the mechanism of photic activation in idiopathic epilepsy. Electroencephalogr Clin Neurophysiol 1950;2:263–87.

Glick SD, Jerussi TP, Cox RD, Fleisher LN. Pre- and post-synaptic actions of Pharmacodyn Ther 1977;225:303–7.

Heyck H, Hess R. Vasomotorische Kopfschmerzen als Symptom larvierter Epilepsien. Schweiz Med Wochenschr 1955;85:573–5.

Hughes JR. Usefulness of photic stimulation in routine clinical electroencephalography. Neurology 1960;10:777–82.

Jeavons PM, Harding GFA. Photosensitive epilepsy. A review of the literature and a study of 460 patients. London: William Heinemann, 1975.

Johnson DD, Jaju AT, Ness L, Richardson JS, Crawford RD. Brain norepinephrine, dopamine and 5-hydroxytryptamine concentration abnormalities and their role in the high seizure susceptibility of epileptic chickens. Can J Physiol Pharmacol 1981;59:144–9.

Kostopoulos G. Physiology and pharmacology studies on synaptic transmission in the mammalian brain. Thesis for Ph.D. Department of Physiology, University of Saskatchewan, 1977:159–70.

Kostopoulos G, Gloor P, Pellegrini A, Siatitsas I. A study of the transition from spindles to spike and wave discharge in feline generalized penicillin epilepsy: EEG features. Exp Neurol 1981;73:43–54.

Meldrum B, Anlezark G, Trimble M. Drugs modifying dopaminergic activity and behaviour, the EEG and epilepsy in *Papio papio.* Eur J Pharmacol 1975;32:203–13.

Meldrum B, Anlezark G. Dopamine agonists in reflex epilepsy. In: Gessa GL, Corsini GU, eds. Apomorphine and other dopaminomimetics. Clinical pharmacology. New York: Raven Press, 1981;2:25–31.

Meldrum BS, Balzano E. Etudes des éffets de l'α-méthylparatyrosine chez le *Papio papio.* Soc Biol 1971;165:2379.

Meldrum BS, Balzano E, Wada JA, Vuillon-Cacciuttolo G. Effects of *L*-tryptophan, *L*-3,4,dihydroxyphenylalanine and tranylcypromine on the electroencephalogram and on photically induced epilepsy in the baboon, *Papio papio.* Physiol Behav 1972;9:615–21.

Meldrum B, Brailowsky S, Naquet R. Approche pharmacologique de l'épilepsie photosensible du *Papio papio.* Actual Pharmacol 1978;30:51–9.

Melsen S. The value of photic stimulation in the diagnosis of epilepsy. J Nerv Dis 1959;128:508–19.

Ménini Ch. Rôle du cortex frontal dans l'épilepsie photosensible du singe *Papio papio.* J Physiol (Paris) 1976;72:5–44.

Naquet R, Catier J, Ménini Ch. Neurophysiology of photically induced epilepsy in *Papio papio.* In: Meldrum BS, Marsden CD, eds. Advances in neurology. New York: Raven Press, 1975;10:107–18.

Phillis JW, Tebecis AK. The responses of thalamic neurons to iontophoretically applied monoamines. J Physiol 1969;193:715–45.

Protais P, Costentin J, Schwartz JC. Climbing behaviour induced by apomorphine in mice: A simple test for the study of dopamine receptors in striatum. Psychopharmacology 1976;50:1–6.

Quesney LF, Gloor P. Generalized penicillin epilepsy in the cat: correlation between electrophysiological data and distribution of 14^C-penicillin in the brain. Epilepsia 1978;19:35–45.

Quesney LF, Andermann F, Lal S, Prelevic S. Transient abolition of generalized photosensitive epileptic discharge in humans by apomorphine, a dopamine-receptor agonist. Neurology 1980;30:1169–74.

Quesney LF, Andermann F, Gloor P. Dopaminergic mechanism in generalized photosensitive epilepsy. Neurology 1981;31:1542–4.

Quesney LF. Dopamine and generalized photosensitive epilepsy. In: Morselli PL et al., eds. Neurotransmitters, seizures and epilepsy. New York: Raven Press, 1981:263–73.

Quesney LF. Pathophysiology of generalized photosensitive epilepsy in the cat. Epilepsia 1984;25(1):61–9.

Quesney LF, Reader T. Role of cortical catecholamine depletion in the genesis of epileptic photosensitivity. In: WONIEP II (Second Workshop on Neurotransmitters in Epilepsy). New York: Raven Press, 1984.

Reader TA. The effects of dopamine, noradrenaline and serotonin in the visual cortex of the cat. Experientia 1978;34:1586–7.

Reader TA. Distribution of catecholamines and serotonin in the rat cerebral cortex: absolute levels and relative proportions. J Neural Transm 1981;50:13–27.

Reader TA, de Champlain J, Jasper H. Catecholamines released from cerebral cortex in the cat: decrease during sensory stimulation. Brain Res 1976;111:95–108.

Reader TA, Ferron A, Descarries L, Jasper HH. Modulatory role for biogenic amines in the cerebral cortex. Microiontophoretic studies. Brain Res 1979;160:217–29.

Roos BE. Decrease in homovanillic acid as evidence for dopamine receptor stimulation by apomorphine in the neostriatum of the rat. J Pharm Pharmacol 1969;21:263–4.

Roth RH. Dopamine autoreceptors: pharmacology, function and comparison with postsynaptic dopamine receptors. Commun Psychopharmacol 1979;3:429–46.

Rowan AJ. The electroencephalographic characteristics of migraine. Arch Neurobiol (Madrid) 1974;37:95–104.

Scollo-Lavizzari G. Prognostic significance of epileptiform discharges in the EEG of non-epileptic subjects during photic stimulation. Electroencephalogr Clin Neurophysiol 1971;31:174.

Smyth VOG, Winter AL. The EEG in migraine. Excerpta Medica International Congress Series 1961;37:136–7.

Wada JA, Naquet R. Examination of neural mechanisms involved in photogenic seizure susceptibility in epileptic Senegalese baboon *Papio papio.* Epilepsia 1972;13:344–5.

Wada JA, Catier J, Charmasson G, Ménini Ch, Naquet R. Further examination of neural mechanisms underlying photosensitivity in the epileptic Senegalese baboon, *Papio papio.* Electroencephalogr Clin Neurophysiol 1973;34:786.

Wada JA, Balzano E, Meldrum BS, Naquet R. Behavioural and electrographic effects of L-5 hydroxytryptophan and D,L-parachlorophenylalanine on epileptic Senegalese baboon *(Papio papio).* Electroencephalogr Clin Neurophysiol 1972;33:520–6.

Ziegler DK, Wong G. Migraine in children: clinical and electroencephalographic study of families. The possible relation to epilepsy. Epilepsia 1967;8:171–87.

27

Migraine and Epilepsy: An Overview

Frederick Andermann

The observations and studies presented in this volume have suggested that migraine and epilepsy are fundamentally different disorders, confirming the clinical impressions already reached during the last century. They are both paroxysmal, with excessive neuronal discharge the hallmark of the former, and spreading depression most likely the basis of the classical features of the latter. A number of relationships between the two disorders have emerged. Some of these appear to be causal, and it is no longer possible to dismiss the relationship between epilepsy and migraine as merely representing the coexistence of the two common disorders or as the effect of cerebral damage caused by presumed vascular complications of migraine.

A common genetic basis for both migraine and epilepsy has long been suspected and it therefore seems appropriate to first consider the evidence for or against such a relationship.

GENETICS AND EPIDEMIOLOGY OF MIGRAINE AND EPILEPSY

In the last quarter century it has been shown that the epilepsies are inherited in a multifactorial manner but that certain EEG characteristics, such as the 3Hz spike and wave or the rolandic spike, may represent autosomal dominant traits with age-dependent manifestation.

The electroclinical features of epileptic seizures and of a number of epileptic syndromes are now well delineated. There has also been progress in our knowledge of the epidemiological aspects of epilepsy. A prevalence of 0.5 to 1% is now generally accepted.

In contrast, there is extreme variability in the diagnostic criteria for migraine which has led to enormous divergence in the prevalence figures quoted by different studies, ranging from 1 to 60%. The definition formulated by the World Federation of Neurology Working Group on Headache is certainly acceptable, but it is difficult to translate it into criteria which can be statistically analyzed. The fluctuation in symptoms over time with the resultant tendency to forget some of them, the concept of "normal headache" quite prevalent in some population groups, and the occurrence of vascular headaches only during special circumstances such as the time of menstruation, are examples of factors which contribute to the difficulties in uniform diagnosis. There is much more agreement regarding the diagnosis of classical migraine, where a clinical marker, the characteristic slow march of the migrainous aura, is present. The finding of a marker for common migraine would, of course, greatly facilitate epidemiological study of this disorder as well.

It is largely for these reasons that it has been difficult to determine whether there is a genetic relationship between migraine and epilepsy. Recently Kraus (1978) conclusively demonstrated that there is no overall increase in migraine in relatives of epileptic patients compared with relatives of control probands and concluded that there was no genetic relationship between the two conditions. Baier and Doose (Chapter 20, this volume), however, found an increased incidence of migraine in first-degree relatives of children with absence attacks, even as compared with first-degree relatives of children with migraine. Giovanardi Rossi et al. (Chapter 21, this volume), despite finding a very high incidence of migraine in their group of patients with benign rolandic epilepsy and in their parents, concluded that migraine and epilepsy did coexist by chance. These studies, the one by Bladin (Chapter 9, this volume) on benign rolandic epilepsy, and the studies on benign occipital epilepsy (Terasaki et al., Chapter 7, Gastaut and Zifkin, Chapter 3, Aicardi and Newton, Chapter 6, this volume) allow us to draw the following conclusions: There seems to be no genetic relationship between migraine and epilepsy in general, however, some forms of epilepsy, such as benign rolandic epilepsy, benign occipital epilepsy and perhaps even primary generalized corticoreticular epilepsy with absence attacks seem to be associated with a high incidence of migraine not only in patients, but also in their parents. Further, well-controlled prospective studies of the occurence of migraine in patients who have clearly defined and specific forms of epilepsy and in their relatives should be carried out. Similar studies, but starting with clearly identified migraine probands, would complement the findings. It may then be possible to assess the incidence of patients with syndromes where the two conditions coexist and appear to be causally related.

PROBLEMS IN CLINICAL DIAGNOSIS

Despite the genetic evidence that fails to show a strong link between migraine and epilepsy as a whole, many observers have been impressed by certain patients where the presence of such a link seems beyond doubt. Sufficient experience has now been gained to propose a number of migraine-epilepsy syndromes. The identification of these syndromes is largely clinical, making it essential to be able to distinguish the features of migraine from those of epilepsy before suggesting that there is a link between them. While this differentiation is usually easy, difficulties may arise with occipital symptoms that may be similar and prolonged in both conditions. In the case of seizures with prolonged visual symptoms, the situation often becomes clearer when brain regions other than the occipital lobe become involved, leading to clonic jerking or other unmistakably epileptic manifestations.

The clinical difficulties posed by some patients with varieties of migraine or epilepsy are reviewed by Panayiotopoulos (Chapter 2, this volume). Differentiating basilar migraine from epilepsy can, at times, be difficult, as occasional cases with abrupt impairment of consciousness and EEG abnormalities have been reported. Apparently, patients with basilar migraine can always be aroused by vigorous stimulation, and impairment of consciousness in such attacks is not as severe as that seen in many epileptic seizures or during coma. These distinctions are important from a diagnostic point of view, considering that impairment of awareness and consciousness during epileptic events may be quite variable (Gloor 1986).

It may also be hard to distinguish between the epigastric symptoms of epilepsy and those of migraine. The epigastric aura of temporal lobe seizures may occasionally be described as painful, though this is much less common compared to the incidence of epigastric pain associated with migraine (Young and Blume, 1983). The occurrence of pain in both these conditions had led to the outdated, confusing, and misleading concept of abdominal epilepsy. When other clearly epileptic symptoms are associated it is easy to distinguish between the epigastric pain of temporal lobe epilepsy and that of migraine.

CLINICAL MIGRAINE-EPILEPSY SYNDROMES

Patients who have both migraine and seizures may present one of several syndromes (Table 27.1): Some have seizures only at the time of a classical migraine aura; a few go on to develop recurrent seizures independent of classi-

---

Table 27.1 Clinical Migraine-Epilepsy Syndromes

1. Epileptic seizures induced by a classical migraine aura
2. Epilepsy with seizures no longer triggered by migrainous aura
3. Epilepsy due to gross cerebral lesions caused by migraine
4. Benign occipital epilepsy of childhood and the spectrum of the occipital epilepsies
5. Benign rolandic epilepsy
6. Malignant migraine, related to mitochondrial encephalomyopathy
7. Migraine attacks following partial complex seizures
8. Alternating hemiplegia of childhood

---

cal migraine attacks. Patients with focal cerebral lesions caused by a vascular occlusion that may be attributed to migraine sometimes develop epilepsy, also.

Migraine appears to be an important risk factor in the development of occipital epilepsy. The spectrum of the occipital epilepsies, ranging from benign occipital epilepsy of childhood to seizures caused by an occipital lesion, seems to show an increased incidence of migraine or vascular headache. The presence of such a spectrum, ranging from the benign with a probably greater genetic component, to the intractable with more striking acquired features, illustrates again the multifactorial nature of the epilepsies. Migraine is also an important feature of benign rolandic epilepsy.

Patients with the characteristic clinical syndrome of mitochondrial encephalopathy, with or without evidence for mitochondrial myopathy, have migraine and a strong family history of migraine and therefore this syndrome appears to be migraine related, too. Some forms of peri-ictal headache are clearly migrainous. Finally, the poorly understood disorder of alternating hemiplegia of childhood has clinical features linking it to migraine, and the patients sometimes develop epilepsy. It may be tentatively regarded as a special migraine-epilepsy syndrome.

Epileptic Seizures Induced by a Classical Migraine Aura

The occurrence of an epileptic seizure triggered by a classical migraine aura is not uncommon. This can occur at any time in life, but appears more often in childhood and adolescence. Much is inferred from the hallucinatory experiences described by affected small children, from observation of their sympathetic dysfunction, and from interpretation of their behavior. The information obtainable from the clinical history improves as the age of the patient increases. The evidence for a causal relationship is much clearer in adolescents, rendering the diagnosis easier in this age group. Conversely, the electrographic abnormalities diminish between childhood and adulthood, likely in relation to cerebral maturation, and as a reflection of the progressive rise of the seizure threshold.

Terzano et al. (Chapter 4, this volume) stress the migrainous character of the headache that follows the seizure, and consider the seizure to be intercalated between the aura and headache phase of the classical migraine attack. They also suggest the presence of a fortuitous association of migraine and epilepsy in some patients. Indeed, this must arise occasionally on purely statistical grounds. Such a fortuitous association however should only be invoked when, despite a clear history and detailed investigation, it is not possible to demonstrate a more definite or perhaps a causal relationship between the two disorders.

Classical, basilar, and confusional migraine attacks may all lead to epileptic events, suggesting that they share certain fundamental mechanisms. The triggering of epileptic events by non-classical migraine remains a matter of speculation, mainly because of the absence of a reliable marker for common migraine. The recurrent problem of diagnosing the nature of headache also arises in relation to some of the benign epilepsies of childhood and in relation to the headache which may precede, accompany, or follow other epileptic manifestations. For the moment, the extent and the significance of the relationship of common migraine to epilepsy can only be surmised.

In the majority of affected children and adults, the tendency for seizures to occur following migrainous events is self-limited. When migraine preventive medication is effective, no additional measures are required; antiepileptic drugs however must be used when there is a tendency for recurrence of seizures and when migraine attacks cannot be adequately controlled.

Bladin and Berkovic (Chapter 12, this volume) describe a boy who had seizures and status epilepticus always ushered in by a prolonged migrainous aura. The child died in status. At autopsy, hippocampal sclerosis on the side of origin of his habitual attacks was found. This patient again highlights the multifactorial nature of these problems, but migraine was convincingly the triggering factor in the development of his seizures. Obviously, there is a very wide range in the severity of migraine-related epileptic manifestations, from the mild and occasional to the intractable and fatal.

Epilepsy with Seizures No Longer Triggered by Migrainous Auras

Some of the patients who initially have epileptic attacks only during a migrainous event may go on to develop seizures spontaneously and independently of the migrainous episodes (Andermann, Chapter 1, this volume). The natural history of such epilepsies requires careful, longitudinal, clinical observation and electrographic study, as well as intelligent and observant medical historians. It is often only possible to reconstruct the sequence of events if careful clinical documentation from earlier years is available. The epilepsy usually has clinical features suggesting an origin in the temporal lobe, a finding not unexpected in view of the predilection of classical migraine for the territory of the posterior circulation, which supplies inferomesial temporal structures. When there is evidence of early occipital involvement followed by temporal lobe epilepsy, such cases suggest the development of secondary epileptogenesis. This may also involve the ripening of independent epileptogenic discharge in the temporal lobe on the side opposite to where the initial events took place. There is no good statistical information available as to the incidence of such a sequence of events. In many patients the evidence is not adequate for firm clinical conclusions, and overenthusiastic correlations must be avoided in such situations.

Epilepsy Due to Gross Cerebral Lesions Caused by Migraine

The occurrence of strokes related to migrainous events has been well documented in the past, and the advent of the C.T. and M.R.I. scans has facilitated the recognition of such lesions (see Dvorkin et al., Chapter 14, this volume, for discussion). Patients with cerebral lesions of this nature may then develop epilepsy and here, too, a causal relationship between the two conditions exists. The finding of otherwise unexplainable field defects, for instance, in patients with epilepsy and a strong personal and family history of classical migraine, may also suggest that the migraine has played an important role in causing the epilepsy. Cases with isolated strokes must be carefully distinguished from those with the characteristic clinical picture of malignant migraine or mitochondrial encephalopathy, where recurrent strokes are an integral part of a progressive syndrome, which will be discussed more fully later in this chapter.

Benign Occipital Epilepsy of Childhood and the Spectrum of the Occipital Epilepsies

Gastaut and Zifkin (Chapter 3, this volume) describe a childhood form of epilepsy in which seizures are characterized by visual symptoms that are often followed by sensory, motor, or psychomotor symptoms and postictal migrainous and visceral manifestations. The EEG usually shows characteristic repetitive occipital paroxysmal activity attenuated by eye opening. Structural occipital lesions are not found. The authors suggest that this syndrome derives at least in part from a constitutional predisposition to such attacks, similar to that proposed for primary generalized epilepsy.

Benign epilepsy with occipital paroxysms belongs among the idiopathic or primary partial epilepsies, and is usually associated with a good prognosis for seizure control with appropriate medication and for eventual disappearance of the attacks. It thus behaves like the better known benign epilepsy of childhood with rolandic spikes, but seems to take longer to resolve. In another paper, Gastaut and Zifkin (1985) have suggested that the pathogenesis of these benign focal epilepsies is related to interactions between a genetic predisposition to epilepsy and local factors of cerebral maturation. They have also noted the similarity between the ages at remission of these two partial epilepsies and the course of electrophysiologic maturation of the relevant sensory systems as determined by evoked response studies in humans.

The cases of benign epilepsy with occipital paroxysms discussed by Gastaut and Zifkin add another condition to the differential diagnosis of transient visual obscuration and headache, especially in children and adolescents. Though postictal migrainous headache is common in their patients, the syndrome itself seems clearly epileptic. The reasons why occipital seizures should be associated with postictal migraine are at present unclear.

The identification of this benign syndrome does not exclude the possibility of similar clinical manifestations occurring in patients with occipital lesions giving rise to a secondary or symptomatic partial epilepsy. Patients with a diffuse encephalopathy and occipital spikes may also manifest such seizures. Aicardi and Newton (Chapter 6, this volume) reviewed the clinical spectrum found in their patients with epilepsy and occipital spike-wave complexes suppressed by eye opening. They found migrainous symptoms in one-half of their patients, again suggesting some relationship between this epileptic disorder and migraine. In two-thirds of their patients the seizures were difficult to control or they had educational problems. They concluded that this striking EEG abnormality occurs in patients with a wide spectrum of symptoms, as well as neurological and intellectual deficits, and that the epilepsy associated with it is by no means always benign.

In a study of patients with migraine and epilepsy Andermann (Chapter 1, this volume) identified a group of children with occipital epilepsy who have a family history of either common or classical migraine, and who may have migraine themselves. These children have a high incidence of acquired factors in their histories and of structural changes on imaging studies. Their epilepsy may be either benign or severe. Their family history suggests that migraine may be a risk factor in the development of occipital epilepsy. This concept is in keeping with current views on the multifactorial etiology of the epilepsies.

Children with occipital epilepsy were divided by Terasaki, Yamatogi and Ohtahara (Chapter 7, this volume) into those with and those without obvious exogenous, causative, or acquired factors. Those without such factors had a striking genetic predisposition to migraine and epilepsy in their families in comparison with the others, suggesting that in the spectrum of the occipital epilepsies of childhood, the greater the genetic factor, the less severe the acquired dysfunction has to be in order for epilepsy to develop and vice versa. These findings are analogous to the biological continuum which exists between the generalized and partial epilepsies (E. Andermann 1982, 1985; Gloor et al., 1982; Metrakos and Metrakos, 1974), and also between the primary and the secondary generalized epilepsies (Gloor 1977, Berkovic et al., in press). They conform to the multifactorial theory of epilepsy as outlined by E. Andermann (1980, 1982, 1985).

In the "non-organic" group of patients reported by Terasaki, Yamatogi and Ohtahara, corresponding to benign occipital epilepsy of childhood, there was a remarkable age-dependent mode of onset with a peak at 7 to 9 years of age, a predominance of girls, partial simple seizures were significantly more common and prognosis was better. Autonomic symptoms were present in 75% and the attacks were followed by headache in half of the children of both groups. The "organic" group had more dysrhythmic EEG's with other spike foci or generalization, and they had an increase in additional, other, seizure types.

This group of studies suggests the presence of a group of children with functional or benign occipital epilepsy and of another group with obvious acquired factors or organic lesions, with overlap between the two forms and the presence of a wide spectrum of involvement between these two extremes. The reason for the striking incidence of migraine in these clinical situations is presumably linked to that for the preferential involvement of the occipital lobe in migraine: whether this relates to cell density and propensity to spreading depression, to the distribution of neurotransmitter activity, or to other factors remains speculative.

Migraine and Benign Rolandic Epilepsy

Benign rolandic epilepsy appears to be a migraine-related disorder, although this association has not been generally recognized. Bladin (Chapter 9, this volume) presents a thoughtful analysis of the reasons why this correlation is sometimes missed. His personal observations which, since they are based on previous awareness of this association, are both prospective and retrospective, show that 80% of patients admit to migraine and this was classical in 13%. Recurrent sympathetic symptoms without headache were present in 10% and another 10% had neither migraine nor "migraine equivalents". A positive family history of migraine was present in two-thirds. Interestingly the patient's headache was usually ipsilateral to the spike focus. Giovanardi Rossi et al. (Chapter 21, this volume) however, who found a similarly high incidence of recurrent headache associated with this condition, concluded, unlike Bladin and other observers (Andermann, personal observations 1986, Watters, personal communication 1984) that these disorders were associated by chance.

The mechanism of benign rolandic epilepsy is poorly understood. The strong genetic basis, tendency for the EEG discharges to shift from side-to-side, universally benign prognosis, as well as the relationship to migraine, sets it apart from the acquired partial epilepsies arising in these areas. Bladin also postulates a relationship to the Landau-Kleffner syndrome, a relationship suggested by other authors as well. There are many analogies between benign rolandic and benign occipital epilepsy, including the probability of finding both a personal and a family history of migraine. Discharge spreading to brainstem structures, as suggested by Gastaut and Zifkin (Chapter 2, this volume), is not likely to explain the headaches in these conditions, particularly those of otherwise symptom-free relatives.

Malignant Migraine: A Syndrome of Severe Classical Migraine, Epilepsia Partialis Continua, and Multiple Strokes Related to Mitochondrial Encephalomyopathy

Over the last 25 years we observed a series of patients who had a family history of classical or common migraine and who had migraine themselves (Dvorkin et al., Chapter 14, this volume). They developed infrequent occipital seizures, or severe, prolonged migraine attacks and, later, episodes of partial status epilepticus. Important focal neurological sequelae, often referable to alternating lesions, then became apparent, usually in the territory of the posterior circulation. Hypodense lesions were well visualized with CT scans and abnormal signals were seen on MRI. The CT changes tended to recede. Cumulative neurological deficits persisted, resulting in increasing disability often consisting of cortical blindness and deafness. Most patients died due to status epilepticus. It recently became apparent that some, but by no means all of these patients had ragged red fibers in muscle biopsies and/or lactic acid elevation in blood and CSF, suggesting that this disorder represented the MELAS syndrome (Mitochondrial Encephalomyopathy with Lactic Acidosis and Stroke-like episodes). The clinical spectrum of mitochondrial disease is currently being defined, and new clinical forms are frequently reported. It seemed clear from the study of these patients with malignant migraine, with or without ragged red fibers or lactic acidosis, that they had a distinctive clinical pattern, not encountered in epilepsy of other causes, and also distinct from patients with migraine who have isolated strokes or from those with hemiplegic migraine.

Within this group of patients, it is impossible to distinguish clinically between those who have ragged red fibers and those who do not, suggesting that these muscular changes are not an obligatory marker of mitochondrial disease. Lactic acid levels were at times elevated both in our patients who had, and in those who did not have ragged red fibers, again suggesting that the absence of such fibers does not exclude the diagnosis of mitochondrial disorder.

It is possible that in some patients the brain rather than other organs is primarily affected; this is borne out by the fact that a neuromuscular component has not been clinically evident in our patients. These cases presented with a history of migraine and severe epilepsy at epilepsy centers, whereas those with prominent muscular features have usually been reported from neuromuscular clinics. It is probably for this reason that a family history of migraine has not been stressed in the patients who presented with more prominent peripheral symptoms.

The cerebral lesions are indicative of ischemia in some, but not in all, confirming that the cerebral pathology in this disorder has not been fully clarified. Further pathological studies of brain and other organs, particularly of the smooth muscle in cerebral blood vessels, are under way. An abnormality of energy metabolism in the smooth muscles of cerebral arteries, or perhaps a small reduction in the inherited number of neural mitochondria leading to hereditary inadequacy of calcium binding ability in these patients (van Gelder, Chapter 24, this volume) could explain this disorder which combines a family history of migraine in relatives with a catastrophic recurrent illness in one or two affected family members. The presence of mild involvement in the mother of one of our patients is compatible with the maternal inheritance demonstrated in other forms of mitochondrial disease (Rosing et al., 1981). Fatigue seems to be a major triggering factor leading to the acute episodes, but the mechanism by which prolonged migraine attacks lead to the catastrophic neurological events is still not clear. Better understanding of the mitochondrial encephalopathies may in turn throw some light on the mechanism of migraine in general.

Ictal and Peri-ictal Headache

The headache which follows generalized tonic clonic seizures is well known and is a classical feature of major seizures. However, it has also long been suspected that headache sometimes occurs as a manifestation of epileptic seizure activity. In Blume and Young's series (Chapter 15, this volume), this association between headache and epilepsy was found predominantly with temporal or occipital epileptic discharges, and they concluded that it could arise through a variety of mechanisms. In occipital cases a relation to migraine could be suspected as discussed above in relation to the spectrum of the occipital epilepsies in childhood (Andermann, Chapter 1, Gastaut and Zifkin, Chapter 3, Aicardi and Newman, Chapter 6, this volume).

When the peri-ictal headache is localized to the area overlying the EEG focus, Blume and Young considered that it could be the result of vascular changes related to the epileptic discharge, but they stress the overall lack of localizing value of headache of this type. We, on the other hand, have found that such head pain represents a valuable lateralizing symptom in patients with known temporal lobe epilepsy.

The predominantly temporal localization of ictal headache is confirmed by the studies of Isler et al. and St-Hilaire et al. (Chapters 16 and 17, this volume). Depth electrode recordings in their cases have shown that the headache occurs during ictal discharge which is usually ipsilateral, and arises from the amygdala and the hippocampus. Because of its abrupt onset and cessation, within the same second as the seizure discharge, and because of its short duration, Isler and his colleagues argue against a vascular and in favor of a neural mechanism for this type of headache. Such a neural mechanism would be analogous to the reaction to injury in other pain-sensitive structures, and would require reexamination of the current view based on Penfield's observations (1954) and Thomas Willis's dogma that the brain is insensitive to pain. However, such brief, severe headaches with sudden onset and cessation also resemble the so called "ice-pick headache," that is probably migraine related and that may have a vascular mechanism. The observations of Isler et al. and of St-Hilaire et al. confirm the clinical suspicion that headache may at times represent an ictal symptom of seizures originating in mesial temporal structures.

Isler and his colleagues consider the more prolonged headaches associated with seizures to be related to vascular factors, for example, reactive hyperemia.

Headache occurring after nonconvulsive complex partial seizures originating in the temporal lobe is described by D'Allessandro et al. (Chapter 18, this volume). In some cases, it took the form of long lasting migraine attacks, though only one-half of the patients had headaches outside the postictal period. This appears to represent yet another migraine-epilepsy syndrome. The recent observation by Binnie et al. (1986) that flunarizine, a calcium channel blocker, which is effective in the preventive treatment of migraine also prevents postictal headache, offers further support for the view that some of these headaches may be of a migrainous nature.

These studies identify several types of pre-ictal, ictal and postictal headaches which may have both localizing and lateralizing value. However, since optimal correlation is possible only when recording from depth electrodes is available, one must guard against drawing conclusions that are too rigid from the clinical history.

Alternating Hemiplegia of Childhood

This is a specific disorder that, by virtue of a positive family history of migraine, appears to have a genetic relationship to this condition. The misery and crying of the children at the beginning of the attacks, the intense sympathetic manifestations particularly obvious in bilateral attacks, and the clinical evidence for involvement of the posterior circulation are certainly suggestive of migraine. However, in early childhood a clear history of migrainous headache is difficult to obtain. Later on, retardation associated with an extrapyramidal syndrome supervenes, again rendering clarification by history from the patient difficult. Epilepsy may also occur but it is often mild and the seizures are easily controlled. Certainly, affected children have a family history of migraine. This was present in all the 7 children we have seen, but how this relates to the characteristic and almost stereotypical clinical picture of alternating hemiplegia remains uncertain. In particular, the progressive deterioration and the appearance of the dystonic and athetotic movement disorders are difficult to account for and have no analogy in other migraine related disorders. The possibility of a mitochondrial disorder must also be considered when autopsy studies become available.

It was the analogy and putative relationship of alternating hemiplegia of childhood to migraine that led to the trial of treatment with calcium channel blockers for this condition. These agents lead to definite improvement but usually not to complete cessation of the attacks (Casaer and Azou, 1984; Andermann et al., 1986). The underlying mechanisms of this specific disease remain unknown.

ELECTROGRAPHIC STUDIES OF OCCIPITAL EPILEPTIC ACTIVITY AND THE EEG CORRELATES OF MIGRAINE

Occipital Spike Wave Paroxysms Blocking with Eye Opening

The characteristic occipital spike and wave or sharp and slow wave discharge recorded in patients with occipital epilepsy was studied by Cirignotta, Lugaresi and Montagna (Chapter 8, this volume). They showed that abolition of central vision rather than darkness, per se, led to both the appearance of these discharges and of the alpha rhythm, confirming the earlier observations made by Panayiotopoulous (1981). This reactivity to eye closure, to complete darkness, and, more specifically, to abolition of central vision appears to represent a basic neurophysiological feature of the visual system, involving both normal rhythms and pathologic discharges arising in the occipital lobe.

Beaumanoir and Grandjean (Chapter 5, this volume) also emphasized the nonspecificity of the occipital sharp and slow wave discharges blocking with visual perception. Such discharges have been identified in children with strabismus, amblyopia, learning or behavior disorder, occipital epilepsy, benign occipital epilepsy of childhood and in association with basilar or classical migraine. Thus, a number of factors, including genetic ones, that affect the occipital lobe can lead to this nonspecific but localizing abnormality that is associated with a wide range of clinical manifestations. Obviously, description of the electrographic features alone is not adequate for assessment of the clinical problem of the patients who show this abnormality.

Interestingly the five patients with basilar migraine, epilepsy, and occipital epileptogenic abnormalities described by Beaumanoir and Grandjean usually developed migraine only after the first epileptic attack. On the other hand, the EEG focus was present before the first migrainous attack and disappeared before the migraine stopped in another group of four patients. The authors conclude that their findings speak against the hypothesis that these occipital spike foci are the result of transient ischemia accompanying the vasoconstrictor phase or to other factors related to the classical aura of the migraine. Despite the lingering uncertainty about the cause and mechanism of the EEG abnormalities, there is little doubt that the migrainous aura triggers epileptic manifestations.

EEG Recording during the Classical Migraine Aura:
Repetitive Spike Discharges Underlie the Transition from
Migraine to Epilepsy; A Mechanism Analogous
to "Spreading Convulsion?"

Only exceptionally has it been possible to record the EEG during a classical migraine aura. Beaumanoir and Jekiel present two such patients and Sacquegna et al., a third (Chapters 10, 11, this volume). The EEG discharges consisting of posterior rhythmic sharp waves or spikes greatly resembled epileptic activity and were considered as such. However, the clinical manifestations in the first two of these patients showed no features which were necessarily epileptic and would have been considered quite typical and not at all unusual for migrainous events. These patients highlight the difficulties in distinguishing between migrainous events and minor occipital seizures discussed by Panayiotopoulos (Chapter 2, this volume). From a practical point of view, it is only the presence of symptoms that are necessarily epileptic that allows distinction between the two. One wonders, however, how often this process of rhythmical cortical spiking occurs in the classical migraine population; it may in fact be quite a typical accompaniment of the aura. Anterior spread or generalization of such discharges probably correlates with the seizures induced by the classical migraine aura (Andermann, Chapter 1, this volume), also described as intercalated attacks by Terzano et al. (Chapter 4, this volume). This transition from migraine to epilepsy is dramatically illustrated by the patient described by Bladin and Berkovic (Chapter 12, this volume) who had unequivocal clinical and electrographic epileptic manifestations during his attacks.

Spreading depression (SD) in the primate proceeds anteriorly but stops at the central sulcus (Lauritzen, Chapter 22, this volume). Under certain experimental conditions (such as repeatedly evoked episodes of SD, pretreatment with pilocarpine or acetylcholine or induction of SD during hypercapnia) spreading depression leads to paroxysmal activity or "spreading convulsion". This may be the underlying mechanism of the repetitive spike discharges recorded during the classical migraine aura in man. In predisposed individuals, this type of activity may cross the central sulcus, involve the precentral gyrus and other regions, and lead to the motor and postural epileptic manifestations which characterize the seizures induced by the classical migraine aura in this migraine-epilepsy syndrome.

The Electroencephalogram during the Headache Phase of Migraine

EEG changes during the headache phase in patients with classical or basilar migraine consist of monomorphic or polymorphic slow waves (Beaumanoir and Jekiel, Chapter 10, this volume). At first they are seen bilaterally even in patients with hemicrania; then they tend to become more unilateral and the area involved progressively diminishes as the headache improves. Such lateralized slow activity was also described following a migraine-induced attack of transient global amnesia and during an episode of confusional migraine by Sacquegna et al. (Chapter 11, this volume). A second pattern associated with the headache phase consists of high-amplitude, monomorphic, slow delta activity over posterior quadrants, blocking with eye opening. On the basis of the morphology of these abnormalities, Beaumanoir and Jekiel concluded that this particular pattern is more likely to be of cortical origin, whereas monomorphic slow waves seen in patients with vegetative or brainstem symptoms may reflect dysfunction of the midbrain structures implicated in basilar migraine.

Photosensitivity in Migraine and Epilepsy

Migraine shares with epilepsy a tendency to excessive and abnormal response to intermittent photic stimulation in the EEG. The classical photoconvulsive spike and wave response induces spike and wave as an afterdischarge, is of high voltage, contains prominent spike components, and may be associated with pattern sensitivity. The photosensitive abnormalities associated with migraine are often less striking, especially in adults. Often there is no afterdischarge, sharp waves, or slow sharp waves, and slow waves are often seen and spike components are not conspicuous. The discharges are also not as rhythmic as those associated with photosensitive epilepsy. Such abnormalities are not uncommonly encountered in EEG laboratories where patients, particularly children with migraine, are frequently recorded. These photosensitive irregularities have generated much interest, and many publications such as those by Weil (1962), Ziegler and Wong (1967), Hess (1982), and others have led to concepts such as that of dysrhythmic migraine, and to attempts to treat migraine with anticonvulsants.

Patients with photosensitive epilepsy are often aware of minor symptoms that correlate well with their EEG abnormalities, but the subjective photosensitive complaints of migraineurs have not been studied systematically until recently. Wilkins and his collaborators (Chapter 23, this volume) have shown that the epileptogenic, photosensitive abnormalities are produced by stimuli with parameters almost precisely the same as those that provoke anomalous visual effects such as hallucinations of color, blurring, distortion, shimmering or headache in people who do not have epilepsy. There is also a correlation between the number of such illusions and the number and nature of headaches that these photosensitive persons suffer. Wilkins's observations bring into perspective the popular view that eyestrain causes headache, which leads most children with headache first to the ophthalmologist or optician before their migraine is diagnosed.

It is very likely that the photosensitivity of epilepsy and migraine have very similar cortical mechanisms and that "the mechanisms whereby visual stimuli induce seizures, illusions, and pain appear to have much in common" (Wilkins, Chapter 23, this volume). Hyperexcitability of the visual cortex may be the basis for these genetically determined phenomena.

Meldrum and Wilkins (1984) have also proposed that "human photosensitivity may be the result of a diffuse minimal failure of intracortical inhibition, possibly one that is GABA-ergic in nature or dopaminergic."

Quesney and his colleagues (see Chapter 26, this volume for discussion), have demonstrated that apomorphine, a dopamine agonist, blocks photosensitive epileptic discharges in patients with primary generalized epilepsy and in patients with various underlying progressive diffuse neuronal diseases. Such a blockade is also found in the photosensitive baboon (*Papio papio*) and in feline generalized penicillin epilepsy. These findings suggest a common mechanism for photosensitivity stemming from a variety of causes and in a variety of species. Epileptic photosensitivity may be related to a cortical deficit of dopaminergic neurotransmission; photic stimulation may facilitate the genesis of spike and wave discharges by enhancing a preexistant, genetically determined state of cortical hyperexcitability.

It is possible, though unproven, that such a dopaminergic mechanism may be involved in the photosensitivity found in patients with migraine as well. Paradoxically, however, valproic acid, the most effective blocker of photosensitivity in man (and the treatment of choice for photosensitive epilepsy) is at times associated with the emergence, or more likely, the aggravation of vascular headache or common migraine.

PATHOPHYSIOLOGICAL CONSIDERATIONS

Neurochemical explanations of the link between migraine and epilepsy are still at a speculative level. Van Gelder (Chapter 24, this volume) suggests that in both epilepsy and migraine there may be a somewhat increased excitatory state of the cortex. A slight increase in glutamate release could result in a lowered seizure threshold, GABA malfunction, and hypersynchronous neuronal discharge. This, in association with acquired cerebral dysfunction, could lead to the clinical manifestations of epilepsy. Such an excess glutamate release and the resultant excitation could be explained in part by a chronic enhanced intracellular Ca^{2+} mobilization. In migraine, such increased cortical excitability would be associated with vascular abnormalities, or hypersensitivity to certain nutritional, endocrine or environmental factors, eventually leading to the clinical manifestations.

Van Gelder, addressing the increased prevalence of migraine and epilepsy in the young, suggests that a hereditary inadequacy in calcium binding ability may be shared by these conditions. The amount of inorganic phosphate available to the cell for mitochondrial sequestration of calcium may become inadequate during growth and puberty and predispose children to the triggering of attacks by any further factors such as diet or hormonal disturbance.

The catamenial aspects of migraine and epilepsy are discussed by Matthew and Abrams (Chapter 25, this volume) who conclude that "estrogen related cyclical menstrual changes and autonomic activation, both influential in migraine and to a lesser extent in epilepsy may influence the functional aspects of neurally released peptides." They find that despite the superficial relationship between ovarian steroids, neuropeptides and some of the physiological changes proposed in migraine and epilepsy, there is no concluding evidence to link the two conditions on the basis of peptidergic dysfunction.

Much new information about the pathogenesis of migraine has been presented in recent years, primarily by the Danish group, and this has been summarized by Lauritzen (Chapter 22, this volume). It appears likely that the spreading oligemia that characterizes the early portion of the classical migraine attack may be related to spreading depression (SD). These processes start predominantly in posterior head regions. One of the possible reasons for this is the high density of neuronal elements in those areas. The biochemical basis for the greater likelihood of SD to occur in certain species and in areas with high neuronal density is still unknown. The oligemia or hypoperfusion spreads anteriorly at a rate of 2 to 3 mm/min, a rate similar to that of SD. The process does not cross primary sulci or areas of abrupt architectonic change of the cerebral cortex. Limitations in EEG recording technique, namely the small area of EEG depression, its short duration, nonsteady state of the condition, and absence of DC tracings may explain why corresponding EEG abnormalities are usually not recorded in uncomplicated attacks of classical migraine (Lauritzen et al., 1981). In some recorded classical auras, however, occipital rhythmic spiking is found as described above. This type of discharge may be more common, or even always present, during the migraine aura. This phenomenon may well prove to be important for our understanding of migraine-epilepsy relationships. The abnormal facilitation of spread of the oligemia or SD to the motor strip or other regions may be responsible for the clinical epileptic seizures which the classical aura triggers.

Later in the migraine attack, during the headache phase, hypoperfusion similar to that which follows SD is present for some hours. Lauritzen (Chapter 22, this volume) suggests that in classical migraine the function of both the blood vessels and the cerebral cortex are perturbed but that disturbance of cortical function is the causal factor.

The absence of significant alterations of blood flow in common migraine is difficult to explain. Genetic evidence suggests that classical and common migraine are closely related. Families with members affected by one or the other are frequently encountered. Obviously the fundamental abnormality which may be expressed in both these clinical forms still eludes us.

CONCLUSIONS

The delineation of eight migraine-epilepsy syndromes provides clarification for the migraine epilepsy relationship encountered in a number of individuals. The prevalence of these disorders, however, remains to be determined. The seizures in some of these conditions are not particularly difficult to control and their recognition should be helpful in establishing a prognosis.

The identification of a relationship between migraine and some of the benign epilepsies of childhood suggests the need for further epidemiological and genetic studies of these entities. The studies presented in this volume illustrate abnormal functioning of the occipital lobe and provide a background for an improved understanding of both occipital epilepsy and occipital function in general.

Photosensitivity may be viewed as a correlate of both epilepsy and migraine. Genetically determined cortical hyperexcitability may be present in both of these conditions. Further study of migraine-epilepsy relationships may provide better understanding of partial epilepsy and it may also provide insights into some mechanisms of generalized epilepsy. From the clinical point of view, however, the need for distinction between the two disorders and for accurate diagnosis remains the most important priority.

Jackson wrote a hundred years ago "I have seen cases intermediate in type between migraine, epileptiform seizures and epilepsy proper ("missing links")". He was referring to the Darwinian evolutionary concept of his time and perhaps foresaw relationships between these conditions which were not, and which are still not, fully identifiable. I think he would have approved of the efforts made by the authors of this book to clarify and unravel the tantalizing relationships between these two disorders that continue to bedevil and plague mankind.

REFERENCES

Andermann E. Multifactorial inheritance in the epilepsies. In: Canger R, Angeleri F, Penry JK, eds. Advances in epileptology: XIth Epilepsy International Symposium. New York: Raven Press, 1980;297–309.

Andermann E. Multifactorial inheritance of generalized and focal epilepsy. In: Anderson VE, Hauser WA, Penry JK, Sing CF, eds. Genetic basis of the epilepsies. New York: Raven Press, 1982;355–74.

Andermann E. Genetic basis of the epilepsy. In: Sakai T, Tsuboi T, eds. Genetic aspects of human behaviour. Igaku-Shoin: Aino Foundation 1985;129–145.

Andermann E, Straszak M. Family studies of epileptiform EEG abnormalities and photosensitivity in focal epilepsy. In: Akimoto H, et al., eds. Advances in epileptology: XIIIth epilepsy international symposium. New York: Raven Press, 1982; 105–12.

Andermann F, Silver K, St-Hilaire MH, Morris N, Lacey DJ, McGreal D, Starreveld E. Paroxysmal alternating hemiplegia of childhood: treatment with flunarizine and other agents. Neurology 1986;36(4):Suppl 1:327.

Berkovic SF, Andermann F, Andermann E, Gloor P. Concepts of absence epilepsies: discrete syndromes or biological continuum? Neurology, in press.

Binnie CD. Aura and postictal headache in epileptic patients treated with flunarzine. Rome: Proceedings of the International Congress on Migraine and Epilepsia; Neural basis and calcium modulation, Functional Neurology, 1986;(in press).

Casaer P, Azou M. Flunarizine in alternating hemiplegia in childhood, letter. Lancet 1984;579.

Gastaut H, Zifkin BG. Classification of the epilepsies. J Clin Neurophysiol 1985;2:313–26.

Gloor P. Generalized cortico-reticular epilepsies: Some considerations on the pathophysiology of generalized bilaterally synchronous spike and wave discharge. Epilepsia 1968;9:249–63.

Gloor P. The EEG and differential diagnosis of epilepsy. In: van Duijn H, Donker DNJ, van Huffelen AC, eds. Current concepts in clinical neurophysiology, The Hague: N. V. Drukkerij, Trio 1977;9–21.

Gloor P. Consciousness as a neurological concept in epileptology: a critical review. New York: Raven Press. Epilepsy and Behavior. Merritt Putnam Sympos. Suppl. 2 to Epilepsia 1986;27:514–26.

Gloor P, Metrakos J, Metrakos K, Andermann E, van Gelder N. Neurophysiological, genetic and biochemical nature of the epileptic diathesis. EEG J [Suppl 35] 1982:45–56.

Hess R. Migraine und epilepsie. Schweiz Med Rundschau 1982;71:1595–99.

Kraus D. Migraine and epilepsy: a case for divorce. M.Sc. thesis, McGill University, 1978.

Lauritzen M, Trojaborg W, Olesen J. EEG during attacks of common and classical migraine. Cephalalgia 1981;1:63–6.

Meldrum BS, Wilkins AJ. Photosensitive epilepsy: integration of pharmacological and psychophysical evidence. In: Schwartzkroin P, Wheal HW, eds. Electrophysiology of epilepsy. London: Academic Press, 1984;51–77.

Metrakos K, and Metrakos JD. Genetics of epilepsy. In: The epilepsies: handbook of clinical neurology. Vinken PJ, Bruyn GW, eds. Amsterdam: North-Holland Publishing Company, 1974;15:429–39.

Panaiyotopoulous CP. Inhibitory effect of central vision on occipital lobe seizures. Neurology 1981;31:1331–33.

Penfield W, Jasper H. Epilepsy and the functional anatomy of the human brain. Boston: Little Brown 1954;749.

Rosing HS, Hopkins LC, Wallace DC, Epstein CM, Weidenheim K. Maternally inherited mitochondrial myopathy and myoclonic epilepsy. Ann Neurol 1985;17:228–37.

Weil AA. Observation on "dysrhythmic" migraine. J Nero Ment Dis 1962;134:277–81.

Young GB, Blume WT. Painful epileptic seizures. Brain 1983;106:537–54.

Ziegler DK, Wong G Jr. Migraine in children: clinical and electroencephalographic study of families, the possible relation to epilepsy. Epilepsia 1967;8:171–87.

Index